BANANAS

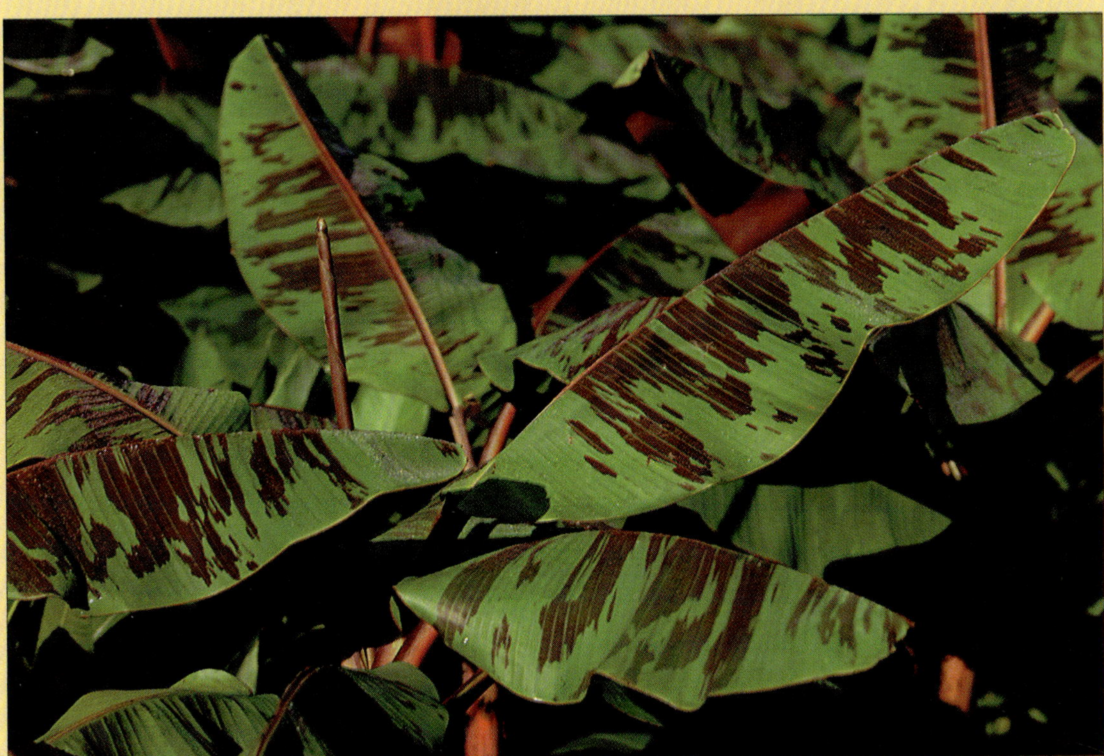

Banana leaves, pseudostem (trunk) and fruiting stem (raceme) grow from the underground rhizome (or pseudobulb's) top surface and the roots grow from the lower surface of the rhizome. The fleshy stems sheathed with huge broad leaves can grow from 2 to 35 feet in as little as 1 year, depending on variety and growing environment. Each pseudostem produces one flower cluster, which develops fruit, then dies. In addition each parent banana plant during its life cycle, will produce as many as 10 suckers which grow into new plants. New pseudostems then grow from the rhizome.

Bananas grow best in a uniformly warm environment and need 9 to 15 months of frost-free conditions to produce a flower stalk. In the subtropics, fruit ripens in 2-3 months. In cooler climates it may take several weeks longer to ripen. Plant growth stops when temperatures drop to 57°F. Stokes Tropicals' Banana Blend (6-2-12) is the best fertilizer source for these fascinating tropical giants.

Banana varieties are available as rooted growing plants in both 4'' and 6'' pots. A growing banana plant will be barerooted and shipped to you in growing condition with living roots. Cultural directions are supplied with each order.

Bananas

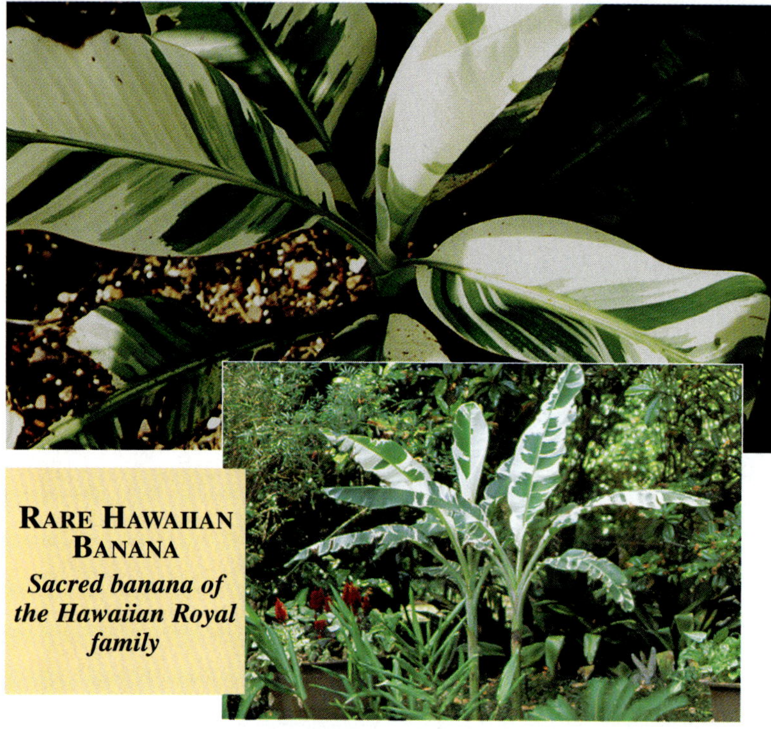

RARE HAWAIIAN BANANA

Sacred banana of the Hawaiian Royal family

AE AE 'Variegated Hawaiian'

When Hawaii was a kingdom, this banana, called 'Koae', was sacred and could only be grown and eaten by the Royal family. A very rare plant! The leaves are a kaleidoscopic pattern of dark green, medium green, and creamy white. Even the fruit is variegated with white linear stripes. Although it is usually cooked, fruit can be eaten out-of-hand. Does best in partial shade, otherwise white portions of leaves may sunburn. Needs acid pH (5.5-6.5) for best growth. Can grow 12' (3.75m) to 15' (4.5m). Very limited supply.
10051 Growing Plant (6" Pot) *$119.95*

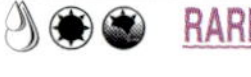 **RARE**

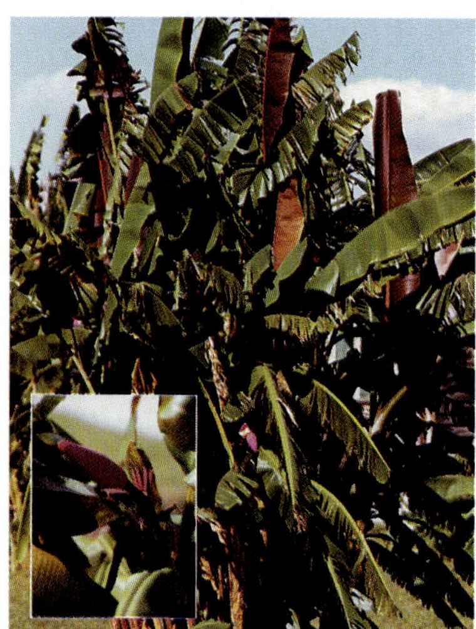

BORDELON

An absolutely magnificent ornamental banana that superficially resembles the 'sumatrana', however the 'Bordelon' grows taller, the leaves are more maroon underneath and it flowers and fruits easily. Fruit is inedible and semi-pendulous. Grows 9'-12' tall. Zone 8 and higher. Discovered growing in Bordelonville, a small Louisiana town, hence the name.
10122 Growing Plant (4" Pot) *$9.95*
10121 Growing Plant (6" Pot) *$14.95*

Visit our Web Site @
www.stokestropicals.com

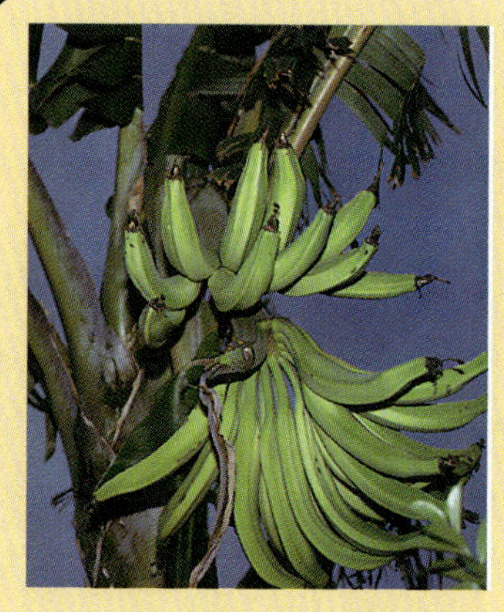

AFRICAN RHINO HORN

A slender, tall plantain that grows 17' (5.1m) to 20' (6m) with huge fingers (bananas) of fruit up to 2' (60cm) long (hence the name rhino horn). Fruit can be cooked green or eaten ripe out-of-hand. Plant is very attractive with red coloration of the pseudostem and leaves.
10102 Growing Plant (4" Pot) *$9.95*
10101 Growing Plant (6" Pot) *$14.95*

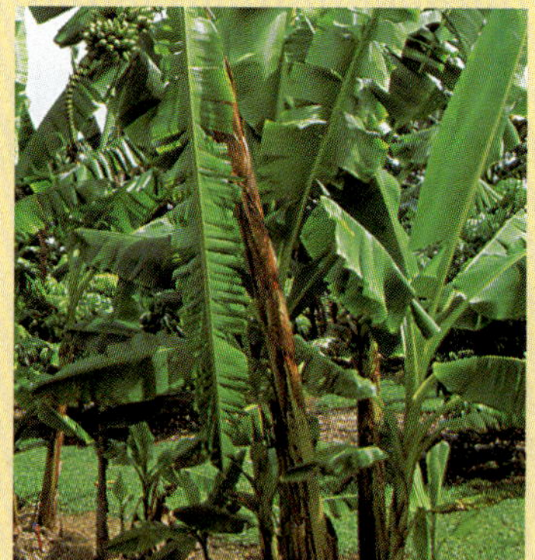

BRAZILIAN

Has also been called the "Brazilian Tall." This excellent landscaping specimen has good wind resistance. 15' (4.5m) to 20' (6m) in height. Solid green with some pink. Small raceme of fruit is extremely sweet. One of our most popular bananas.
10152 Growing Plant (4" Pot) *$9.95*
10151 Growing Plant (6" Pot) ...*$14.95*

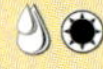

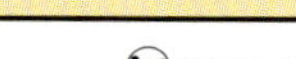

2

Full Sun   Part Sun   Shade   Extra Water   Fragrant   Cut Flower   New

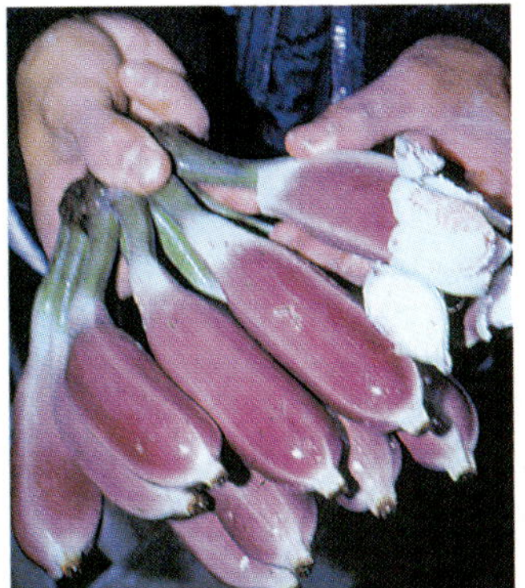

'Burmese Blue'

A truly outstanding new ornamental and edible banana from the Golden Triangle area of Burma, Thailand and Laos. Some local hill tribes cook the banana fruit and eat it. Other hill tribes consider it poisonous. Maybe those hill tribes that eat it spread the word to the other hill tribes that it is poisonous so that they have more to eat? The main attraction is its blue-skinned fruit. 12'-14'. Zone 9 and higher.

10172 Growing Plant (4" Pot)....................$9.95
10171 Growing Plant (6" Pot).................$14.95

Ⓝ ♨ ☀ ◖ **RARE**

Photo from *Plants and People of the Golden Triangle: Ethnobotany of the Hill Tribes of Northern Thailand* with permission from Edward F. Anderson.

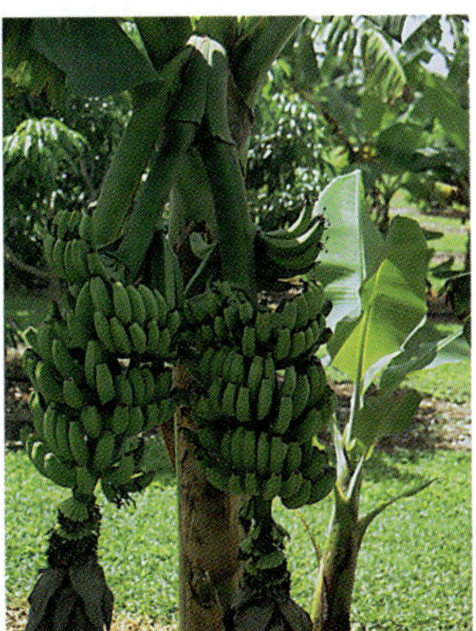

DOUBLE (MAHOI)

Dwarf plant, 5' (1.5m) to 7' (2.1m) in height. A very rare and extremely unusual plant that produces two or more bunches of very tasty sweet bananas on the same plant after suckering of the mother plant. Excellent container plant. A must for serious collectors. A dwarf cavendish mutation. Mahoi means twins in Hawaiian.

10252 Growing Plant(4" Pot).....................$9.95
10251 Growing Plant(6" Pot)...................$14.95

♨ ☀

ALL STOKES TROPICALS' PLANTS ARE EASY-TO-GROW.

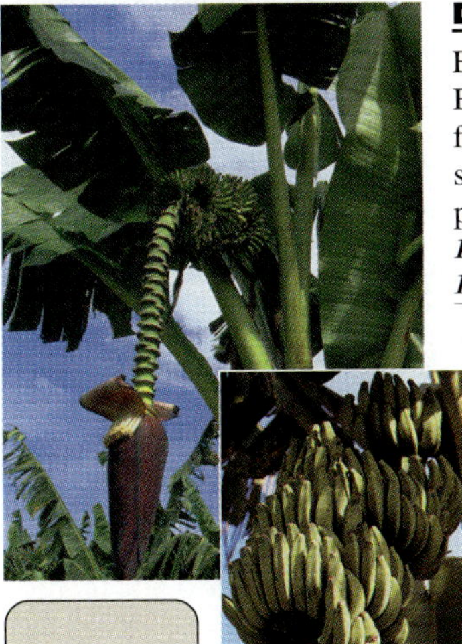

DWARF BRAZILIAN

Excellent flavored fruit similar to regular Brazilian. Plant has racemes of medium-size fruit. Grows to 8' (2.4m). Solid green with some pink in pseudostem. Strong, hardy plant. Good wind resistance.

10302 Growing Plant(4" Pot).....................$9.95
10301 Growing Plant(6" Pot)...................$14.95

♨ ☀

All bananas, unless noted, are hardy in Zone 9 and higher planted outside in ground with virtually no protection. In lower Zones, hardy with special protection. If you can prevent the rhizome (bulb) from freezing the plant will come back the following spring.

TO PLACE AN ORDER: *CALL:*
1-800-624-9706
FAX: **(337) 365-6991**
E-Mail: **info@stokestropicals.com**

BANANA FERTILIZER PAGE 130

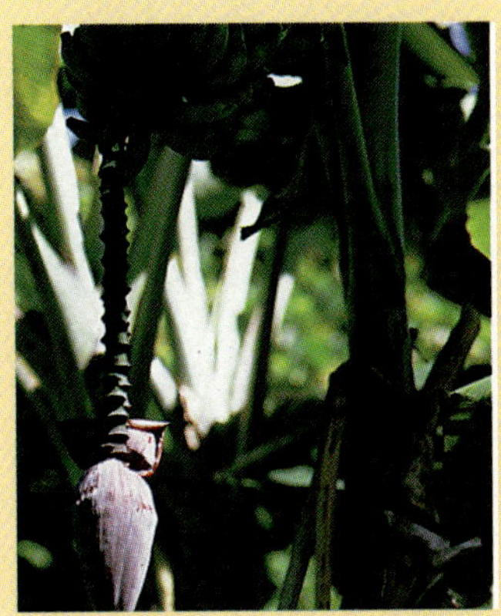

CARDABA

Very beautiful variety that has blue-green colored fruit that is short and fat. Pulp is bright white. A plantain from Thailand. 12' (3.6m) to 14' (4.2m) in height. Particularly good for cooking and making tostones.

10202 Growing Plant (4" Pot).....$9.95
10201 Growing Plant (6" Pot)...$14.95

♨ ☀

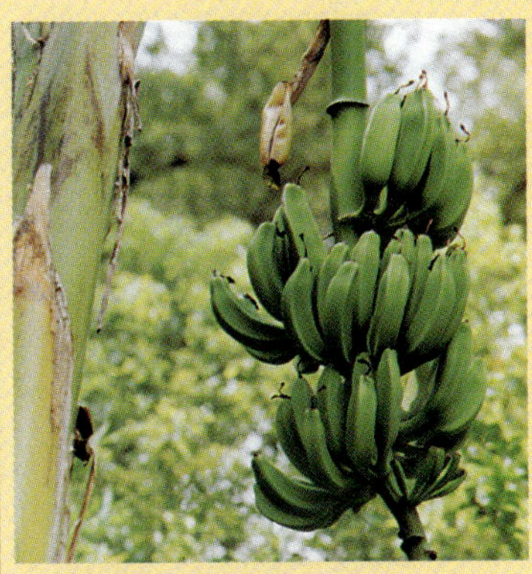

DWARF ORINOCO

Wonderful small 5' (1.5m) to 6' (1.8m) plant with large racemes of fruit. Thick skinned fruit that can be cooked or eaten out-of-hand. Good cold tolerance and wind resistance. Plant is a nice solid green color. Fruit almost square in cross section. Heavy bearer.

10402 Growing Plant (4" Pot).....$9.95
10401 Growing Plant (6" Pot)...$14.95

♨ ☀

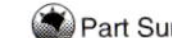
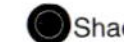
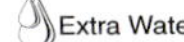

☀ Full Sun   ♨ Part Sun   ● Shade   ♨ Extra Water   ☀ Fragrant   ✂ Cut Flower   Ⓝ New

🌴
3

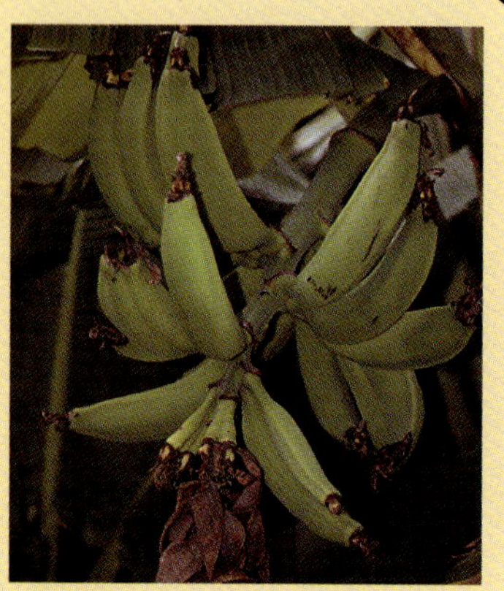

DWARF PUERTO RICAN PLANTAIN

A very commonly eaten cooking banana grown throughout the island of Puerto Rico. A dwarf attractive plant growing 6'-8' tall. Zone 9 and higher.

10422 Growing Plant (4" Pot).....$9.95
10421 Growing Plant (6" Pot)...$14.95

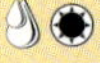

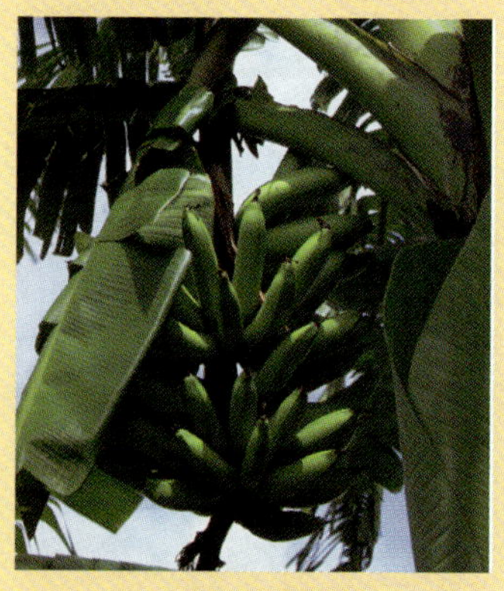

EBUN MUSAK

Outstanding specimen. One of few banana varieties with fruit that ripens green. 10' (3m) to 12' (3.6m) in height. Green plant with lots of chocolate brown color in pseudostem. 4" (10cm) to 6" (15cm) pointed fruit. Nickname is "Crocodile Fingers". Introduced from Borneo.

10502 Growing Plant (4" Pot).....$9.95
10501 Growing Plant (6" Pot)...$14.95

DWARF RED

One of the most beautiful banana plants. A strong, vigorous plant which produces a medium-size bunch of bananas that are a brilliant red and gold upon ripening. Fruit is very aromatic with creamy orange pulp. The dwarf matures at 6' (1.8m) to 8' (2.4m). Takes 20-30 months to bear fruit first time, then every year thereafter. Sometimes the red will mutate from red to all green resulting in Dwarf Green Red.

10452 Growing Plant (4" Pot) $9.95
10451 Growing Plant (6" Pot) $14.95

Orders Placed Through Our Web Site Receive a 15% Discount

ELE ELE 'Black Hawaiian'

A very different Hawaiian variety that has almost blackish leaf sheaths, petioles, and midribs. A tall plantain type growing 20' (6m) to 25' (7.5m) producing large bunches of orange-fleshed fruit that tastes best cooked. The fruit is not black, but the pseudostem is blackish. The stem is sturdy and the overall appearance of the plant is that the entire pseudostem is dark brown or black. Leaves are green. The fruit turns yellow as it ripens and tastes between a plantain and a banana. The fruit is so delicious, it was declared taboo to the commoners by the ancient Hawaiian kings. The plant grows well in most conditions and stands up well to the wind. A must for collectors.

10552 Growing Plant (4" Pot)...$9.95
10551 Growing Plant (6" Pot)...$14.95

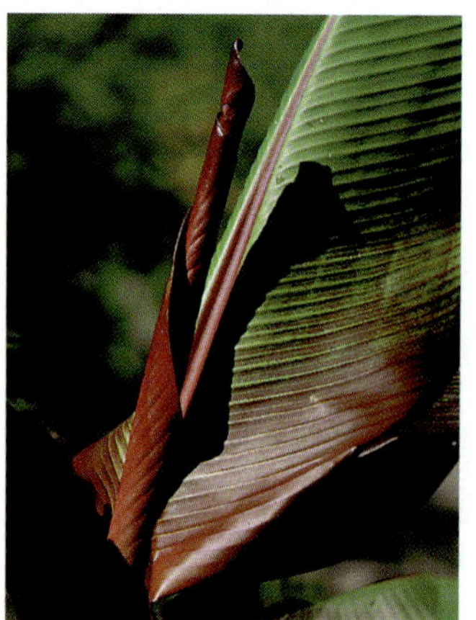

ENSETE MAURELII

Red Abyssinian "banana". Fantastically colorful plant with red leaf surfaces and red leaf axils. Looks hand painted. Huge leaves that can grow 10' (3m) to 15' (4.5m) long and 1.5' (45cm) wide. Plant grows to 18' in warm climates. In Zone 9 rarely reaches 8'. Cold hardy in Zone 9 and higher. Grows well in full sun to partial shade. Fast growing and non-clumping. Does not sucker like other bananas. Does great in containers.

10602 Growing Plant (4" Pot) $9.95
10601 Growing Plant (6" Pot) $14.95

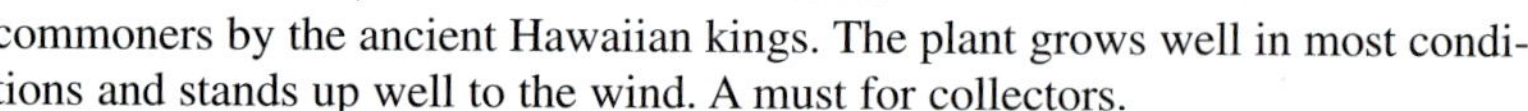

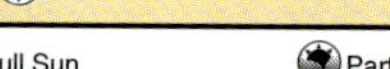  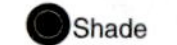 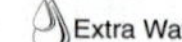 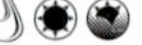 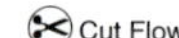

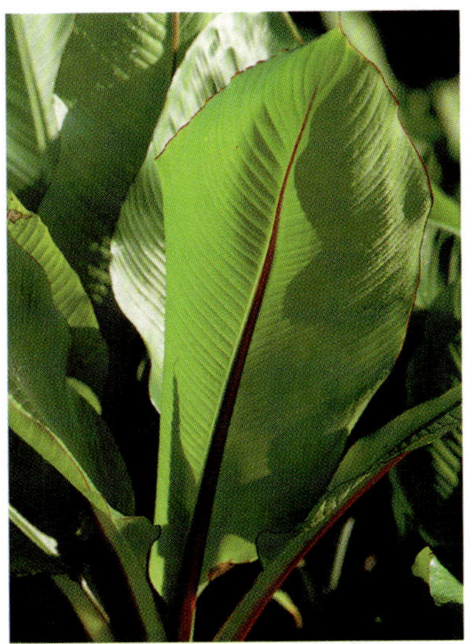

ENSETE VENTRICOSUM 'Red Stripe'

A super looking plant with red midrib on underside of leaves. Grows to 20' (7m) in warm areas. Huge 10' (3m)- 15' (4.5m) leaves up to 1.5' (45cm) wide. Grows in partial shade to full sun. Makes a good interior specimen when space allows. In Zone 9 rarely reaches 12'. Perennial in Zone 9 and higher. Very fast growing and non-clumping. Does not produce suckers.

10702 Growing Plant (4" Pot) $9.95
10701 Growing Plant (6" Pot) $14.95

Save $20 by ordering a Banana Collection. See page 16-17.

FHIA-03 'Sweet Heart'

Another great tasting dessert banana that was developed by the federal experiment station in Honduras. Reaches 10-12' in height. Exhibits tolerance to disease. Has great potential as a new commercial variety. Zone 9-10.

10772 Growing Plant (4" Pot) $9.95
10771 Growing Plant (6" Pot).....$14.95

ALL STOKES TROPICALS' PLANTS ARE EASY-TO-GROW.

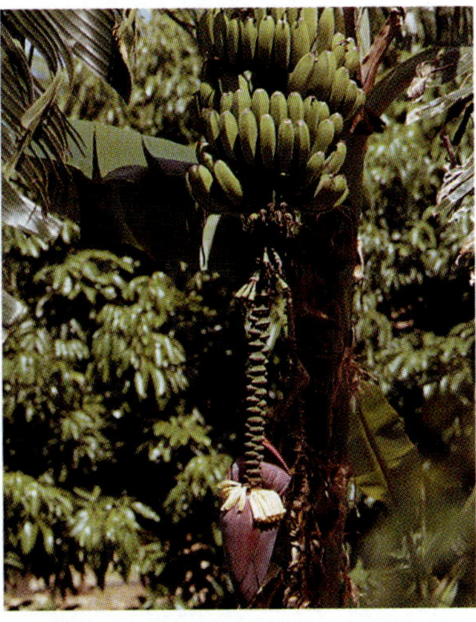

GIANT CAVENDISH

A Central American commercial variety that can be found in American supermarkets. A tall plant that grows 17'-20' Produces large racemes of excellent tasting fruit. Not as wind tolerant as some but does well in protected areas.

11131 Growing Plant (6" Pot)...............................$29.95

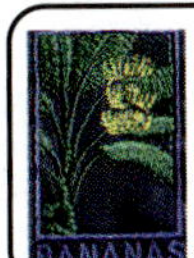

Merchandise using Banana logo available. See pp. 133-134.

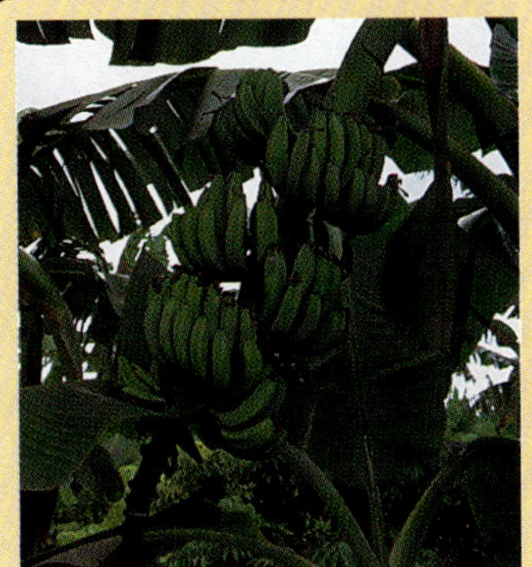

FHIA-01 'Goldfinger'

New variety developed at the FHIA Research Station in Honduras. Medium size plant 12' (3.6m) to 14' (3m) with broad leaves and outstanding fruit production. Cold tolerant and disease resistant. May be the next grocery store variety. Developed to be commercial export banana. Very strong plant with stout base. Excellent taste.

10752 Growing Plant (4" Pot) $9.95
10751 Growing Plant (6" Pot)....$14.95

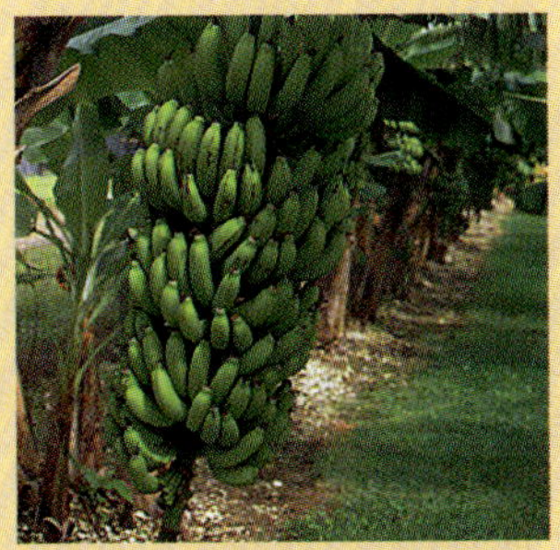

GRAND NAIN

Outstanding banana variety that is the current commercial variety ("Chiquita") from Central America. Large racemes of fruit (up to 150 lbs in the tropics; in U.S. 50 lbs) produced on a 6' (1.8m) to 8' (2.4m) plant. Very attractive for its landscaping potential and good wind resistance. Solid green in color.

10802 Growing Plant (4" Pot) $9.95
10801 Growing Plant (6" Pot) ..$14.95

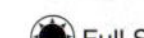 Full Sun   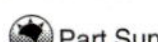 Part Sun   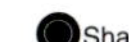 Shade   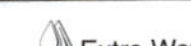 Extra Water   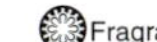 Fragrant   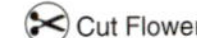 Cut Flower   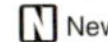 New

5

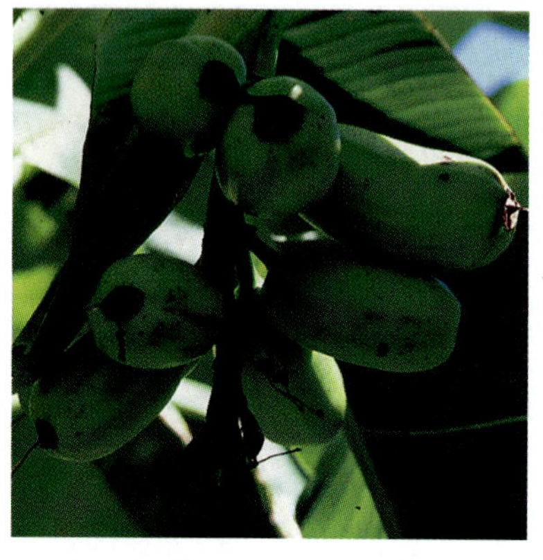

HUA MOA

Unusual looking bananas grow on this 10' (3m) to 12' (3.6m) solid green plant. The fruit gets up to 4" (10cm) in diameter and looks like short fat bananas. The fruit can be eaten ripe, fried or baked, with an excellent taste. This plant is believed to have a South Pacific heritage.

10852 Growing Plant (4" Pot) $9.95
10851 Growing Plant (6" Pot) $14.95

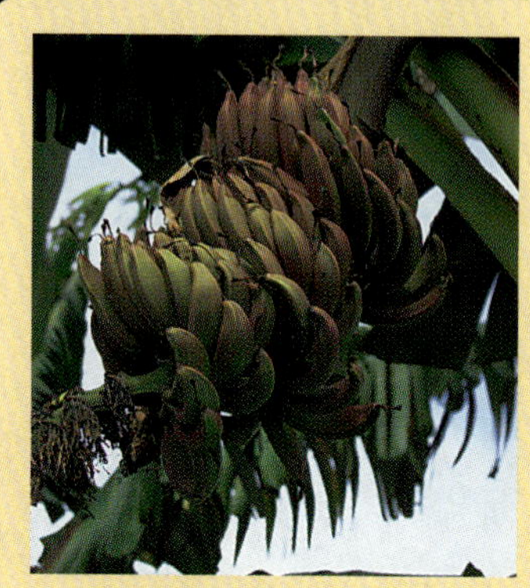

KRU

A rare recent import from New Guinea. Experts consider Kru to be one of the most delicious tasting bananas. Grows to a sturdy 10' (3m) - 12' (3.6m). A must for serious collectors. Also, one of the most beautiful plants with its deep shades of red on pseudostem. Fruit is also a mix of red and green shades.

11002 Growing Plant (4" Pot) $9.95
11001 Growing Plant (6" Pot) ...$14.95

ICE CREAM
'Blue Java'

Fruit looks exotic and when fully ripe, looks like ice cream, tastes like vanilla custard. Skins are silvery blue before ripening, then pale canary yellow. Grows 12' (3.7m) to 15' (4.5m) tall. A very popular banana variety. One of the very best tasting varieties.

10952 Growing Plant (4" Pot).......$9.95
10951 Growing Plant (6" Pot).....$14.95

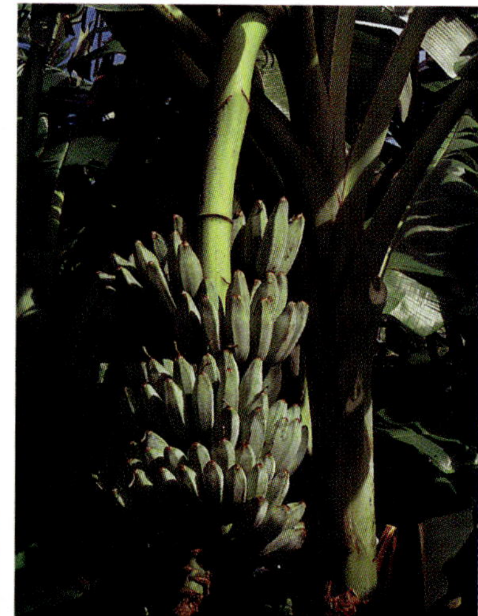

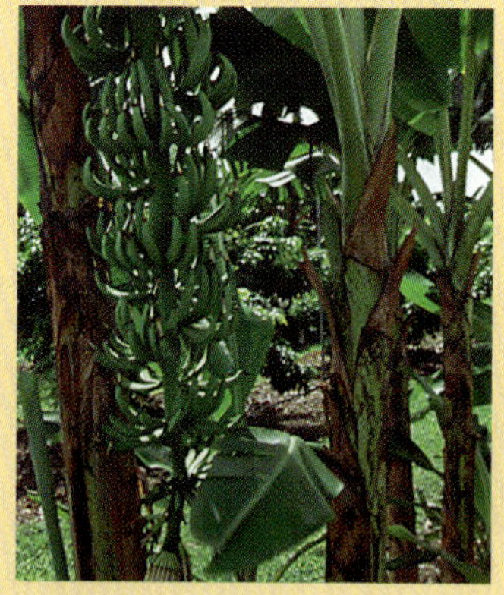

MUSA ACUMINATA
'Dwarf Cavendish'

A fantastic banana because of its size. This dwarf banana only grows to 6' (1.8m). The plant has broad leaves and produces tasty 5" sweet yellow fruit. Excellent for greenhouses and for containers. An old popular variety that originated in the Canary Islands.

11102 Growing Plant (4" Pot)........$9.95
11101 Growing Plant (6" Pot).......$14.95

MONKEY FINGER

Very unusual banana. A must for serious collectors. Grows 18' (5.4m) to 20' (6m). Long raceme 5' (1.5m) - 6' (1.8m) of fruit, with long skinny, tart tasting bananas. A real conversation piece.

11052 Growing Plant (4" Pot) $9.95
11051 Growing Plant (6" Pot) ...$14.95

**ALL STOKES TROPICALS' PLANTS
ARE EASY-TO-GROW.**

Full Sun   Part Sun   Shade   Extra Water   Fragrant   Cut Flower   New

TO ORDER CALL **1-800-624-9706**/24 HRS. OR VISIT OUR WEB SITE: www. stokestropicals.com

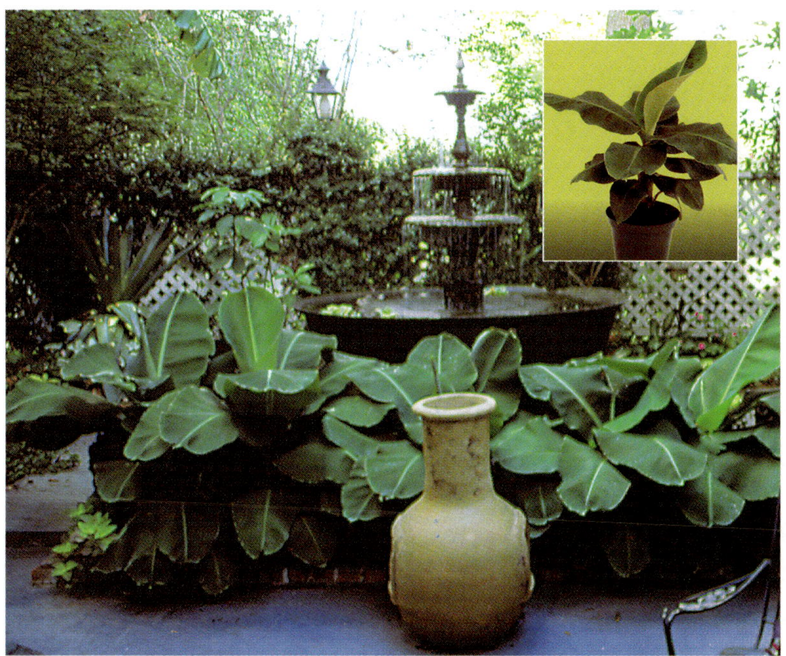

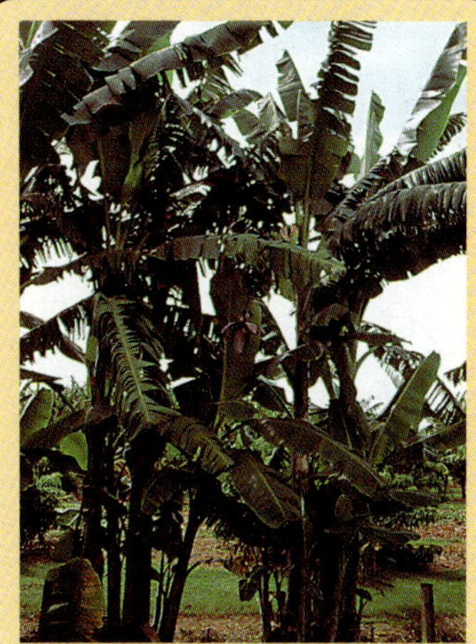

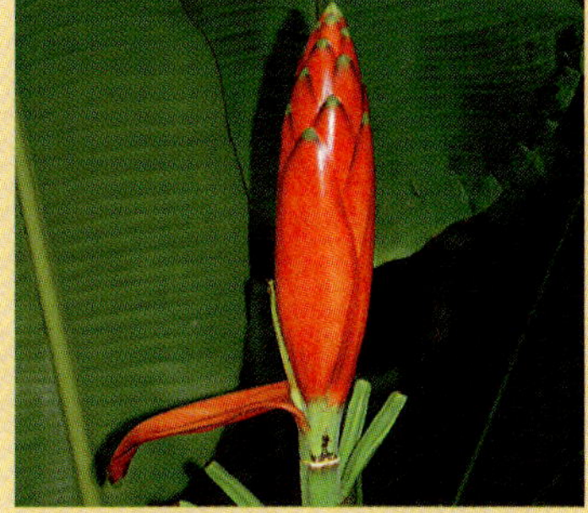

MUSA ACUMINATA 'Super Dwarf Cavendish'

Forget about huge banana plants that need a lot of room. This unique "super dwarf" allows for growing inside the home, on the porch, or close confines of a patio. Has a very symmetrical and compact appearance: 2'-4' in height. Can produce tasty fruit inside or out. Has been used as ground cover around base of palms which provide strong vertical elements. Easy to grow in containers down to 8" in diameter. Because of its size, our most versatile banana. Zone 8 and higher.

11122 Growing Plant (4" Pot) $9.95
11121 Growing Plant (6" Pot) $14.95

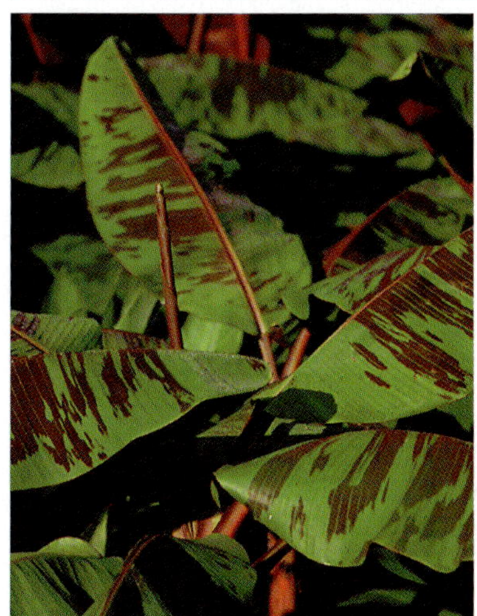

MUSA ACUMINATA 'Sumatrana' (ZEBRINA, BLOODLEAF, OR ROJO)

A strikingly beautiful 6' (1.8m) to 10' (2.4m) red and green ornamental plant grown for its foliage. Leaves appear to be stained with burgundy wine. Unmatched for containers and small areas. Does great inside or outside. Makes dramatic statement when planted in masses. Great interior plant for high light areas.

12002 Growing Plant (4" Pot) $9.95
12001 Growing Plant (6" Pot) ...$14.95

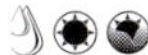

MUSA BALBISIANA

A very impressive plant that is tall and majestic. One of the original parent species of all the present day edible bananas. The other parent species is acuminata. Balbisiana is a seeded species and is more plantain-like than acuminata. Grows 14'-15' tall. Zone 9 and higher.

11142 Growing Plant (4" Pot)......$9.95
11141 Growing Plant (6" Pot)....$14.95

MUSA BECCARII

A strikingly beautiful ornamental banana species. Inflorescence closely resembles that of *Musa uranoscopus*, but not as large. Plant is a tall 10' (3m) to 12' (3.6m) slender species with long slim leaves. Makes an outstanding cut flower. Inflorescence deep red with greenish-yellow tips. A great container plant.

11201 Growing Plant (6" Pot) ...$59.95

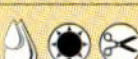

Full Sun   Part Sun   Shade   Extra Water   Fragrant   Cut Flower   New

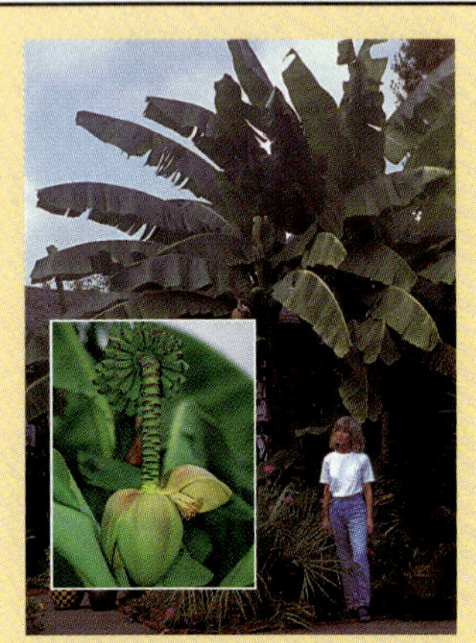

MUSA BASJOO 'Japanese Fiber Banana'

Our most exciting banana. The basjoo is the world's cold hardiest banana. It is hardy planted in ground to -3°F. and, with protective mulching, down to -24° F. Has long, slender, bright green leaves. Grows to 8'-9' in containers and 18' in the ground. Its inflorescence is one of the most beautiful of all bananas. Now literally every U.S. state can grow a banana outside in certain microclimates. Zone 5 and higher. Leaves and pseudostem will freeze if not protected but underground rhizome survives. Our #1 seller.

11152 Growing Plant (4" Pot)......$9.95
11151 Growing Plant (6" Pot)....$14.95

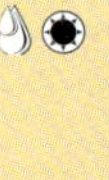

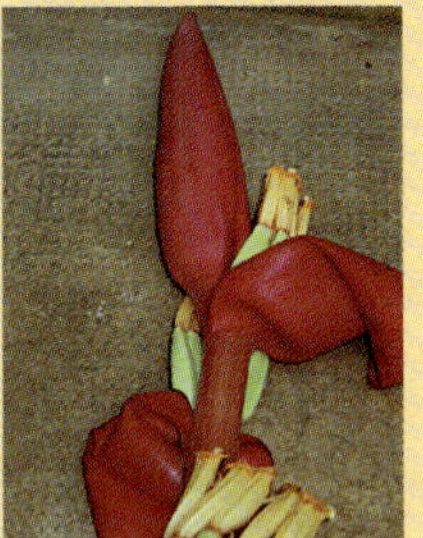

MUSA ORNATA 'African Red'

A new magnificent ornamental specimen from Western Africa. What a great flower. 7'-10'. Zone 9 and higher.

11322 Growing Plant (4" Pot) $9.95
11321 Growing Plant (6" Pot) ...$14.95

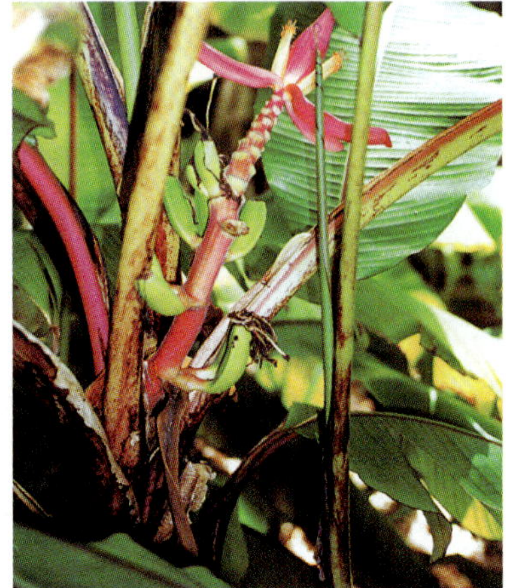

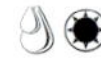

MUSA MANNII

A dwarf ornamental species with pseudostems 3' (90cm) to 4' (1.2m) high. Pseudostem is tinged in black. Broad oblong leaves, glossy green with red midrib. Short erect inflorescence 6" (15cm) long with male bracts light crimson in color. Originally from Assam. Rare.

11302 Growing Plant (4" Pot)..........$9.95
11301 Growing Plant (6" Pot)........$14.95

MUSA ORNATA 'Bronze'

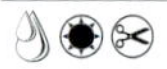

A majestic plant 5' (1.6m) - 9' (2.7m) with light green leaves and stems with pink overtones. The plant will reach its upper limit of growth when planted in the ground in warm climates. The plants growth will be limited to the lower growth range when planted in a container, given less light, and grown in cooler climate. Produces a beautiful orange-bronze inflorescence. A magnificent ornamental plant for small areas and containers. Landscape only, fruit not edible.

11402 Growing Plant (4" Pot)..........$9.95
11401 Growing Plant (6" Pot)........$14.95

MUSA ORNATA 'Lavender Beauty'

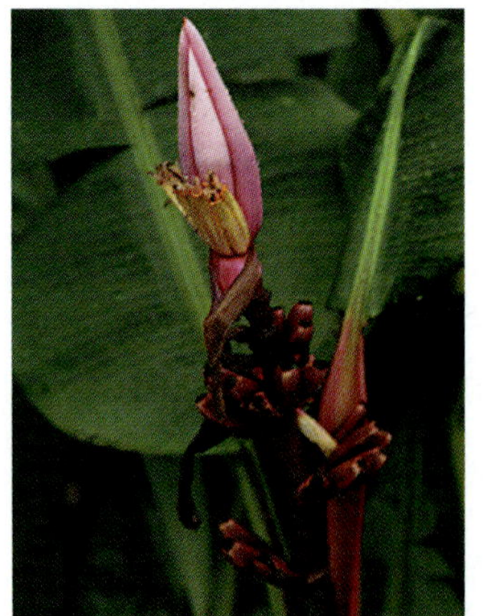

A wonderful plant 5' (1.6m) to 9' (2.7m) with light green leaves and stems with pink overtones. The plant will reach its upper limit of growth when planted in the ground in warm climates. Growth will be limited when planted in a container, given less light, and grown in cooler climate. Produces small pink lavender flowers followed by delicate maroon-colored ornamental bananas. A great ornamental plant for small areas and containers. Landscape only, fruit not edible.

11352 Growing Plant (4" Pot) $9.95
11351 Growing Plant (6" Pot) $14.95

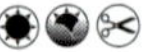

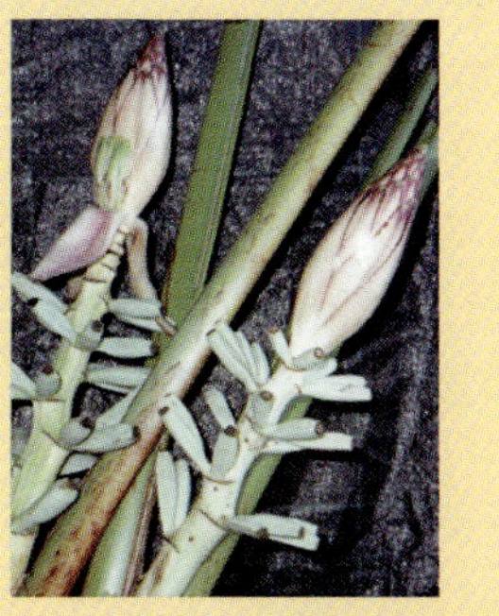

MUSA ORNATA 'Leyte White'

Similar to Musa ornata "Standard Lavender" in appearance but larger, grows 9' to 12' (3.75m) and suckers well. Flower bracts make good cut flower. Bracts are tight artichoke like and tinged with magenta. Small decorative ivory bananas, non-edible. May be named after Leyte Island in the Philippines. The plant will reach its upper limit of growth when planted in the ground in warm climates. Growth will be limited when planted in a container, given less light, or grown in cooler climate. A magnificent ornamental plant for small areas and containers.

11501 Growing Plant (6" Pot) ...$49.95

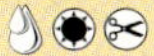

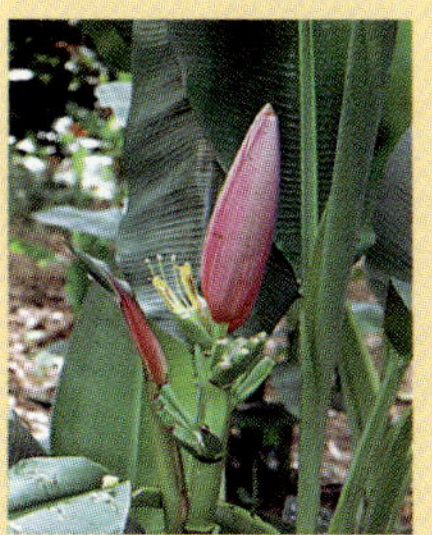

MUSA ORNATA 'Macro'

An outstanding natural hybrid from Costa Rica. Developed from 'Standard Lavendar' ornata that was hummingbird pollinated. When seed were planted, the plant with the largest inflorescense was termed 'Macro'. Grows 5'-9'. Zone 9 and higher.

11572 Growing Plant (4" Pot) $9.95
11571 Growing Plant (6" Pot) ...$14.95

MUSA ORNATA 'Milky Way'

A slim beautiful plant 5' (1.6m) to 9' (2.7m) with dark green leaves that have beautiful red midribs. The plant will reach its upper limit of growth when planted in the ground in warm climates. The plant's growth will be limited to the lower growth range when planted in a container, given less light, and grown in cooler climate. Absolutely gorgeous flower bracts that are milky white with small white bananas. White inflorescence really makes a dramatic statement against its graceful dark green leaves. A magnificent ornamental plant for small areas and containers. Landscape only, fruit not edible.

11551 Bareroot (6" Pot)...$59.95

MUSA ORNATA 'Royal Purple'

A great new plant 5' (1.6m) to 9' (2.7m) with light green leaves. Will reach its upper limit of growth when planted in the ground in warm climates. Growth will be limited when planted in a container, given less light, and grown in cooler climate. Bracts have a bluish hue. Easily distinguishable from the "Standard Lavender". A nice ornamental plant for small areas and containers. Landscape only, fruit not edible.

11602 Growing Plant (4" Pot) $9.95
11601 Growing Plant (6" Pot) $14.95

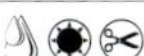

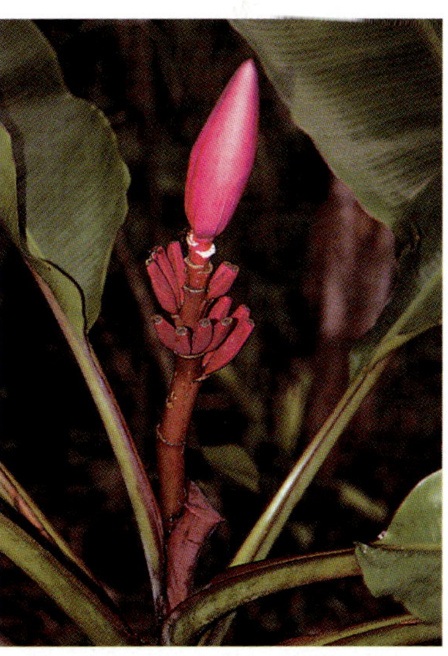

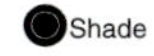

MUSA ORNATA 'Standard Lavender'

A slim stately plant 9'-12' with light green leaves and stems with pink overtones. The plant will reach its upper limit of growth when planted in the ground in warm climates. The plants growth will be limited to the lower growth range when planted in a container, given less light, and grown in cooler climate. Produces a pink lavender flower followed by delicate light green bananas. A magnificent ornamental plant for small areas and containers. Landscape only, fruit not edible.

11451 Growing Plant (6" Pot)...................$19.95

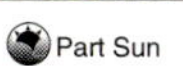

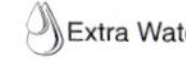

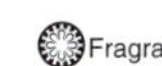

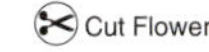

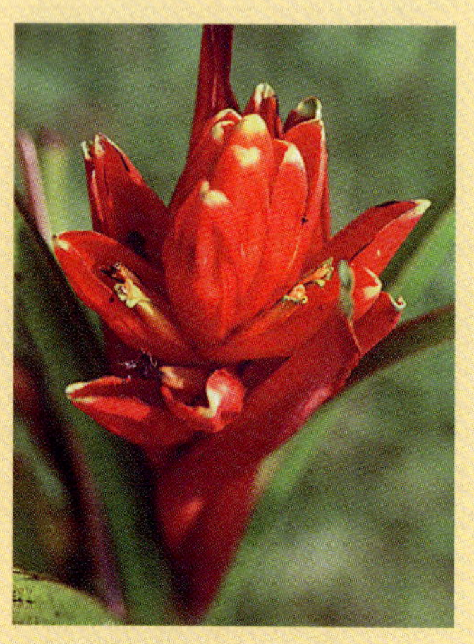

MUSA URANOSCOPUS
'Red Flowering Thai Banana'

Formerly called Musa coccinea. Undoubtedly the most beautiful inflorescence of any banana. Starting as tightly held reddish-orange bracts with yellow tips the inflorescence gradually opens over a 3 to 6 month period, becoming more beautiful daily. Plants grow 6' to 10'. Makes a great container plant. Requires pH below 6 for best growth and flowering. Medium shade to full sun. Native of Burma, Cambodia, Thailand, and Viet Nam. No fruit but marvelous flowers for cutting. Can be planted in large clumps for borders and as backgrounds.

11252 Growing Plant (4" Pot) $9.95
11251 Growing Plant (6" Pot) ...$14.95

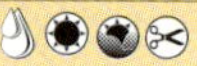

F FACTOIDS

A bunch of bananas consists of a peduncle (stem) and hands of fruit. Each hand of fruit consists of fingers (individual fruit).

Between 200 to 500 distinct banana varieties are known today.

MUSA VELUTINA

Very attractive ornamental variety that produces an erect pink blossom followed by small fuzzy pink bananas. Fruit is self-peeling when ripe. Has many seeds that are like buckshot. Good choice for small areas and containers. Grows 5' (1.5m) to 7' (2.1m). Blooms and produces ornamental fruit every year even following hard freezes. Every patio or deck should have a velutina.

12302 Growing Plant (4" Pot).........$9.95
12301 Growing Plant (6" Pot) $14.95

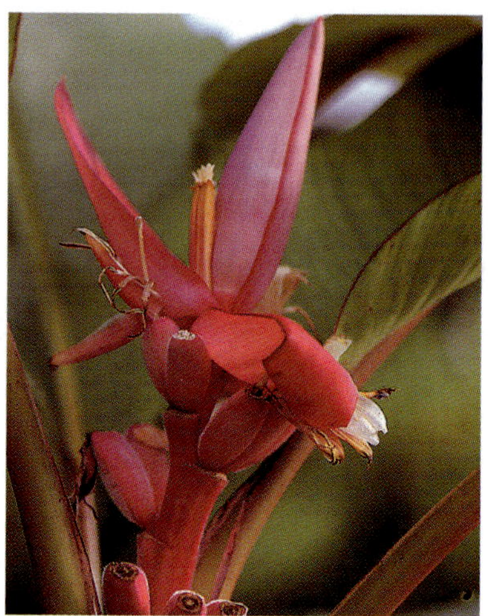

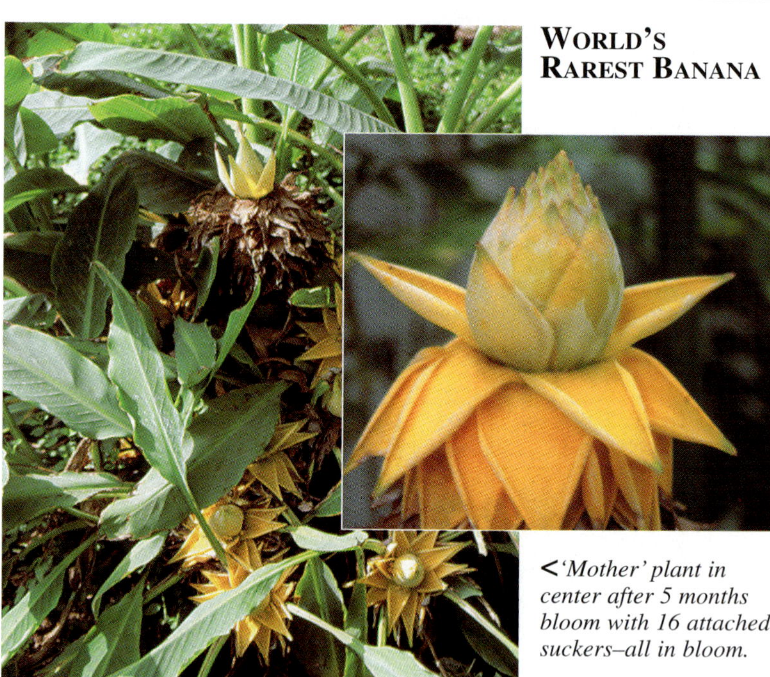

WORLD'S RAREST BANANA

< 'Mother' plant in center after 5 months bloom with 16 attached suckers–all in bloom.

MUSELLA LASIOCARPA 'Chinese Yellow'

World's rarest banana–from Yunnan Province, China. Less than 10 plants in U.S. in 1997. Its butter-yellow inflorescence is unmatched in show. Bracts are stiff and waxy, lasting for several months. On some plants 2 or 3 inflorescences are produced. Plant is very cold hardy, down into teens fahrenheit. Zone 7 and higher. Clumps tightly, does not run. Prices drastically reduced as a result of micropropagation. (Originally priced at $275.)

11652 Growing Plant (4" Pot) $9.95
11651 Growing Plant (6" Pot) $14.95

RARE

Full Sun   Part Sun   Shade   Extra Water   Fragrant   Cut Flower   New

TO ORDER CALL **1-800-624-9706**/24 HRS. OR VISIT OUR WEB SITE: www. stokestropicals.com

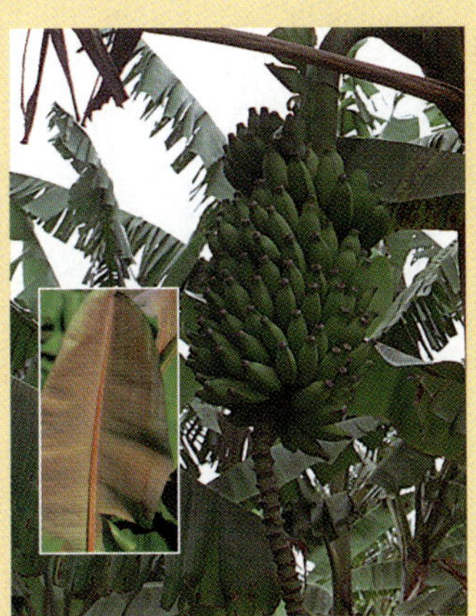

MYSORE

Tall, 14' (4.2m) to 16' (4.8m), plant with a dark brown patchy trunk that is wind resistant, vigorous and produces very thin-skinned sweet fruit. Green leaf with red midrib. Undersides of leaves have pinkish, waxy coating. Probably the best producing of the "lady finger" bananas. Most popular variety in India. One of our best tasting bananas.

11702 Growing Plant (4" Pot) $9.95
11701 Growing Plant (6" Pot) ...$14.95

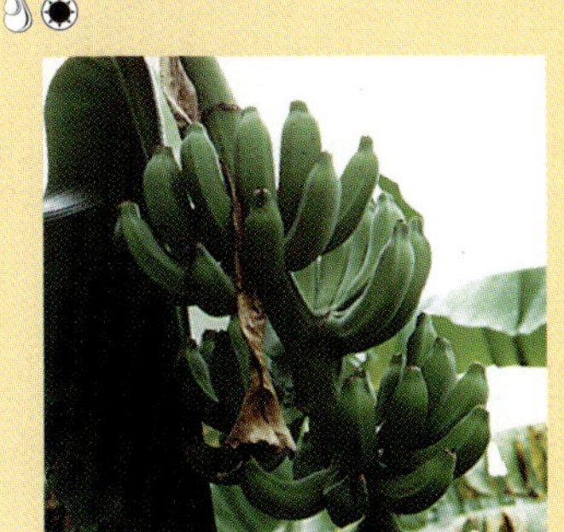

PISANG RAJA

A large variety up to 18' (5.4m) that produces medium size bunches of very good fruit that have a slightly "fuzzy" peel. Tolerates cold and wind better than most. Probably from Indonesia. Pisang is the Malay word for banana.

11902 Growing Plant (4" Pot) $9.95
11901 Growing Plant (6" Pot) ...$14.95

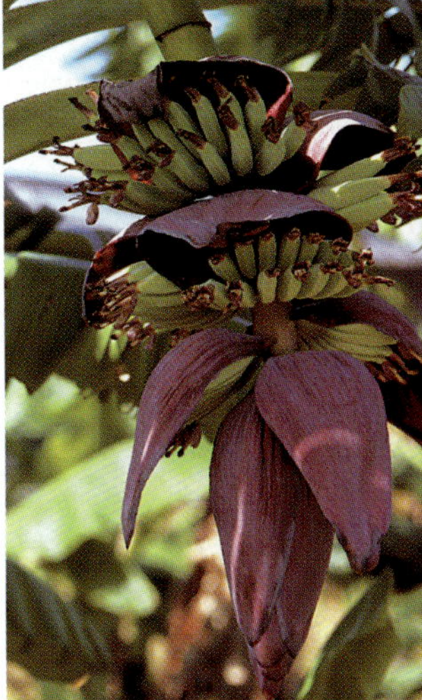

NAMWAH

A very tasty dessert banana from Thailand. Grows 10'-14'. Zone 9 and higher.

11732 Growing Plant (4" Pot) $9.95
11731 Growing Plant (6" Pot) $14.95

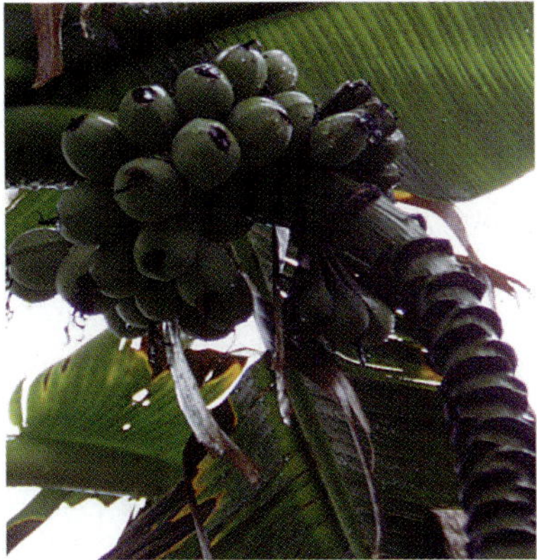

PITOGO

A most unusual banana. Solid green pseudostem 10' (3m) to 12' (3.6m) in height. Bananas resemble tennis balls in size and shape; they are more round than long. Excellent flavor. A must for serious collector.

11802 Growing Plant (4" Pot) $9.95
11801 Growing Plant (6" Pot) $14.95

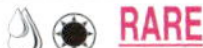 **RARE**

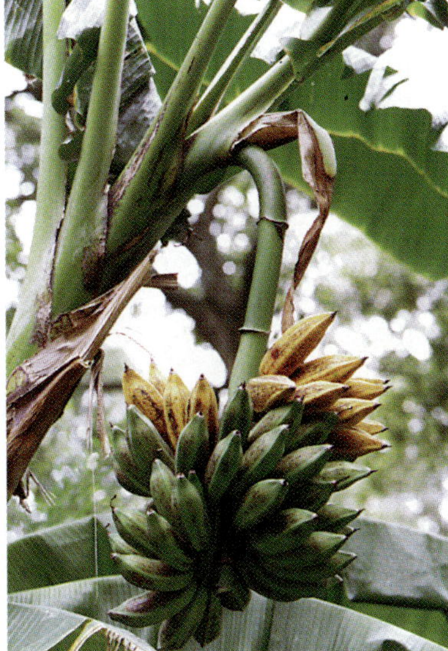

ORINOCO

Hardy vigorous plant that clumps easily, producing a very tropical effect. Produces large racemes of angular fruit that can be eaten out-of-hand or cooked. Relatively cold hardy. Easy to grow. Produces fruit nearly every year in Zone 9. Tall plant from 16' to 19'. Responds well to heavy fertilizer and lots of water. One of the most common bananas growing along the U.S. Gulf Coast.

11752 Growing Plant (4" Pot) $9.95
11751 Growing Plant (6" Pot) $14.95

STOKES TROPICALS' BANANA BLEND FERTILIZER

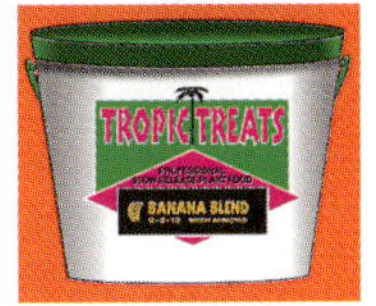

Controlled Release Fertilizer (3-Month Formula)
ANALYSIS 6-2-12 w/minors.

Uniquely formulated for best growth of Bananas. This total nutrient formula provides complete balance of all major and minor elements.

6000 (1 lb. Bucket) $6.00
6001 (4 lb. Bucket) $17.00

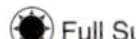 Full Sun 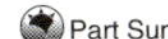 Part Sun 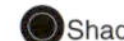 Shade 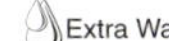 Extra Water 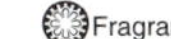 Fragrant 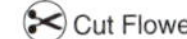 Cut Flower N New

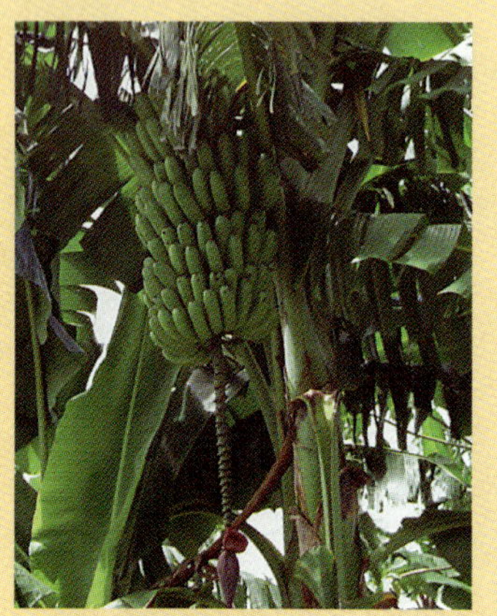

POPOULU

A popular Hawaiian plantain variety. Fruit can be eaten out-of-hand or cooked. The flesh is a salmon pink and has a very pleasing subacid apple-like taste. The plant is slender to 14' (4.2m) and likes some shade. In Hawaiian, "popoulu" means "ball-shaped like breadfruit".
11812 Growing Plant (4" Pot) $9.95
11811 Growing Plant (6" Pot)....$14.95

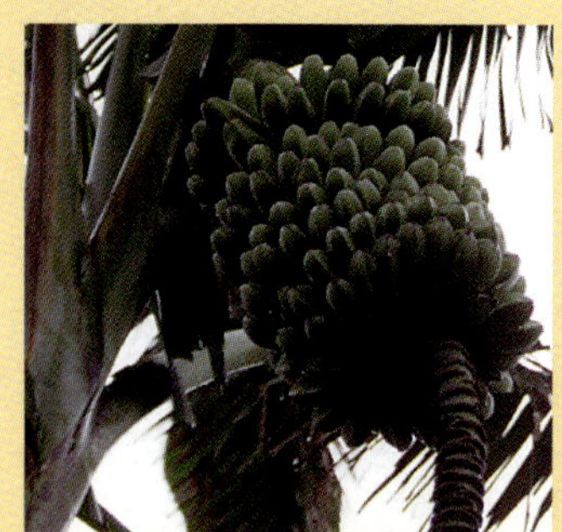

SABA

Large plant 18' to 21' tall with pseudostem 18" to 20" in diameter, widely grown in the Philippines. Plant has dark green color and is often grown for shade as well as fruit. Relatively cold tolerant and wind resistant. Very good cooking banana. Also excellent to eat out-of-hand when very ripe.
12052 Growing Plant (4" Pot) $9.95
12051 Growing Plant (6" Pot) ...$14.95

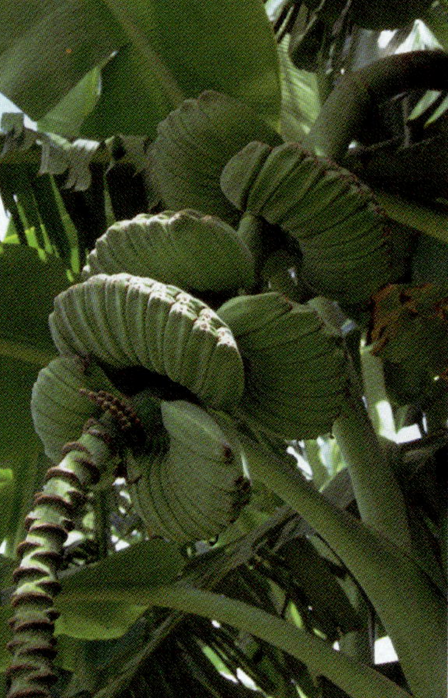

PRAYING HANDS

A beautiful deep green plant with rigid stem 10' (3m) to 12' (3.6m) and leaf structure. Unique fruit with hands of fruit fused together in pairs. Delicious tasting fruit, may be cut from stem and sliced horizontally and eaten with a spoon. A must for serious collectors. When very ripe, can be delicately peeled one fruit from the other. A real conversation piece.
11852 Growing Plant (4" Pot) $9.95
11851 Growing Plant (6" Pot) $14.95

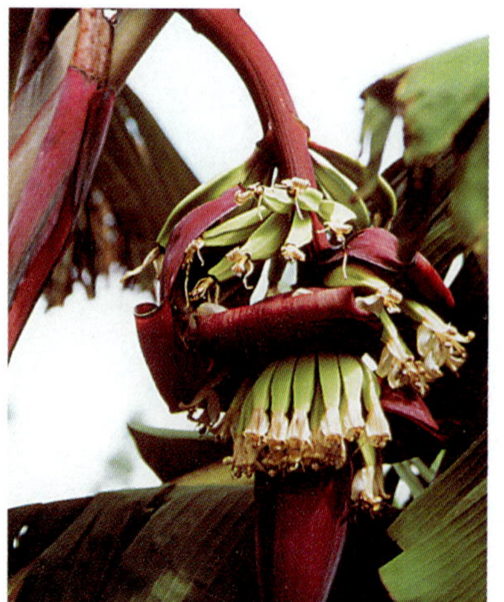

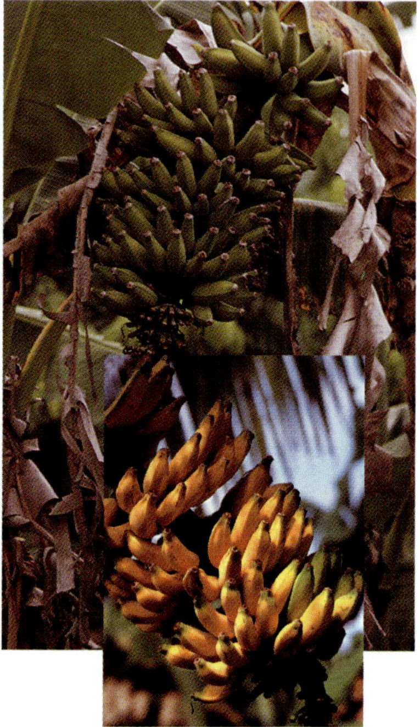

RAJA PURI

One of India's favorites. Smallish, 6' (1.8m) to 8' (2.4m); relatively cold hardy and wind resistant. Very sweet medium size fruit. First choice of homeowner for landscaping. Very stout base. Easy to grow. One of our best tasting bananas.
11952 Growing Plant (4" Pot) $9.95
11951 Growing Plant (6" Pot) $14.95

RED IHOLENE

Without a doubt, the most beautiful of the banana plants. It has leaves with a burgundy-colored underside and an exquisite reddish-pinkish pseudostem. Grows to 10'-12'. Like the White Iholene it is from Hawaii and has slightly drier fruit than the dessert bananas, but can be used for cooking or eating out-of-hand. Also has very distinctive characteristic of fruit starting out pale yellow. One must be careful to not pick fruit too early based on its color alone.
11962 Growing Plant (4" Pot) $9.95
11961 Growing Plant (6" Pot) $14.95

'1780'

The '1780' is almost certainly a cavendish with a very tasty edible fruit. The importance of this plant is that its origin can be traced back to the Caribbean island of Hispaniola in 1780. It was shipped from there to Laura Plantation (40 miles up the Mississippi River above New Orleans, Louisiana) where it has grown continuously in a mat since 1780, hence the name.

12072 Growing Plant (4" Pot) $9.95
12071 Growing Plant (6" Pot) $14.95

Orders Placed Through Our Web Site Receive a 15% Discount

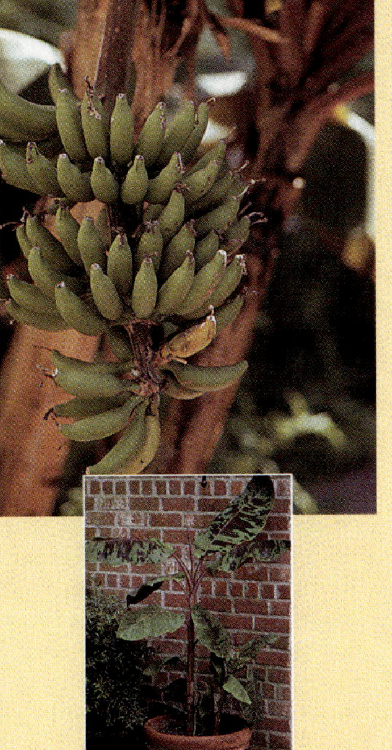

TALL RED

A beautiful, strong, vigorous plant that produces a medium size bunch of bananas that are a brilliant red and gold upon ripening. Fruit is very aromatic with creamy orange pulp. The "tall" matures at 16' (4.8m) to 18' (5.4m). Takes 20-30 months to bear fruit first time, then every year thereafter. Sometimes the red will mutate from red to all green. Then it is called the Tall Green Red. It just happens and there is nothing that can be done to prevent it.

12202 Growing Plant (4" Pot) $9.95
12201 Growing Plant (6" Pot) $14.95

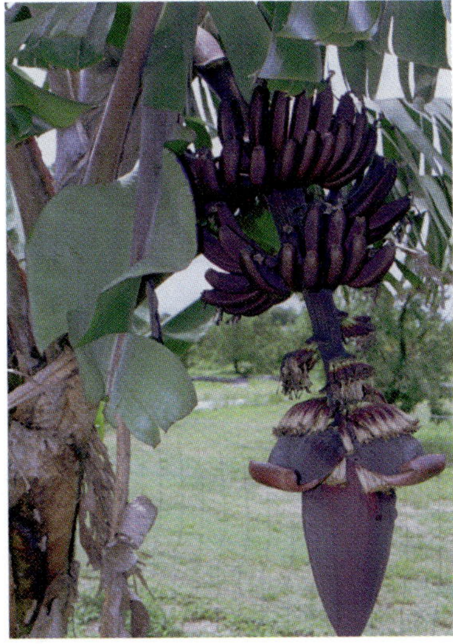

SUMATRANA X GRAND NAIN CROSS 'X Cross'

Very unusual hybrid with the leaf coloring of the Sumatrana and the growth habit of the Grand Nain. Plant is short and stout 7' (2.1m) to 10' (3m) with wide maroon variegated leaves that make it a prized landscape specimen. Has small seedless fruit that are very tasty. Sometimes referred to as 'x cross.'

12102 Growing Plant (4" Pot) $9.95
12101 Growing Plant (6" Pot) ...$14.95

THOUSAND FINGERS

Beautiful solid green plant that grows 10' (3m) to 12' (3.6m) tall and produces sweet 1½" (3.5cm) tiny bananas too numerous to count. Raceme of fruit can be as long as 8' (2.4m). A most unusual banana. A must for serious collectors. Quite a conversation piece.

12252 Growing Plant (4" Pot) $9.95
12251 Growing Plant (6" Pot) $14.95

FACTOID

Early Indonesian and Arab traders took bananas to Africa. In the 16th century the Spanish distributed bananas to the farthest warm reaches of their empire. Bananas came to North America directly from Europe by way of the Caribbean and Central and South America.

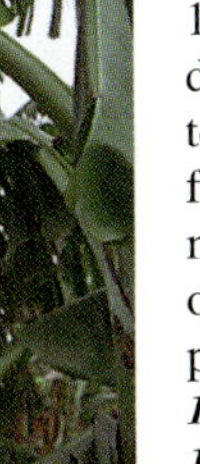

Visit our Web Site :
www.stokestropicals.com
E-mail us: info@stokestropicals.com

Full Sun   Part Sun   Shade   Extra Water   Fragrant   Cut Flower   New

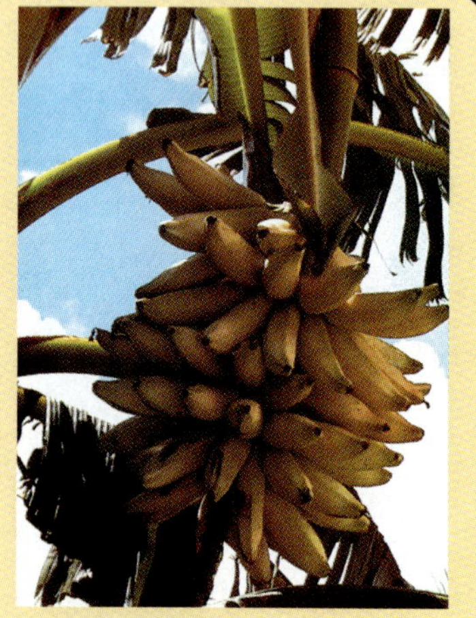

WHITE IHOLENE

A beautiful medium size 14' (4.2m) to 16' (4.8m) banana plant that is light green in color with waxy flakes of excess chitin that give it a whitish look. Undersides of leaves are light maroon. The White Iholene is actually a reverted green sport of the Red Iholene. The Iholene group is very interesting in that the newly emerged bananas are light yellow. When the fruit matures it darkens to a light orange color with pulp the same color. The fruit is like a cross between a plantain and a banana, so it can be eaten out-of-hand or cooked. The Iholenes mature their fruit quickly in 7 to 8 weeks. They appear to be more cold sensitive than most other bananas.

12352 Growing Plant (4" Pot) $9.95
12351 Growing Plant (6" Pot) ...$14.95

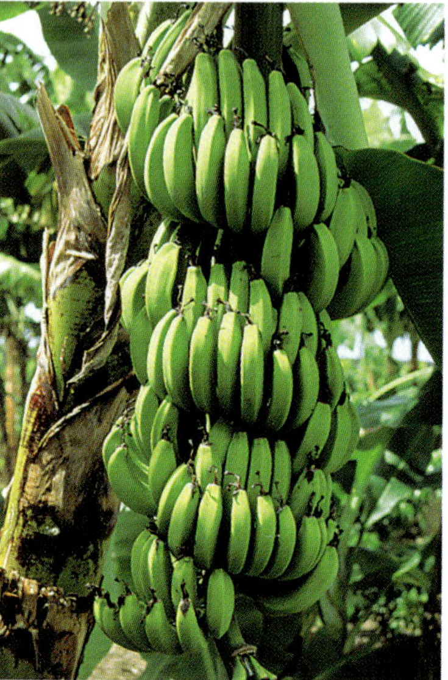

WILLIAMS HYBRID

A great looking variety, growing 6'-8'. A delightful cavendish type with very nice tasting fruit. One of the bananas of commerce. Relatively wind resistant and cold tolerant. Produces large bunches of fruit.

12332 Growing Plant (4" Pot) $9.95
12331 Growing Plant (6" Pot) $14.95

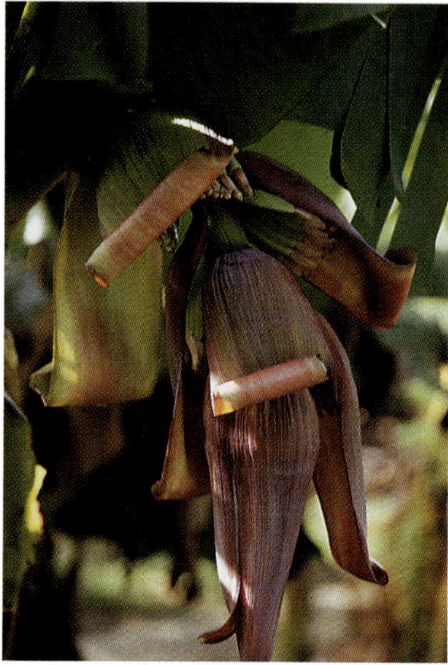

ZAN MORENO

A great new addition to the dwarf edible dessert bananas. Grows 6'-8'. Zone 9 and higher.

12362 Growing Plant (4" Pot) $9.95
12361 Growing Plant (6" Pot) $14.95

FACTOIDS

- One banana is about 75 calories on average.
- Bananas are about 75% water.
- Bananas have almost no fat.
- Bananas are rich in Vitamin C, B6 and Potassium.
- A ripe dessert banana may contain up to 21% sugar.

Banana Collections

Save $20 on each collection.

Beginner's Collection (5)—Dwarf Cavendish, Dwarf Red, Kru, Mysore, Raja Puri

Best Eating Collection (5)—Grand Nain, Ice Cream, Brazilian, Mysore, Goldfinger

Best Cooking Collection (5)—Hua Moa, Saba, Orinoco, Cardaba, African Rhino Horn

Best Ornamental Collection (5)—Velutina, Uranoscopus, Sumatrana, Ornata "Bronze", Ensete maurelii

Best Sellers Collection (5)—Musa Basjoo, Musella lasiocarpa, Sumatrana, Raja Puri, Super Dwarf Cavendish

Ornata Collection (5)—Standard Lavender, Bronze, Royal Purple, Macro, Lavender Beauty

Dwarf Collection (5)—Dwarf Red, Dwarf Cavendish, Dwarf Brazilian, Dwarf Orinoco, Super Dwarf Cavendish

Giant Collection (5)—Pisang Raja, Orinoco, Saba, Tall Red, Brazilian

Exotic Collection (5)—Monkey Finger, Double, Thousand Finger, Ebun Musak, Praying Hands

Rare Collection (5)—Musella lasiocarpa, Musa mannii, Ae Ae, Red Iholene, Ele Ele

(See pages 16-17.)

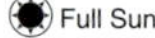 Full Sun   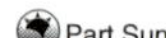 Part Sun   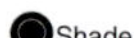 Shade   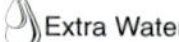 Extra Water   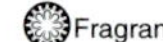 Fragrant   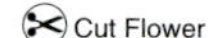 Cut Flower   N New

FAQ

FREQUENTLY ASKED QUESTIONS ABOUT BANANAS

What is the best tasting banana?

A difficult question to answer. Just as beauty is in the eyes of the beholder, taste is in the mouth of the beholder. According to many taste buds, the Mysore, Raja Puri and Ice Cream bananas are the best. But every dessert banana is someone's favorite.

What is the best cooking banana?

Another difficult question. For 'tostones', (fried plantains), the Hua Moa or Dwarf Puerto Rican get high ratings. For sweet plantains, (Maduros), the Giant Plantain and Saba are rated tops.

If I could get only one kind of banana, which one would you recommend?

A hard question to answer. But based on customer orders, the Raja Puri is our most popular eating banana and the Musa basjoo is our most popular ornamental. Our most popular dwarf is the Super Dwarf Cavendish. Our most popular cooking banana (plantain) is the Hua Moa.

How large will my plant (all kinds) grow?

A very difficult question to answer. There are so many variables that affect plant growth. The finished size is based on the genetic instructions of the plant and is influenced by soil type, moisture levels, optimum light conditions, ground planted or container planted (and container size), pruning, fertilization, altitude, growing temperatures (maximum, minimum and average), humidity and latitude. Growing a tropical plant in the North is different from growing the same plant in the South. In the North a shade plant in the South may be able to thrive in fall, winter, or spring sun. Plants in the ground always grow bigger than those planted in a container. We provide a range of heights in our plant descriptions; consider the lower height for containers and the greater height for in-the-ground plantings. With a little experimentation on your part you can find the ideal growing habitat for your lovely tropical plant. And if you need help just call us at 1-337-365-6998, M-F, between the hours of 9:00 and 4:00 Central Time.

Will my plant survive if it arrives with brown (or yellow) or damaged leaves?

Your plants will almost certainly arrive with brown, yellow or damaged (bent or broken) leaves. Uprooting your selected tropical plants from their optimum growing environment, cleaning them, spraying them for potential pests, dipping rhizome, or roots in fungicide, then packing them inside a dark box, surrounding them by shredded paper and/or banding to box, then shipping via truck and/or airplane to you with greatly varying temperatures and humidities (none of which are optimum), then waiting for you on your doorstep or at your post office, and then waiting for you to unpack and plant it and place it back into its optimum environment. Is it any wonder that some leaves and stems are damaged, brown or yellow? The wonder is that a tropical plant, or any plant for that matter, could survive such treatment. However our plants have been shipped all over the world with very good survival success. If planted promptly upon receipt in the correct type of potting soil and placed in the correct light conditions and not over-watered or over-fertilized they will revive quickly and put out new growth to replace yellowed or damaged leaves. The single factor that kills most plants is over watering. Plant roots need oxygen; they cannot get oxygen with roots standing in water unless they are water plants. The second most common cause of killing a plant is too much fertilizer. If a plant does not have a good leaf system and a good root system it cannot take a lot of water or full strength fertilizer. Start out slowly until you see the plant responding favorably by putting out new green leaves and developing a good root system. Too much care can be the death knell for an otherwise healthy plant.

Why won't my banana plant flower and fruit?

When I get this question, the first thing I ask is how long have you had it? Bananas need 9-15 consecutive months of non-freezing temperatures to flower and another 2-3 months to fruit. So if you are growing it outside in ground you should be in zone 10 or higher or if in zone 9 you need a mild winter. The second thing I ask is, do you have it in full sun? Bananas need full sun. The third question is are you fertilizing it well? Bananas are heavy feeders and they need a fertilizer high in potassium (K) such as our Stokes Tropicals' Banana Blend (6-2-12). Bananas are also heavy drinkers. So with 9-15 months of non-freezing weather, plenty of sun, plenty of high K fertilizer, and plenty of water you'll get flowers and soon-to-follow fruit.

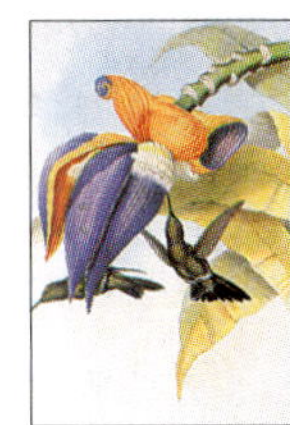

All bananas, unless noted, are hardy in Zone 8 and higher planted outside in ground with virtually no protection. In lower Zones they are hardy with special protection. If you can prevent the rhizome (bulb) from freezing, the plant will come back the following spring.

BANANA COLLECTIONS

(Save $20 off listed prices by purchasing collection)

Bananas

BEGINNER'S COLLECTION 5

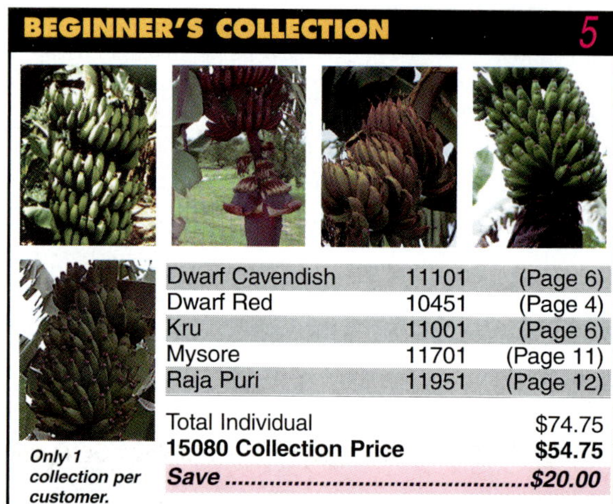

Dwarf Cavendish	11101	(Page 6)
Dwarf Red	10451	(Page 4)
Kru	11001	(Page 6)
Mysore	11701	(Page 11)
Raja Puri	11951	(Page 12)
Total Individual		$74.75
15080 Collection Price		**$54.75**
Save		*$20.00*

Only 1 collection per customer.

BEST EATING COLLECTION 5

Grand Nain	10801	(Page 5)
Ice Cream 'Blue Java'	10951	(Page 6)
Brazilian	10151	(Page 2)
Mysore	11701	(Page 11)
FHIA-01 'Goldfinger'	10751	(Page 5)
Total Individual		$74.75
15040 Collection Price		**$54.75**
Save		*$20.00*

Only 1 collection per customer.

BEST COOKING COLLECTION 5

Hua Moa	10851	(Page 6)
Saba	12051	(Page 12)
Orinoco	11751	(Page 11)
Cardaba	10201	(Page 3)
African Rhino Horn	10101	(Page 2)
Total Individual		$74.75
15050 Collection Price		**$54.75**
Save		*$20.00*

Only 1 collection per customer.

BEST ORNAMENTAL COLLECTION 5

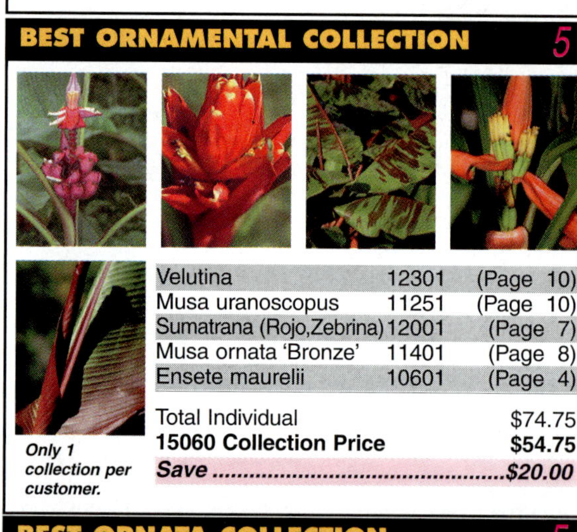

Velutina	12301	(Page 10)
Musa uranoscopus	11251	(Page 10)
Sumatrana (Rojo, Zebrina)	12001	(Page 7)
Musa ornata 'Bronze'	11401	(Page 8)
Ensete maurelii	10601	(Page 4)
Total Individual		$74.75
15060 Collection Price		**$54.75**
Save		*$20.00*

Only 1 collection per customer.

BEST SELLERS COLLECTION 5

Musa basjoo	11151	(Page 8)
Musella lasiocarpa	11651	(Page 10)
Sumatrana (Rojo, Zebrina)	12001	(Page 7)
Raja Puri	11951	(Page 12)
Super Dwarf Cavendish	11121	(Page 7)
Total Individual		$74.75
15090 Collection Price		**$54.75**
Save		*$20.00*

Only 1 collection per customer.

BEST ORNATA COLLECTION 5

Musa ornata 'S. Lavender'	11451	(Page 9)
Musa ornata 'Bronze'	11401	(Page 8)
Musa ornata 'Royal Purple'	11601	(Page 9)
Musa ornata 'Macro'	11571	(Page 9)
Musa ornata 'Lavender B.'	11351	(Page 8)
Total Individual		$79.75
15070 Collection Price		**$59.75**
Save		*$20.00*

Only 1 collection per customer.

DWARF COLLECTION 5

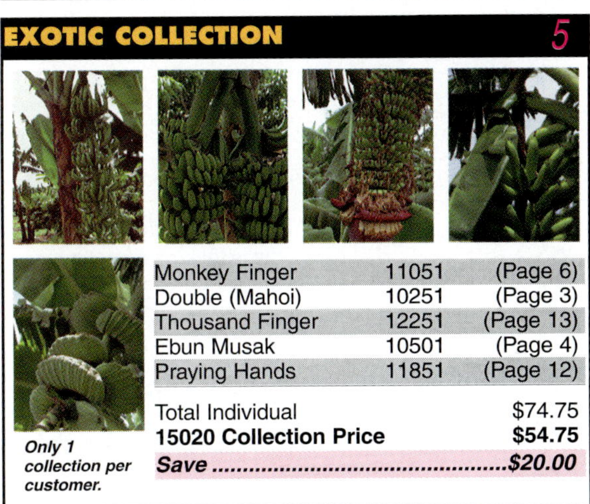

Dwarf Red	10451	(Page 4)
Musa acuminata 'Dwf Cav.'	11101	(Page 6)
Dwarf Brazilian	10301	(Page 3)
Dwarf Orinoco	10401	(Page 3)
Super Dwarf Cavendish	11121	(Page 7)

Total Individual	**$74.75**
15000 Collection Price	***$54.75***
Save	*$20.00*

Only 1 collection per customer.

GIANT COLLECTION 5

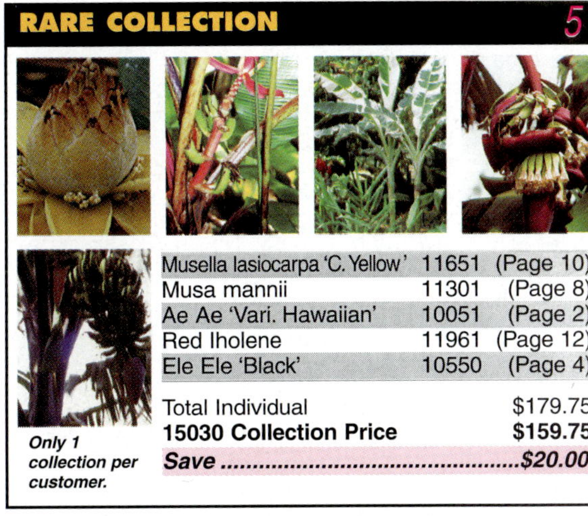

Pisang Raja	11901	(Page 11)
Orinoco	11751	(Page 11)
Saba	12051	(Page 12)
Tall Red	12201	(Page 13)
Brazilian	10151	(Page 2)

Total Individual	**$74.75**
15010 Collection Price	***$54.75***
Save	*$20.00*

Only 1 collection per customer.

EXOTIC COLLECTION 5

Monkey Finger	11051	(Page 6)
Double (Mahoi)	10251	(Page 3)
Thousand Finger	12251	(Page 13)
Ebun Musak	10501	(Page 4)
Praying Hands	11851	(Page 12)

Total Individual	$74.75
15020 Collection Price	**$54.75**
Save	*$20.00*

Only 1 collection per customer.

RARE COLLECTION 5

Musella lasiocarpa 'C. Yellow'	11651	(Page 10)
Musa mannii	11301	(Page 8)
Ae Ae 'Vari. Hawaiian'	10051	(Page 2)
Red Iholene	11961	(Page 12)
Ele Ele 'Black'	10550	(Page 4)

Total Individual	$179.75
15030 Collection Price	**$159.75**
Save	*$20.00*

Only 1 collection per customer.

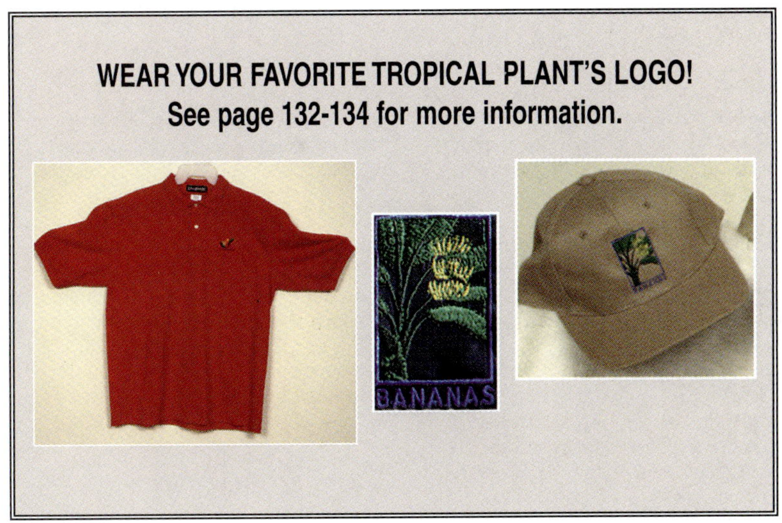

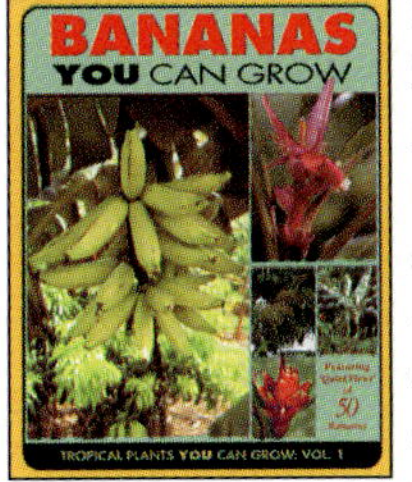

BANANAS YOU CAN GROW

By James W. Waddick & Glenn M. Stokes 2000 129 pp. See Page 129 for a detailed description.

71125 .... **$19.95**

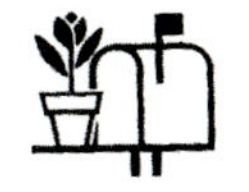

We are proud to be a member of the **Mail Order Gardening Association**

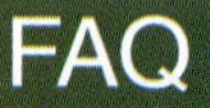

FAQ

FREQUENTLY ASKED QUESTIONS ABOUT OUR GUIDE/CATALOG

Will I get a guide/catalog next year?
If you have ordered from us in the last 24 months or have membership in certain professional societies and/or organizations, you will receive a guide/catalog. We update our mailing list annually and if you haven't ordered from us in the last 24 months you will be removed from our mailing list. However if you want to get back on our active mailing list you could purchase plants, products or a guide/catalog at any time.

DEFINITIONS

What is a rhizome?
A rhizome is the enlarged underground stem that contains food reserves and from which grows the roots and above ground stem and leaves. <u>Rhizomes are available only from about December 15 to about May 1.</u> This is because they are dormant at this time only. Rhizomes are stored until temperatures warm up, at which time they may be planted.

What is a growing plant?
A growing plant is one that is actively growing with a good root system and a good above ground stem and leaves. In order to ship a healthy growing plant to you, we gently remove plant from soil, wrap sphagnum moss or newspaper around root system, secure and carefully pack in a cardboard box and ship to you. Upon receipt you just need to plant at the same level it was growing (see markings on stem), into a well-drained, loose potting mix and water lightly. After growth resumes (new growth is seen) you can fertilize with a half strength fertilizer. Then in one month, use full strength fertilizer as recommended. Just follow cultural directions carefully that come with the plant. Rhizomes will be growing plants after May 1st. Growing plants of "long-day" plants (Curcumas, Globbas, Kaempferias, Zingibers, Siphonochilus, Cannas) are available from May/June thru October. Growing plants of bananas, heliconias, certain gingers (Hedychiums, Alpinias, Costus, Monocostus) hibiscus, Siamese lucky plants, and bougainvilleas are available all year.

What is a rooting plumeria cutting?
It is a cutting that we have specially prepared for you. It takes us 4-10 weeks, depending on time of year and variety, to fully root a cutting. We then simply remove the rooting cutting from its growing medium, gently pack to prevent roots from drying, and ship to you. You should then replant at same level (see band on stem), in a well-drained soil mix either directly into the ground or into a container. Water lightly and fertilize with a half strength fertilizer at sign of first new growth. <u>Don't keep too wet</u> and follow cultural directions that come with plant. We take orders for rooting plumeria cuttings all year. And we ship them from <u>March 1st to November 1st.</u>

ORDERING & SHIPPING & EXPORT

What is the best time of the year to order tropical plants?
There is no best time. It depends on where you live and where you are going to grow them. If you live in U.S.D.A. zone 10 and higher, there won't be any freezes to worry about so you can get plants and plant them at any time of the year. If you have a greenhouse or you intend to grow them inside your home you can also get them at any time of the year no matter where you live. And if you order rhizomes in winter or spring when they are dormant they can be safely stored for future planting.

How do you ship your plants?
Unless you otherwise specify, we ship by U.S. Postal Service Priority, which generally takes 3-5 days to arrive anywhere in the U.S.A. If you require even faster service, we will ship via U.S. Postal Service Express, U.P.S. or FedEx for an additional charge. For our overseas customers we ship via air (U.S. Postal Service Express, U.P.S., FedEx, or Airborne Express) for actual cost of shipping.

Do you ship to foreign countries?
Yes, we do. Please see "Ordering/Shipping Instructions" and "Terms of Sale" under "Foreign Orders" on our order form. We have had excellent results with our plants going to foreign countries. Our foreign customers frequently tell us how good our plants look upon arrival.

How long will it take to get my plants?
As mentioned above, you can get them as quick as you want --- even next day by U.P.S., Fed Ex or U.S. Postal Service Express. This costs a little more. Ordinarily, in the continental U.S. you would get your plants within 3-5 days by U.S. Postal Service Priority.

Do you ship plants any time of the year?
Yes, we do–depending on availability of plant material and time of year. Of course, if the particular plant you order is dormant and is in the rhizome stage, we can't supply you with a growing plant. And we can't supply you with rhizomes when they are growing plants. And we won't ship plants into areas where temperatures are well below freezing because of risk of freezing unless customer assumes all risk.

CREDIT CARDS & GUARANTEES

Do you accept credit cards?
Yes, we accept all major credit cards: MasterCard, Visa, American Express and Discover/Novus. We also accept personal checks and money orders. Sorry we can't ship C.O.D.

Are your plants and other products guaranteed?
Yes, they are. If you are not completely satisfied with our products, just <u>notify us within 10 days</u> and return merchandise to us and we'll refund your money, replace merchandise, replace with something else of equal

Continued on page 23

BOUGAINVILLEAS

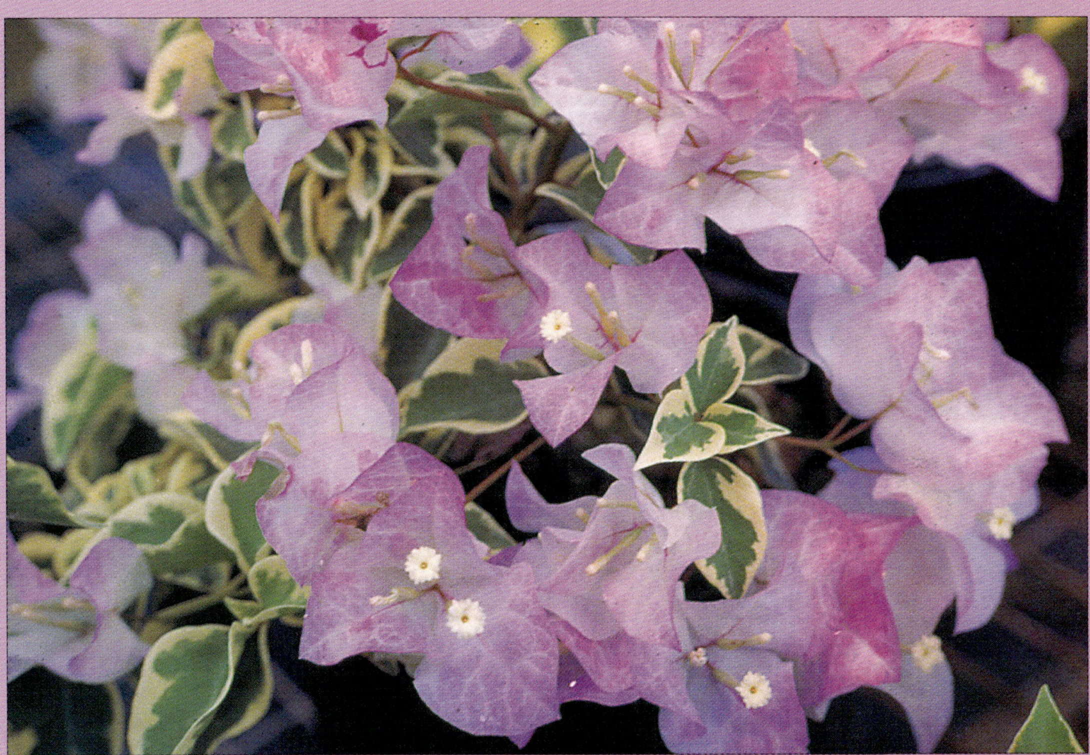

Bougainvillea—one of the most tropical, exciting and deliciously colorful of all tropical plants. A wonderful vining plant that has a rainbow of colored bracts. In zones 10 and 11 they are permanent perennials; in zone 9, they can be considered a returning perennial. In lower zones, they can be greenhoused or protected from freezing temperatures when grown outside in containers or in ground. Bougainvilleas come from South America and have small tubular, short-lived flowers in clusters near ends of stems. Large, brilliantly colored long-lasting bracts surround flowers. The variegated forms do not grow as large as the non-variegated types. Plants can be maintained as shrubs by frequent pruning of the spreading canes. Since plants bloom on new wood, pruning is not detrimental to flower production. Bract colors include white, yellow, orange, pink, numerous shades of red, magenta, purple...just about every color except blue. The majority of bougainvillea cultivars are year-round bloomers in cycles of about three months or so. Fertilizing sparingly throughout the growing season will encourage new growth, which in turn is when the flowering occurs. Our Heliconia Blend fertilizer (9-3-6 with minors) has proved excellent for bougainvillea. The little extra nitrogen (9) provides for just enough new growth and the lesser ratio of phosphorous and potassium (3 and 6 respectively) work perfectly for maximum flower production. Our Tropical Foliage Blend (9-3-6) is our liquid fertilizer that can be sprayed on. It also does an excellent job. When this is combined with Pro-TeKt (0-0-3), our liquid silicon supplement, you can maximize flower production. A good loose, humus soil is best. Feeding and tip pruning should be done at the end of each bloom cycle. The two most important considerations in successfully growing bougainvilleas are sun and good drainage. They do not like soggy or wet feet and they refuse to bloom in the shade. We have chosen 15 of the best and newest cultivars in this fantastic genus of plants.

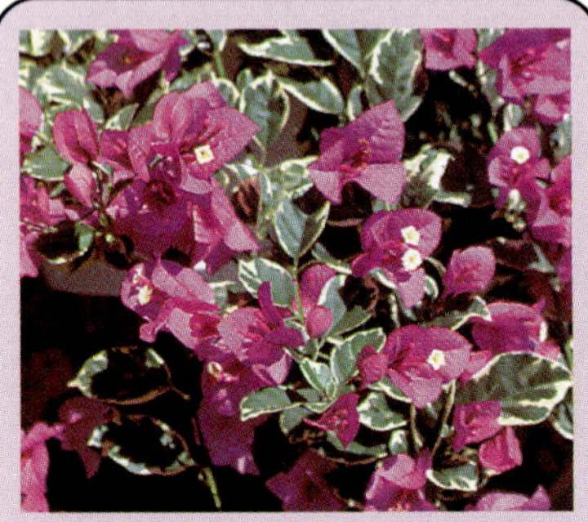

BLUEBERRY ICE

A fantastic new variegated bougainvillea with lavender blue bracts. A great addition to the "Ice" series. One should have all three: Raspberry Ice, Orange Ice and Blueberry Ice to electrify the garden landscape with color from both leaf and flower. Blueberry Ice is probably the easiest to flower and is a semi-dwarf. Likes full sun and not too much water. Zone 10 and higher outside.

86010 Growing Plant (4" pot)......$9.95

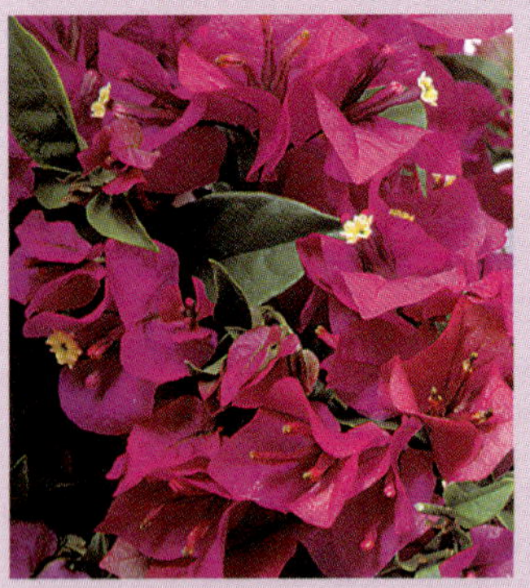

HELEN JOHNSON

A great looking semi-dwarf. Beautiful intense magenta bracts against dark green leaves are marvelous. Has a great growing habit and is considered thornless because it only develops a soft immature thorn. Does well as a bush or in hanging basket.

86020 Growing Plant
(4" pot) $9.95

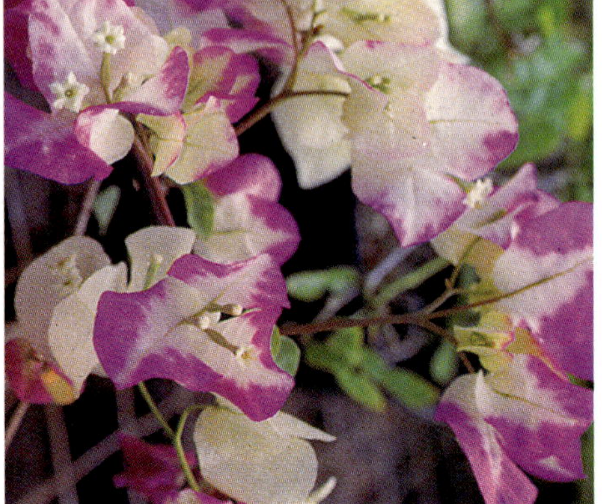

DELTA DAWN >

A smashing new bougainvillea with showy variegated leaves displaying golden bracts flushed with pink. One of the most beautiful of all the bougainvilleas. Full sun and not much water. Zone 10 and higher outside; any zone inside.

86025 Growing Plant
(4" pot) $10.95

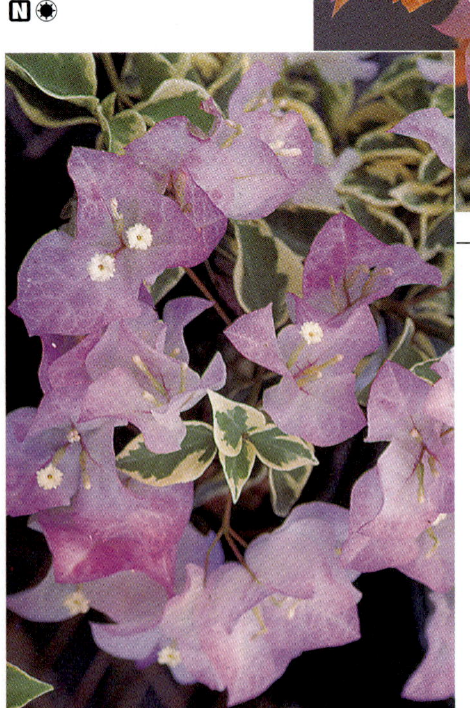

COCONUT ICE

An uncommon African cultivar, featuring pleasant combinations of white and pink bracts – with colors appearing alone or in combination on the same bract. And in addition has wonderful variegated leaves. Full sun and not much water. Zone 10 and higher outside; any zone inside.
86015 Growing Plant
(4" pot) $10.95

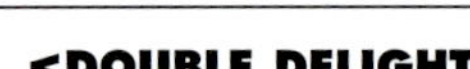

<DOUBLE DELIGHT

A majestic bud sport from 'Barbara Karst'. Looks like a variegated form of Imperial Delight. Bracts open whiteish then blend to different intensities of pink. Compact form, therefore good in hanging baskets. Full sun and not much water. Zone 10 and higher outside; any zone inside.

86045 Growing Plant
(4" pot) $10.95

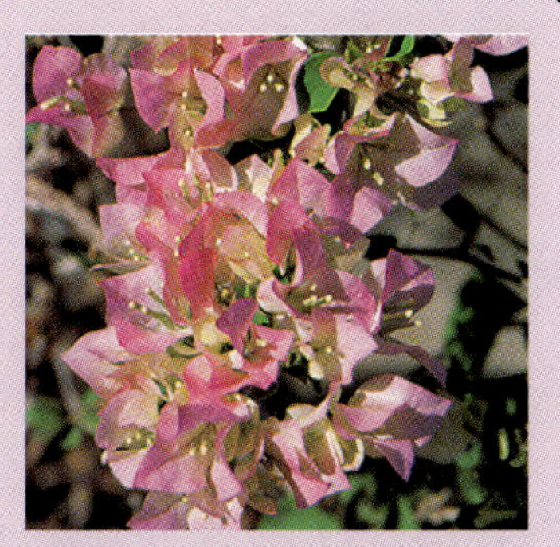

IMPERIAL DELIGHT

A stunning new bougainvillea cultivar that is a semi-dwarf. It's bracts are white suffused with a mixture of strawberry, plum, and peach coloring. Once you grow and bloom this plant you will want more and your friends will too. Just plant in a pot or in the ground and it will thrive—no pruning, fuss, or bother. Likes high light, a little water, and a little fertilizer. Zone 10 and higher outside.
86040 Growing Plant (4" pot)......$9.95

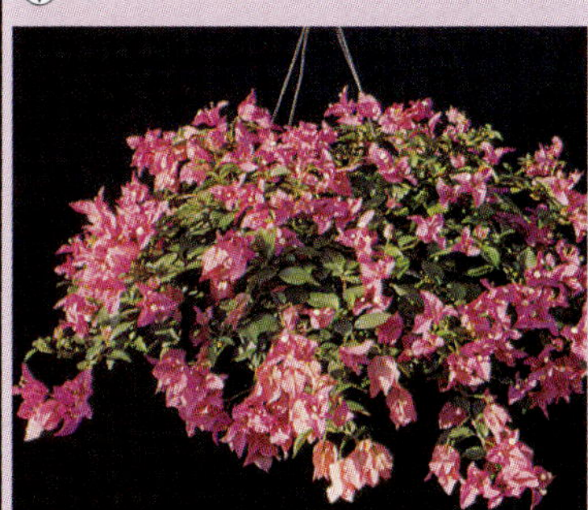

LADY CASIMIR

A dramatic new semi-dwarf bougainvillea cultivar with an amazing creeping growth habit that makes it ideal for basket or pot culture. A super plant for hanging baskets, it just flows over the side and becomes flush with pinkish-lavender colored bracts. Needs no pruning, no special care, just high light, a little water and a little fertilizer. Zone 10 and higher outside.
86060 Growing Plant (4" pot)......$9.95

LADY MARY BARING

Old cultivar that is being rediscovered. May have first occurred as bud sport in India from 'Golden Glow'. Buttery yellow that fades to a beige color as bracts age. Does not turn orangey, vigorous grower. Flowers for long periods several times a year. Full sun and not much water. Zone 10 and higher outside; any zone inside.
85250 Growing Plant (4" pot) $10.95

MAJIC

One of the most outstanding bougainvillea cultivars that we have found. The same plant produces three different striking colors of bract: white, magenta, and a bicolored white-magenta. Yes, some bracts are half-white and half-magenta. The leaves are highly variegated with about equal amounts of yellow/white surface area and green surface area. Even when it is not blooming, you have a marvelous variegated plant in full display. A rather compact grower that doesn't outgrow its welcome. You will be delighted with our favorite bougainvillea. Does well as bush, hanging basket, trellis, or standard.
86030 Growing Plant (4" pot) $9.95

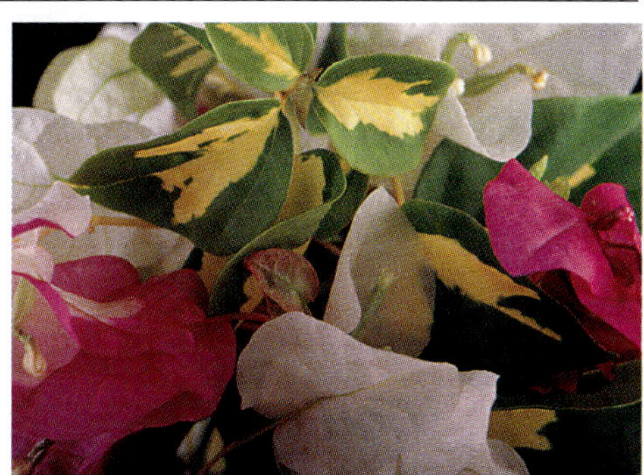

MARDI GRAS

What a great looking bougainvillea! A very compact variegated leaf form with massive flushes of pink and orange bracts that give it a festive Mardi Gras look. Full sun and not much water. Zone 10 and higher outside; any zone inside.
86035 Growing Plant (4"pot) $10.95

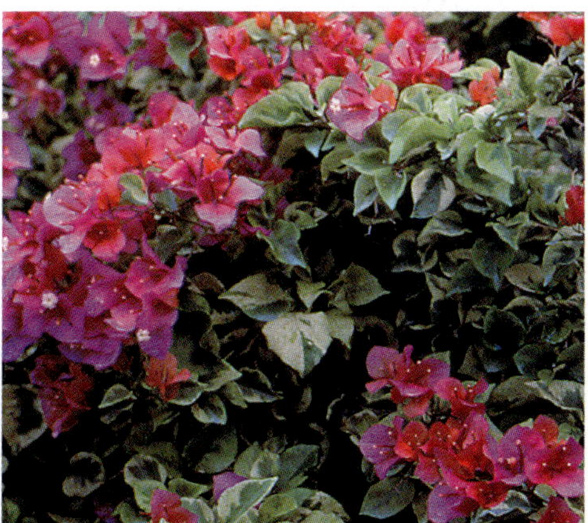

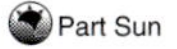 Full Sun   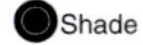 Part Sun   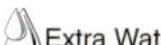 Shade   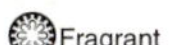 Extra Water   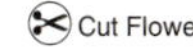 Fragrant   Cut Flower   New

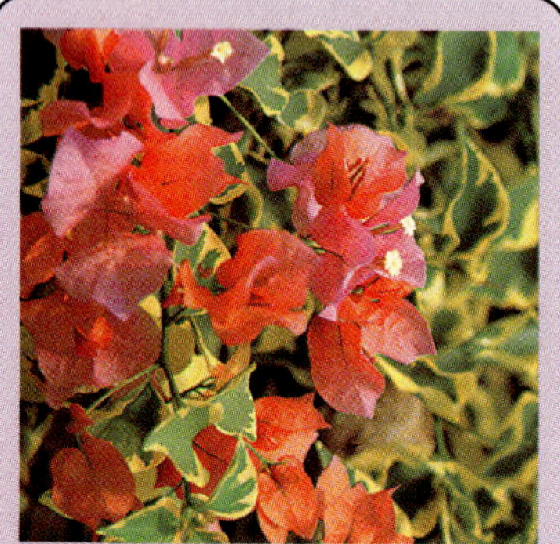

ORANGE ICE

From Thailand, another fantastic new variegated cultivar with transparent tangerine orange bracts. Similar to 'Raspberry Ice', except for color of bracts, but is much easier to bloom. Orange Ice is not an aggressive grower making it easy to manage. The highly variegated foliage provides a continuous display even when not in bloom. Does well as bush, hanging basket, or trellis. Blooms throughout the year. Zone 10 and higher in ground.
86050 Growing Plant (4"pot).......$9.95

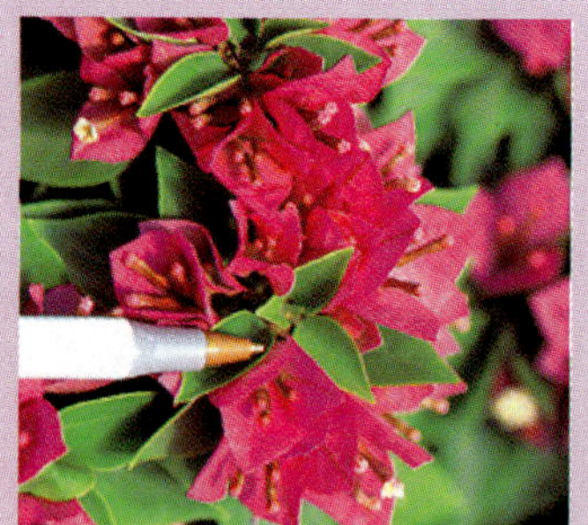

PINK PIXIE

This remarkable dwarf variety is free blooming with wonderful deep pink dwarf bracts and leaves. It is an excellent container plant because of its small size and ease to grow. It lends itself to being a bonsai and topiary subject. You will absolutely love this plant. Can be grown inside with strong light. Does well as a bush.
86070 Growing Plant (4"pot).......$9.95

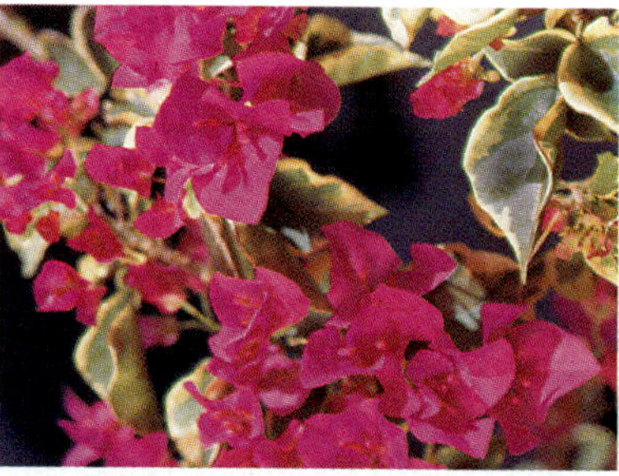

RED FANTASY

A fantastic looking bougainvillea. A sport of Maureen Hatten, with brilliant red bracts surrounded by green and gold variegated leaves. Full sun and not much water. Zone 10 and higher outside; any zone inside.
86055 Growing Plant (4" pot) *$11.95*

SAVITEE

Another dramatic variegated leaf form, similar to Raspberry Ice, but color of bracts are hot pink instead of red. Full sun and not much water. Zone 10 and higher outside; any zone inside.
86065 Growing Plant (4" pot) $11.95

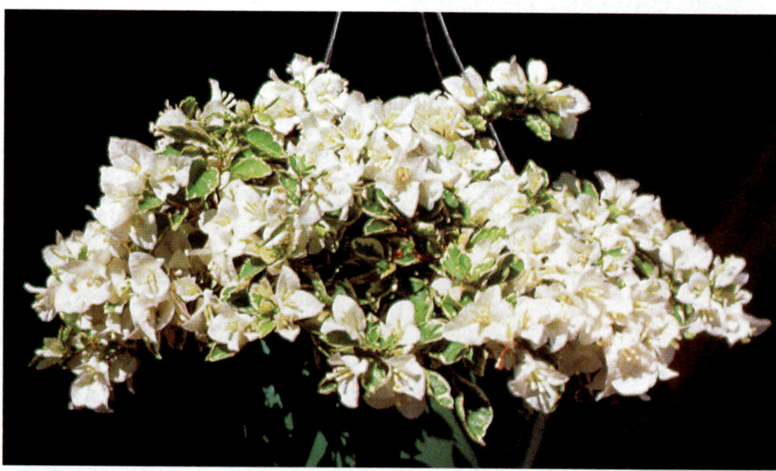

WHITE STRIPE

A variegated beauty with white variegated foliage and lily white bracts. A real charmer with a blast of medium-sized white bracts framed by green and white variegated foliage. Great in hanging baskets. Full sun and not much water. Zone 10 and higher outside; any zone inside.
86075 Growing Plant (4" pot) *$10.95*

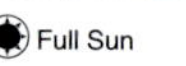 Full Sun   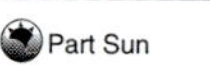 Part Sun   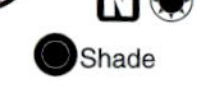 Shade   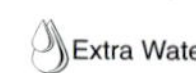 Extra Water   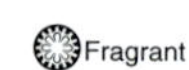 Fragrant   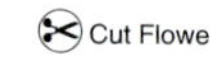 Cut Flower   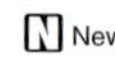 New

VARIEGATED BOUGAINVILLEA COLLECTION 3

Majic	86030	(Page 21)
Orange Ice	86050	(Page 22)
Blueberry Ice	86010	(Page 20)

Catalog price	$29.85
86090 Collection Price	**$24.85**
Save	**$5.00**

Only 1 collection per customer.

SPECIAL VARIEGATED COLLECTION 5

Coconut Ice	86015	(Page 20)
Delta Dawn	86025	(Page 20)
Double Delight	86045	(Page 20)
Savitee	86065	(Page 22)
White Stripe	86075	(Page 22)

Catalog Price	$55.75
86095 Collection Price	**$45.75**
Save	**$10.00**

Only 1 collection per customer.

FAQ

Continued from page 18

or greater value, or give you credit for future purchase. The choice is yours. We want you to be a satisfied customer.

U.S.D.A. PLANT HARDINESS ZONES

What is my U.S.D.A. plant hardiness zone?

For your convenience, we have a map on page 131 and you will be able to determine your zone. Zones are 10°F apart, for example, zone 9 is 20-30°F and zone 10 is 30-40°F. What this means is that the average minimum winter temperature falls between these numbers. To further divide these zones, they are broken down into "A"s and "B"s – with 9A being 20-25°F and 9B being a warmer 26-30°F, on average. It should be remembered that these zones are approximations based on averages. In any one year, the winter temperatures could be well above or well below the average for the zone. Also there are many ameliorating factors: altitude, winds, humidity, etc. Plus no geographical area is uniform in climatic conditions. What really exists is a spectrum of microclimates. It is the microclimate that determines a plants' growth and survival.

CONTAINERS & GROWING INDOORS

Can your tropicals plants be planted in containers?

Yes, all our tropical plants will grow and thrive in containers. In fact, we grow all our plants in containers.

Can your tropical plants be grown indoors?

The answer is yes. All our plants can be successfully grown indoors the year-round if you have enough space and the correct lighting. All our plants can be overwintered by bringing inside to a greenhouse, foyer, solarium, basement or other suitable interior space to avoid freezing. Grow lights may be required.

GIFT CERTIFICATES
Do you sell gift certificates?

Yes, we do. And they make wonderful gifts. They come as a beautiful certificate in $25.00 denominations. They can be redeemed at anytime by the holder for anything we carry in our guide/catalog. And they don't expire.See page 134 for details.

BEST EATING, MOST FRAGRANT, BEST KIND

What is the best tasting banana?

A difficult question to answer. Just as beauty is in the eyes of the beholder, taste is in the mouth of the beholder. According to our taste buds, the Mysore, Raja Puri and Ice Cream bananas are the best. But every dessert banana is someone's favorite. And every cooking banana is someone's favorite.

What is the best cooking banana?

Another difficult question. For "tostones" (fried plantains), the Hua Moa or Dwarf Puerto Rican get high ratings. For sweet plantains (Maduros), the Giant Plantain and Saba are rated tops.

What is the most fragrant plumeria?

This is hard to say because nearly all of the hybrid plumerias are fragrant. One of the most fragrant is the Dwarf Deciduous. And all the Moragnes are very fragrant. What you really need to do is pick out the fragrance you like the most, such as, coconut, frangipani, lemon, citrus, or other and make your choice accordingly.

What is the most fragrant ginger?

This is pretty easy to answer: the white butterfly, Hedychium coronarium. Nearly all of the Hedychium species and hybrids are fragrant. In general, the whiter the flower, the more fragrant. And the redder the flower, the less fragrant. There are certain other ginger flowers that are fragrant: Alpinia henryi, Kaempferia rotunda, Siphonochilus aethiopicus, Siphonochilus decora, Siphonochilus kirkii, Siphonochilus carsonii and Costus afer. And there are many gingers in the genera Zingiber, Curcuma and Alpinia that have aromatic leaves, stems and/or rhizomes.

Continued on page 24

Bananas

FAQ *Continued from page 23*

If I could get only one kind of banana, which one would you recommend?

A hard question to answer. But based on customer orders, the Raja Puri is our most popular eating banana and the Musa basjoo is our most popular ornamental. Our most popular dwarf is the Super Dwarf Cavendish. Our most popular cooking banana (plantain) is the Hua Moa.

If I could get only one kind of plumeria, which one would you recommend?

This is a pretty easy question to answer. The Dwarf Pink would be our choice because it is a true dwarf never getting any taller than 6 feet, and this is after 8 or 10 years. It is evergreen, that is, doesn't lose its leaves. It flowers all year if not exposed to freezing temperatures. And it can even flower indoors in high light. Plus because of its slow growth, 6" or so per year, it lends itself to being containerized.

GETTING STARTED IN TROPICALS, HOW LARGE, SHIPPING DAMAGE

What is the easiest way to start growing a particular group of tropical plants, such as, gingers, bananas, heliconias, plumerias, hibiscus, bougainvilleas, or cannas?

That's easy to answer. We have chosen collections in each of these groups. In some of the larger groups of plants, we have selected a "beginner's collection". A collection will not only save you money but will give you a nice variety to get started with. If you do well with your initial collection, then you can expand to more plants of the same group or you could try your luck with other groups.

How large will my plant grow?

A very difficult question to answer. There are so many variables that affect plant growth. The finished size is based on the genetic instructions of the plant and is influenced by soil

type, moisture levels, optimum light conditions, ground planted or container planted (and container size), pruning, fertilization, altitude, growing temperatures (maximum, minimum and average), humidity and latitude. Growing a tropical plant in the North is different from growing the same plant in the South. In the North a shade plant in the South may be able to thrive in fall, winter, or spring sun. Plants in the ground always grow bigger than those planted in a container. When we provide a range of heights in our plant descriptions; consider the lower height for containers and the greater height for in-the-ground plantings. With a little experimentation on your part you can find the ideal growing habitat for your lovely tropical plant. And if you need help just call us at 1-318-365-6998, M-F, between the hours of 9:00 and 4:00 Central Time.

Will my plant survive if it arrives with brown (or yellow) or damaged leaves?

Your plants will almost certainly arrive with brown, yellow or damaged (bent or broken) leaves. Uprooting your selected tropical plants from their optimum growing environment, cleaning them, spraying them for potential pests, dipping rhizome, or roots in fungicide, then packing them inside a dark box, surrounding them by shredded paper and/or banding to box, then shipping via truck and/or airplane to you with greatly varying temperatures and humidities (none of which are optimum), then waiting for you on your doorstep or at your post office, and then waiting for you to unpack and plant it and place it back into its optimum environment. Is it any wonder that some leaves and stems are damaged, brown or yellow? The wonder is that a tropical plant, or any plant for that matter, could survive such treatment. However our plants have been shipped all over the world with very good survival success. If planted promptly upon receipt in the correct type of potting soil and placed in the correct light conditions and not over-watered or over-fertilized they will revive quickly and put out new growth to replace yellowed or dam-

aged leaves. The single factor that kills most plants is over watering. Plant roots need oxygen; they cannot get oxygen with roots standing in water unless they are water plants. The second most common cause of killing a plant is too much fertilizer. If a plant does not have a good leaf system and a good root system it cannot take a lot of water or full strength fertilizer. Start out slowly until you see the plant responding favorably by putting out new green leaves and developing a good root system. Too much care can be the death knell for an otherwise healthy plant.

FLOWERING & FRUITING

Why won't my banana plant flower and fruit?

When I get this question, the first thing I ask is how long have you had it? Bananas need 9-15 months of non-freezing temperatures to flower and another 2-3 months to fruit. So if you are growing it outside in ground you should be in zone 10 or higher or if in zone 9 you need a mild winter. The second thing I ask is, do you have it in full sun? Bananas need full sun. The third question is are you fertilizing it well. Bananas are heavy feeders and they need a fertilizer high in potassium (K) such as our Stokes Tropicals' Banana Blend (6-2-12). Bananas are also heavy drinkers. So with 9-15 months of non-freezing weather, plenty of sun, plenty of high K fertilizer, and plenty of water you'll get flowers and soon-to-follow fruit.

Why won't my plumeria bloom?

My first question is, do you have it growing in full sun? Plumerias need full sun. Then I ask, are you fertilizing it with a high phosphorus (P) fertilizer? To encourage blooming a fertilizer such as, Stokes Tropicals' Plumeria Blend (8-14-10) is ideal. Rooted plumeria cuttings can bloom the first year if they are terminal and contain enough plant auxin. And all plumeria cuttings should flower in the 2nd or 3rd year with proper sunlight, fertilizer, and care.

ALL STOKES TROPICALS' PLANTS ARE EASY-TO-GROW.

CANNAS

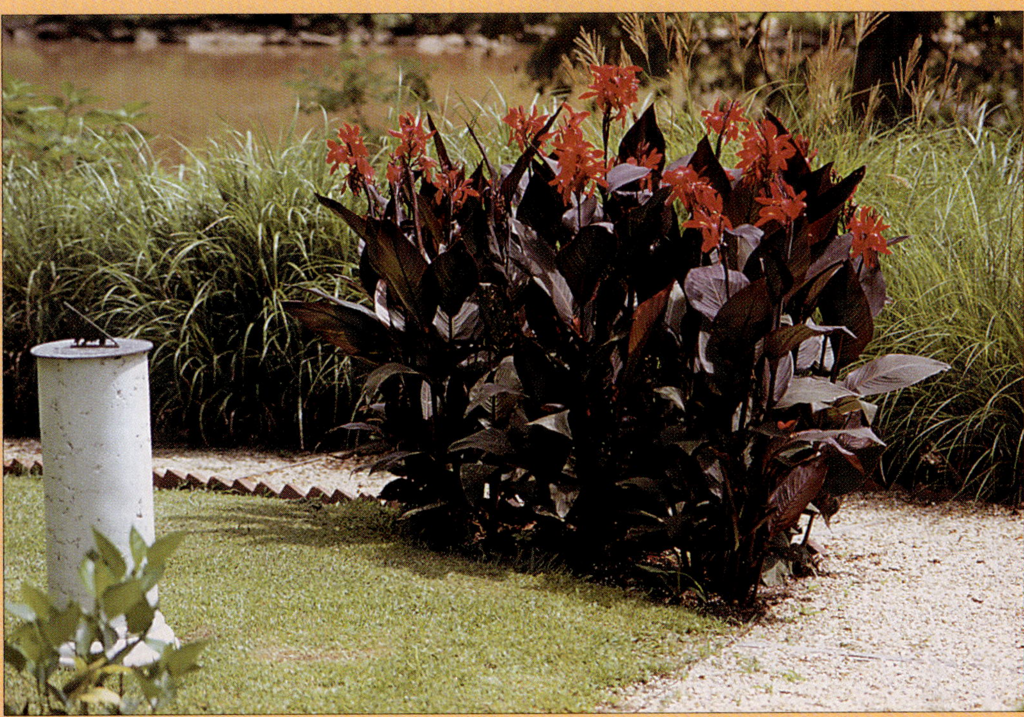

Cannas are a herbaceous perennials closely related to gingers, bananas, heliconias and birds of paradise. Cannas do well over most of the U.S. provided there is plenty of summer heat. Cannas grow from rhizomes (bulbs). They are easy to plant and easy to grow. Their flowers come in a wide variety of colors including red, orange, yellow, pink and fuchsia. They have long, heliconia or banana-like leaves giving them a very tropical look. Cannas should be treated like other tropical plants; plant in spring after chance of last frost and dig before first hard freeze in fall. The bulbs can be stored over winter in a cool dry place like caladiums, dahlias, gladioli, or other bulbs. Of course in zone 10 and higher they will thrive and flower all year. In zones 8 and 9, leaves will freeze back but "bulb" will overwinter safely in ground, if well drained. Cannas do best in full sun, but will do nicely in partial shade. There are basically 3 sizes of Cannas: tall (6-7'), medium (4-6'), and dwarf (2-4'). Cannas can be used as accent plants, borders, or in beds. They also make great container plants. They are easy to grow and maintain, just water well once a week. A balanced fertilizer should be applied monthly during the growing season. Our Plumeria Blend (8-14-10) works extremely well on cannas. And since it is a 3-month slow release formula it can be applied once every 3 months. Also our Flowering Tropical Blend (7-9-5) liquid fertilizer works splendidly with Cannas. And to make it work even better use our Pro-Tekt (0-0-3).

Because of their succulent leaves, cannas can be attractive to moths and butterflies. The resulting caterpillars can be picked off or controlled with safe insecticide treatments. Cannas are easy to keep pristine looking by removing spent flowers and seedpods and trimming unsightly leaves. Also bees, butterflies, moths and hummingbirds are attracted to canna flowers.

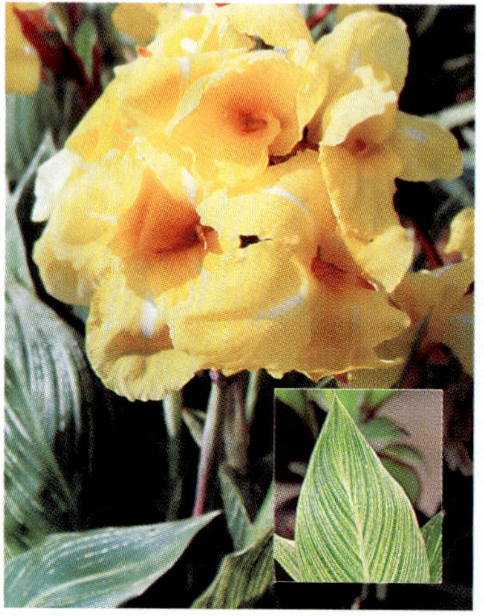

BANGKOK YELLOW

A dwarf canna with foliage that is outstanding—green leaves with white striping. Its' red bud opens into a clear yellow flower that has a white throat. Grows very well in water. An amazing variegated plant that has to be seen to be believed.

88100 Rhizome *$5.95*
88101 Growing Plant (6" pot) *$9.95*

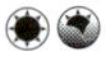

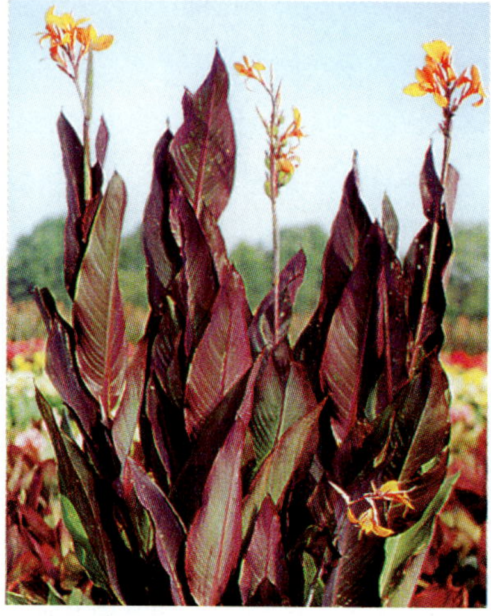

INTRIGUE

Exceptionally tall burgundy and green sword-shape foliage growing from 6-9 ft. in height. Many small light yellow/salmon colored (orchid-shaped) blossoms. Tolerates moderate shade but prefers full sun. Very prolific growing habit that produces lush background foliage in first year of growth.

88240 Rhizome...............................*$6.95*
88241 Growing Plant (6" pot)....*$10.95*

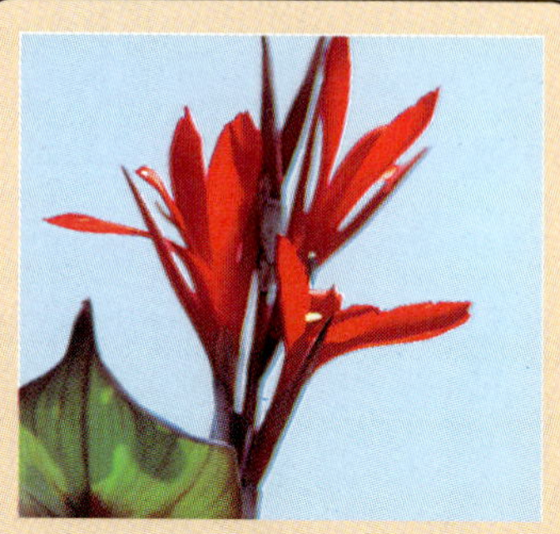

INDIA PRINCE

A nice dark green leaved plant lightly suffused with maroon when young. Permanent maroon edge remains on leaf. Flower bearing stem is dark maroon with slim bright scarlet red flowers. A fast growing, medium size plant, 3'-4'. Makes attractive spiny red seed capsules.

88000 Rhizome...............................*$4.95*
88001 Growing Plant (6" pot)......*$8.95*

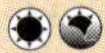

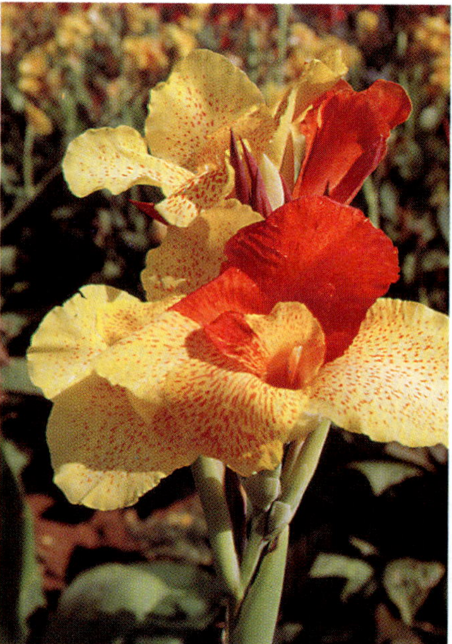

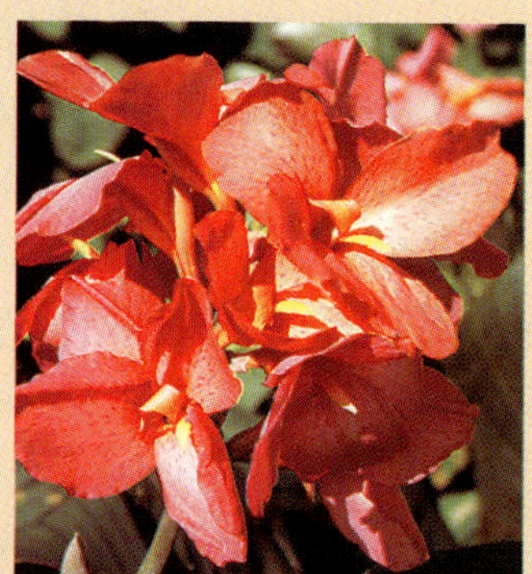

CLEOPATRA

Medium height plant. Most of the petals are yellow with red speckles but can be marked with solid red ranging from a streak to a full petal. Dark green foliage is marked with bronze-red variegation varying from a streak to a full leaf. Grows very well in water.

88200 Rhizome *$7.95*
88201 Growing Plant
(6" pot)...............................*$11.95*

DAWN PINK

A wonderful new canna with dark burgundy foliage and large beautiful pink flowers. A dwarf plant growing to 3 feet or less. Self-cleaning bloom.

88300 Rhizome...............................*$5.95*
88301 Growing Plant (6" pot)......*$9.95*

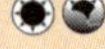

Visit our Web Site :
www.stokestropicals.com
E-mail us:
info@stokestropicals.com
All Orders Placed Through Our
Web Site Receive a 15%
Discount

**STOKES TROPICALS' PLANTS THAT
WILL GROW IN WATER:**
• Alpinia aquatica
• Hedychium coronarium
• Hymenocallis littoralis variegata
• Canna 'Bangkok Yellow'
• Canna 'Cleopatra'

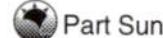 Full Sun   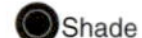 Part Sun   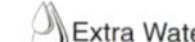 Shade   Extra Water   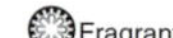 Fragrant   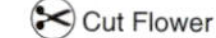 Cut Flower   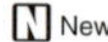 New

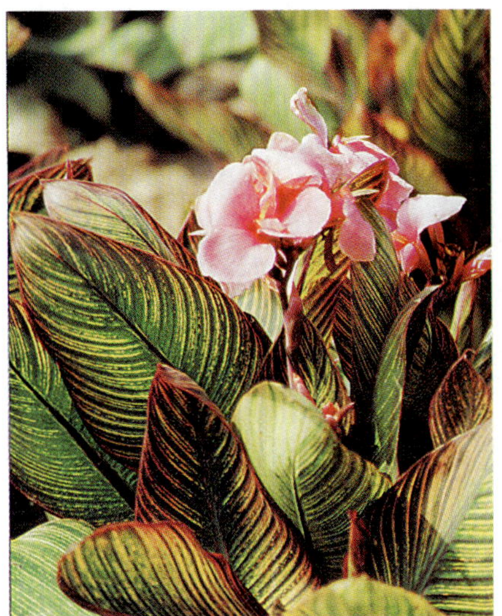

PINK SUNBURST

One of the most dramatic South African cannas that we have seen. Broad picturesque leaves that are variegated with yellow striping. Leaf edges are washed with a deep wine red that combines with the yellow and creates a festive rainbow of colors. Exquisite large pink flowers with dark pink centers perfectly compliment the leaves. Dwarf plant growing only 2¹/₂'-3'.

88350 Rhizome $11.95
88351 Growing Plant (6" pot)..$15.95
88352 Growing Plant (4" pot)..$13.95

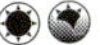 **RARE**

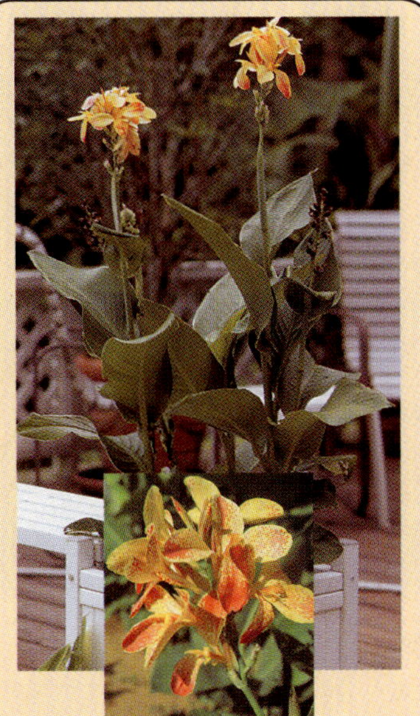

PRETORIA

Medium height. Wonderful variegated leaves with yellow and green stripes. Beautiful orange flowers displayed on a reddish orange stem. Tolerates moderate shade but prefers full sun.

88400 Rhizome......................$7.95
88401 Growing Plant (6" pot).$11.95

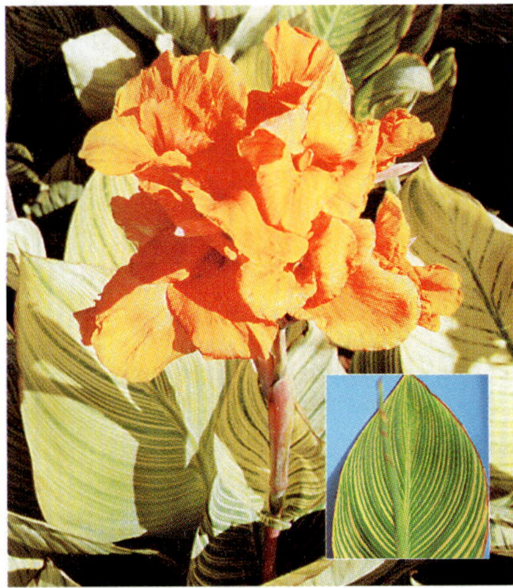

SAVE $6.95 Save on our fantastic new cannas by buying a collection. See page 28.

SUNRISE / SUNSET

Dwarf. Nice solid green foliage. Buttery cream-colored petals with pink/orange speckles and splashes. A real show stopper–nothing like it. Vanda orchid like flowers.

88500 Rhizome..............................$6.95
88501 Growing Plant (6" pot)....$10.95

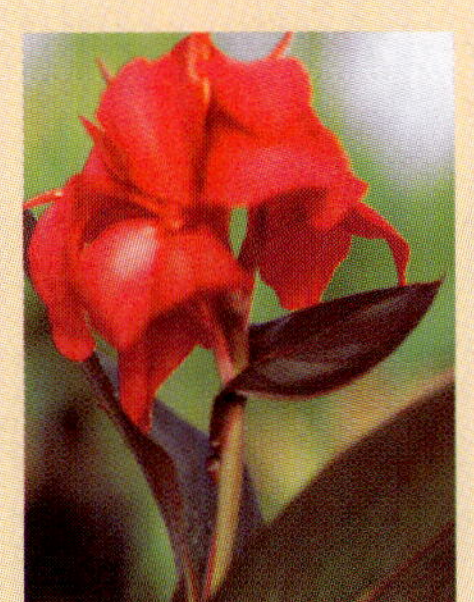

RED FUTURITY

An absolutely beautiful burgundy-leafed plant with outstanding medium dark red florets. Medium growing 3'-3¹/₂'. Supply limited.

88440 Rhizome $6.95
88441 Growing Plant (6" pot)......................$10.95

RED WINE

A new seedling variety that is one of the most outstanding looking cannas ever. It has luscious red flowers on red wine-colored foliage. Plant is short 2¹/₂'-3' and is very floriferous. A dynamite new canna. If you could have only one canna, this might just be the one.

88460 Rhizome..............................$8.95
88461 Growing Plant (6" pot)....$12.95

ALL STOKES TROPICALS' PLANTS ARE EASY-TO-GROW.

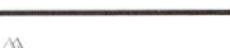 Full Sun   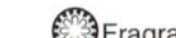 Part Sun   Shade   Extra Water   Fragrant   Cut Flower   New

TO ORDER CALL **1-800-624-9706**/24 HRS. OR VISIT OUR WEB SITE: www. stokestropicals.com

Cannas

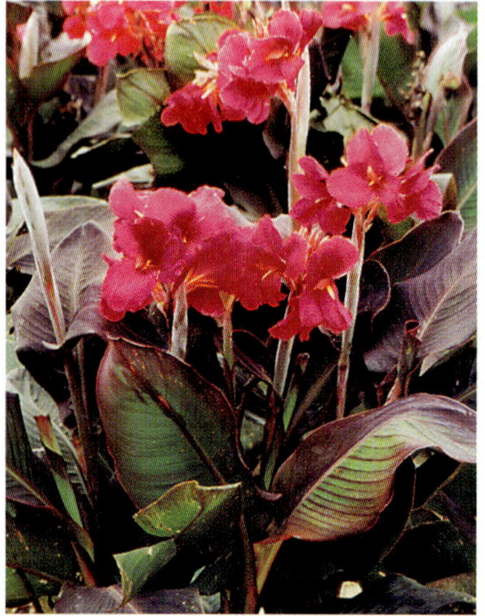

WINE 'N ROSES

Huge deep rose blossoms are proudly displayed on beautiful ovate burgundy leaves that are tinted with green. Flowers are nested at the very tip of the 3'-3½' plant.

88700 Rhizome *$6.95*
88701 Growing Plant (6" pot) *$10.95*

ALL STOKES TROPICALS' PLANTS ARE EASY-TO-GROW.

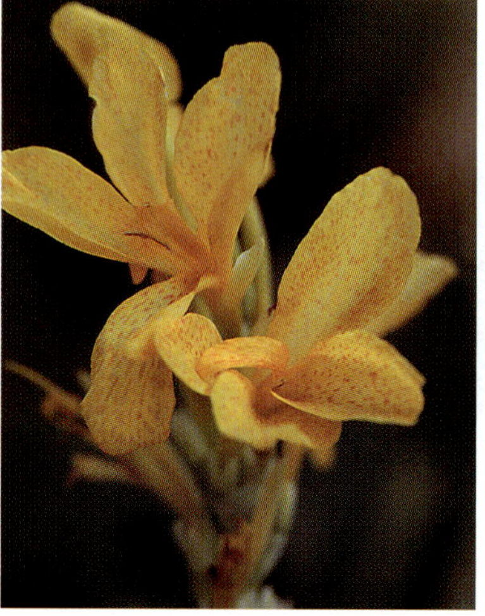

YELLOW LEOPARD

A new seedling variety that is a true dwarf canna growing only 12"-18" tall. Magnificent looking lemon yellow flowers that exhibit small maroon circles, hence, the name Yellow Leopard! Makes a great ground cover or as an understory plant. Zone 8 and higher.

88750 Rhizome *$11.95*
88751 Growing Plant (6" pot) *$15.95*

FACTOIDS

The hard black seeds of Cannas are used for Buddhist rosaries. The word Canna means "help from Buddha".

In Columbia and Ecuador, the "roots" are eaten as food and the leaves are sometimes used for thatching. Cannas were first hybridized by M. Anee in Paris (collected from Chile) in 1846. Also hybridized later in Italy. First "modern" Canna with large "flowers" appeared in 1890 in Italy.

✂ *Comments from customers:*

I came to your site looking for one plant that I could not remember the name of. Then found a world of beauty. Thank you for it. It's a real find,–the plants are all so wonderful. I will shop with you from now on...

GLORIA
DALLAS, TEXAS

CANNA COLLECTIONS

(Save $6.95 off listed prices by purchasing entire collection)
(Rhizomes only)

RARE CANNA COLLECTION:

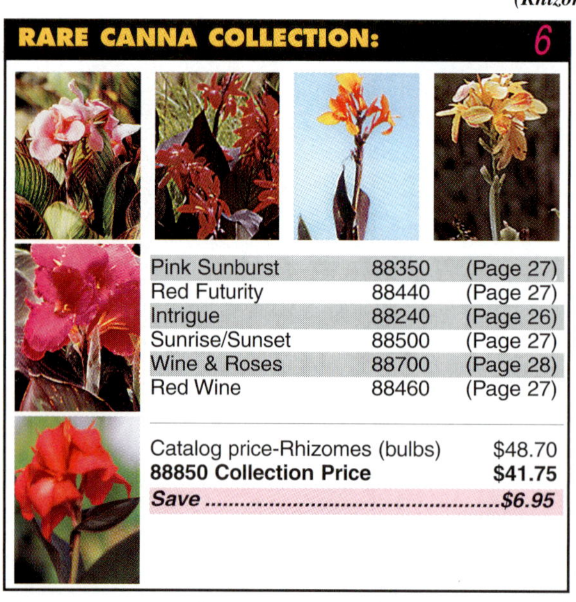

Pink Sunburst	88350	(Page 27)
Red Futurity	88440	(Page 27)
Intrigue	88240	(Page 26)
Sunrise/Sunset	88500	(Page 27)
Wine & Roses	88700	(Page 28)
Red Wine	88460	(Page 27)
Catalog price-Rhizomes (bulbs)		$48.70
88850 Collection Price		**$41.75**
Save		*$6.95*

SUPREME CANNA COLLECTION:

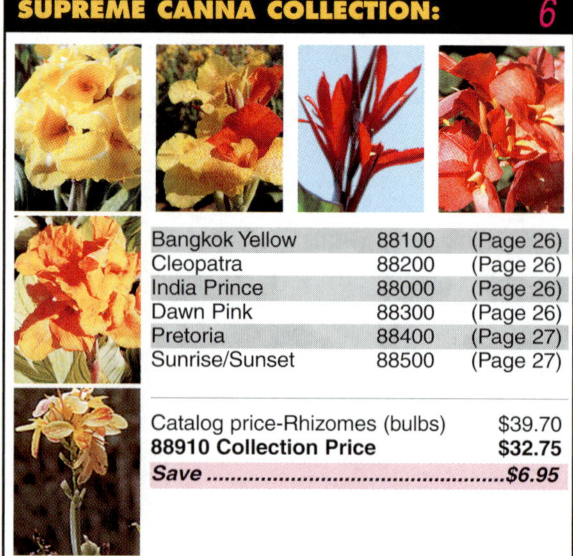

Bangkok Yellow	88100	(Page 26)
Cleopatra	88200	(Page 26)
India Prince	88000	(Page 26)
Dawn Pink	88300	(Page 26)
Pretoria	88400	(Page 27)
Sunrise/Sunset	88500	(Page 27)
Catalog price-Rhizomes (bulbs)		$39.70
88910 Collection Price		**$32.75**
Save		*$6.95*

☀ Full Sun   🌤 Part Sun   ● Shade   💧 Extra Water   ✳ Fragrant   ✂ Cut Flower   N New

TO ORDER CALL **1-800-624-9706**/24 HRS. OR VISIT OUR WEB SITE: www. stokestropicals.com

GINGERS

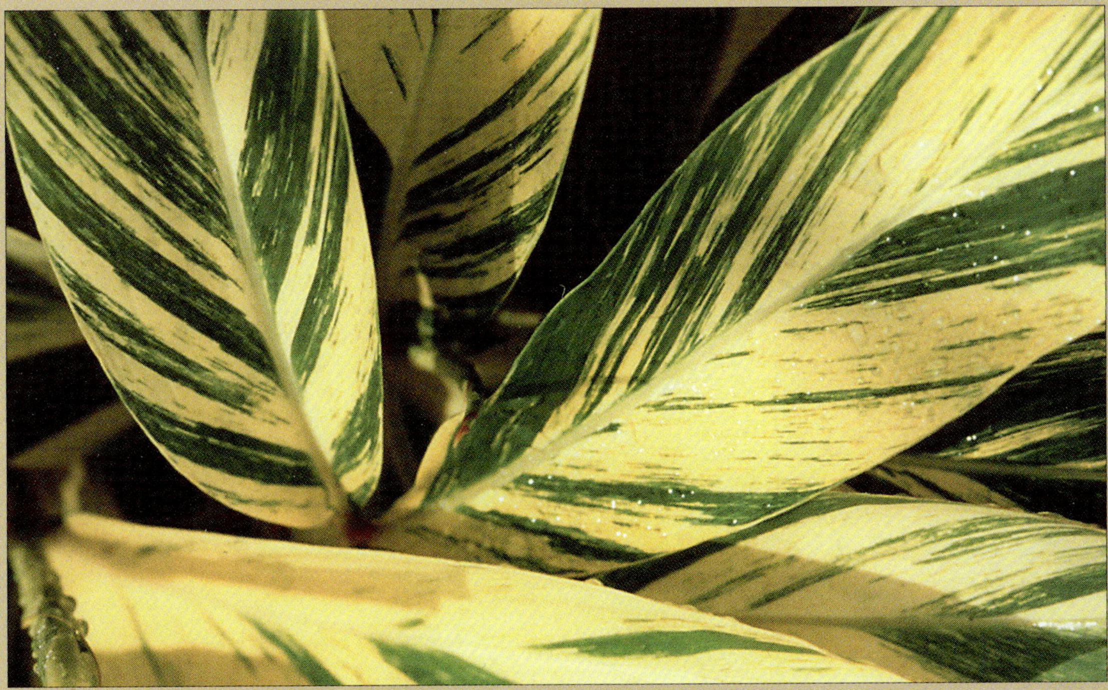

GINGERS enjoy a special position in the botanical kingdom with their elegance in form and texture, sparkling color and amazing symmetry. The word ginger conjures up images of an exotic oriental food flavoring. However edible ginger is only one of approximately 1,300 species of the very diverse Zingiberaceae family. Gingers are classed as a herbaceous perennial and have enjoyed popularity as an ornamental plant in Asia and the Far East for centuries. Only recently have they become known as outstanding ornamentals in the U.S.

Gingers as a group add outstanding exotic foliage and exotic flowers to the landscape. Gingers are wonderful plants for southern climates and protected northern climates. In both areas gingers are finding favor as interior landscape plants and most do very well in containers. Gingers are heavy feeders and drinkers during the growing season. Most do best in partial shade; however some thrive in full sun, others in full shade. So gingers provide plants for all light conditions. Many species enter dormancy in response to shorter days, cool temperatures, or dry conditions.

Rhizomes (the underground stem) survive in a dormant condition beneath the soil surface during cold or dry conditions.

Most common kinds of gingers:

ALPINIAS—Come in all sizes from small to large. Leaves are frequently fragrant. Most bear large clusters of stunning blooms. Like medium to full sun. Many can overwinter without special care. All make good pot plants.

COSTUS—Called 'spiral' gingers. Have true stems and spirally- arranged foliage. Many are grown for cut flowers and flowers attract hummingbirds. Medium to full sun. Flower petals open from a cone on the terminal end of stems.

CURCUMAS—Broadleaf plants with colorful flowers. Go dormant after first frost. Enjoy medium to full sun, and sandy soil. Many make excellent cut flowers. Vary from short to tall plants.

GLOBBAS—Small shade plants of 2 feet or less. All have attractive foliage and some have attractive small, usually yellow, flowers. Flowers are very different from other gingers. Most are called 'dancing girls' because of flower shape. Some species make good cut flowers.

HEDYCHIUMS—Called 'butterfly' gingers. Short to tall plants with colorful and fragrant flowers. Go dormant after first hard frost. Enjoy medium to full sun.

KAEMPFERIAS—Called 'peacock' gingers. Low growing plants with decorative, and often variegated leaves. Perfect as a ground-cover, especially in shade. Many have purple or lavender flowers. Plants are dormant all winter. Make wonderful house plants.

SIPHONOCHILUS—A small genus of African gingers. Only a few species of this genus are in cultivation in the U.S. They are small and attractive plants, some resembling small Alpinias or Hedychiums in form and others are stemless and resemble Curcumas. Most have large attractive flowers and bloom in spring. All prefer light shade.

ZINGIBERS—Many species have large cones that release a thick juice when squeezed. Group includes edible ginger, shampoo ginger and beehive ginger. Most species are great foliage plants. Can grow in medium to full sun.

Gingers

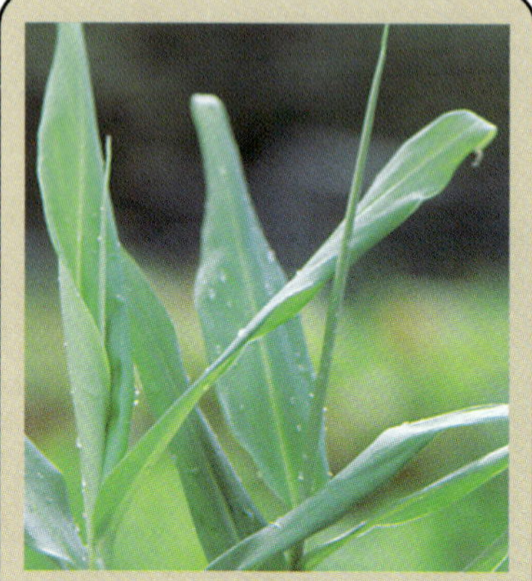

ALPINIA AQUATICA

Originally from China, this ginger is one of the few gingers known to grow in water. It creeps from the shore in mats with fibrous roots. The plant has small pink-lined flowers. It grows to 7' (2.1m). Zone 8 and higher. Great for water gardens.

31000 Rhizome............................$14.95
31001 Growing Plant (6" pot) ...$21.95

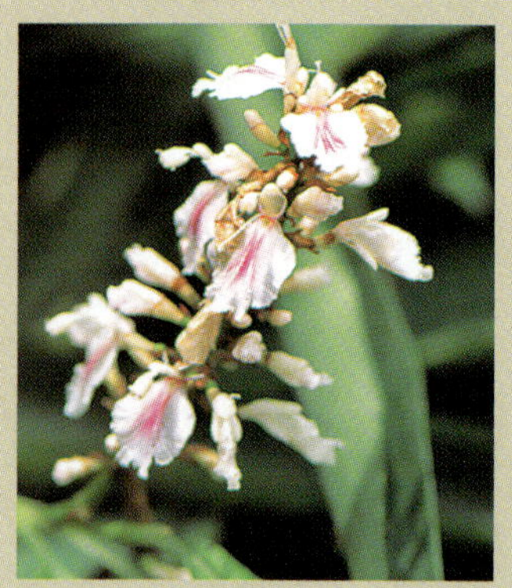

ALPINIA HENRYI
'Sweet Dragon'

A tall plant 5'-6' tall with broad, hairy leaves. It has large spikes of the flowers in the spring that are creamy with many dark red lines. These flowers are remarkable because, unlike other Alpinias, they have a powerful honeylike fragrance. Probably Zone 9 and higher.

31070 Rhizome............................$19.95
31071 Growing Plant (6" pot)....$26.95

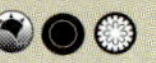

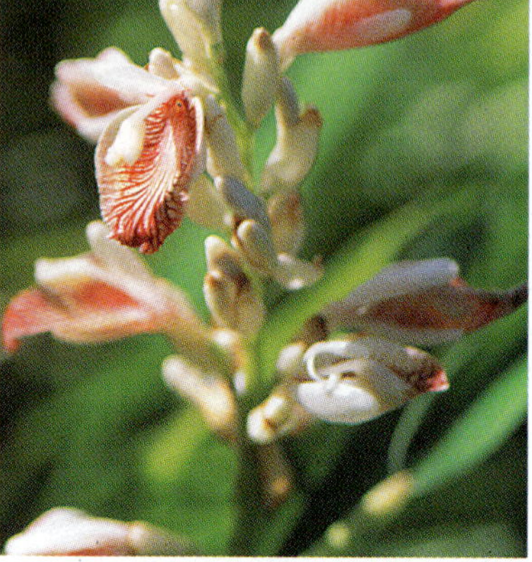

ALPINIA COERULEA

A wonderful new addition to our Alpinia line. Dark green leaves on reedlike stems to 6' (1.8m). Leaves have wine-red undersides. Small white flowers with purple modified stamens are followed by deep blue berries. Quite an outstanding plant. Medium sun. Zone 9 and higher. Origin Queensland, Australia.

31030 Rhizome $17.95
31031 Growing Plant (6" pot) $22.95

ALPINIA CALCARATA
'Snap Ginger'

A great looking medium height (4'-5') ginger, originally from India. A very vigorous grower that is cold hardy. Produces, on old growth, a nice raceme of white and maroon flowers that superficially resemble snapdragon flowers. Medium sun. Zone 8 and higher.

31010 Rhizome $10.95
31011 Growing Plant (6" pot) $17.95

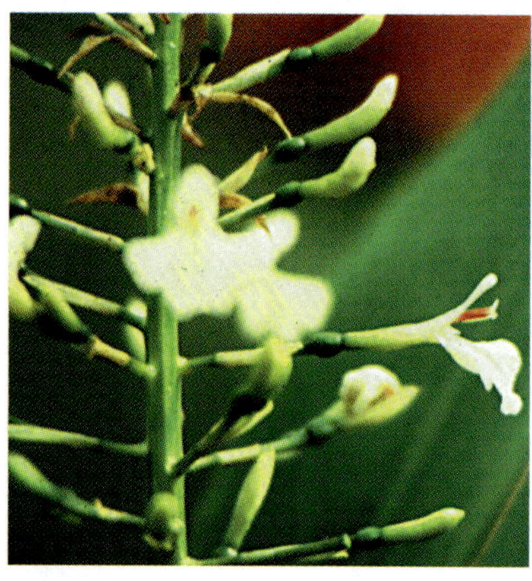

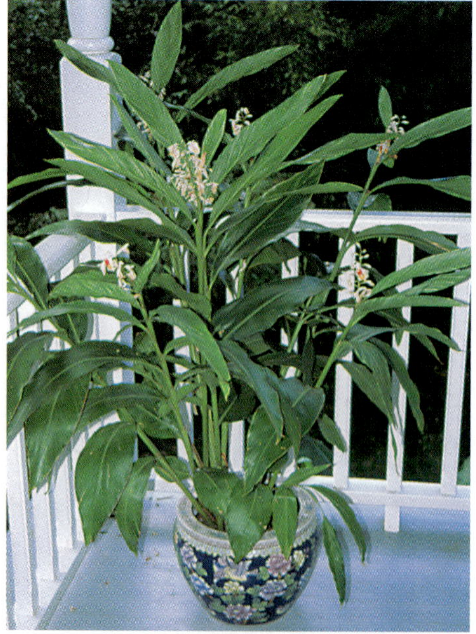

ALL STOKES TROPICALS PLANTS CAN BE CONTAINER GROWN.

Indoor tropical plants are lovely embellishments for any room or interior space and they add a touch of elegance for your courtyard, porch or garden.

Pictured on the left is an Alpinia formosana 'Pinstripe' growing in a container.

Full Sun   Part Sun   Shade   Extra Water   Fragrant   Cut Flower   New

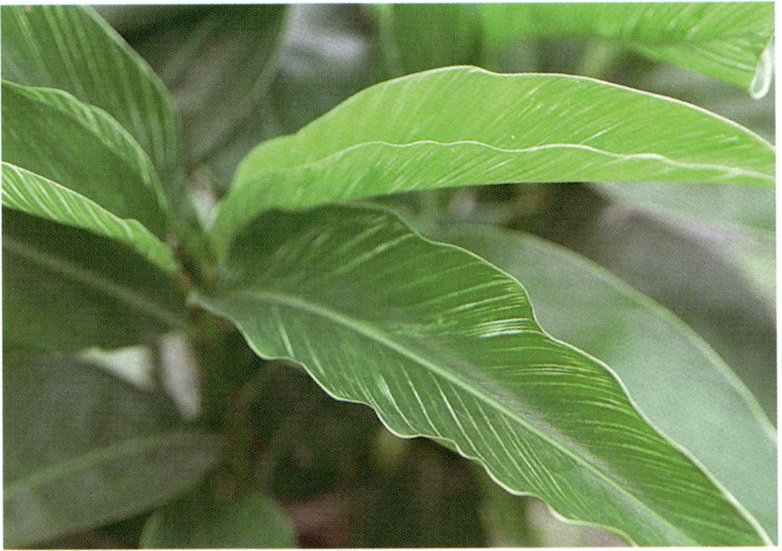

ALPINIA FORMOSANA 'Pinstripe'

An outstanding foliage plant. Produces a large inflorescence of white and red flowers following warm winter or if protected or greenhoused. Grows to 5' (1.5m) in medium to full sun. Zone 7 and higher. Makes great interior plant. One of our most popular and versatile gingers. Very hardy. Has tolerated temperatures down to 10°F.

31050 Rhizome..$6.95   *6($34.95) Save 16%*
31051 Growing Plant (6" pot)..................$12.95

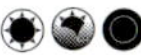

Rhizomes are available only from about December 15th to May 1st . Because they must be planted when temperatures are warm; they cannot be kept in dormancy as a rhizome. After May 1st rhizomes will be growing plants. Growing plants of long-day plants (Curcumas, Globbas, Kaempferias, Zingibers, Siphonochilus) are available from May/June through October. Growing plants of bananas, heliconias, certain gingers (Hedychiums, Alpinias, Costus, Monocostus), hibiscus, Siamese lucky plants, bougainvilleas and others are available all year.

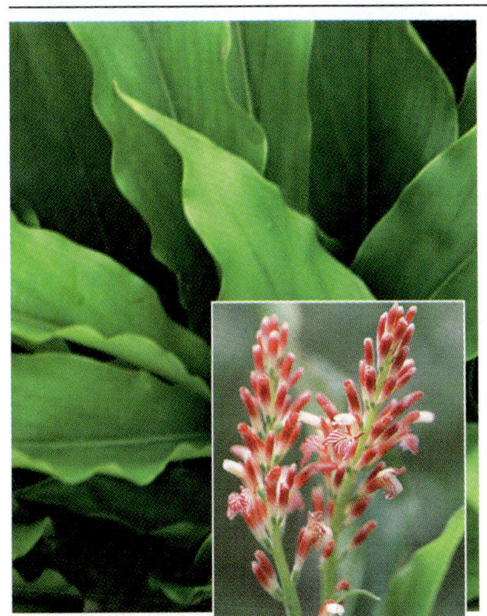

ALPINIA JAPONICA 'Kinisiana' 'Peppermint Stick'

A great-looking landscape plant with long wavy leaves that are fuzzy underneath. Small red and white striped flowers with a spiked inflorescence add to attractiveness of this ginger species. Main feature is foliage. It blooms in Zone 8 on old growth, and is one of the hardiest gingers in cultivation. It grows to 2' (60cm) in shade. Zone 7b and higher.

31100 Rhizome $5.95
6($28.95) Save 19%
31101 Growing Plant (6" pot) $10.95

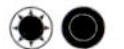

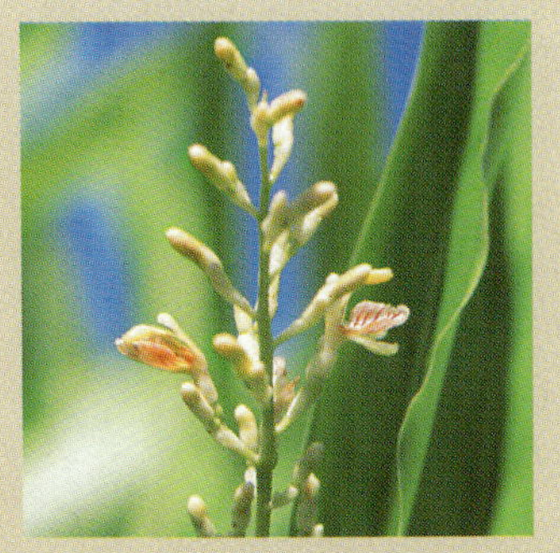

ALPINIA GALANGA 'Spice Ginger'

A beautiful flowering ginger that is favored for its spicy rhizomes that are a major ingredient in Thai and Asian cooking. It is also called 'Galanga major,' 'Galangal,' 'Laos Root,' and 'Siamese Ginger.' It is the only Alpinia to bloom every year even following a freeze. A great looking foliage plant with delightful-looking flowers. Grows 5'-6' in full to medium sun. Zones 8 and higher.

31230 Rhizome.............................$9.95
6($45.95) Save 17%;
31231 Growing Plant (6" pot)....$16.95
31232 Growing Plant (4" pot)......$6.95

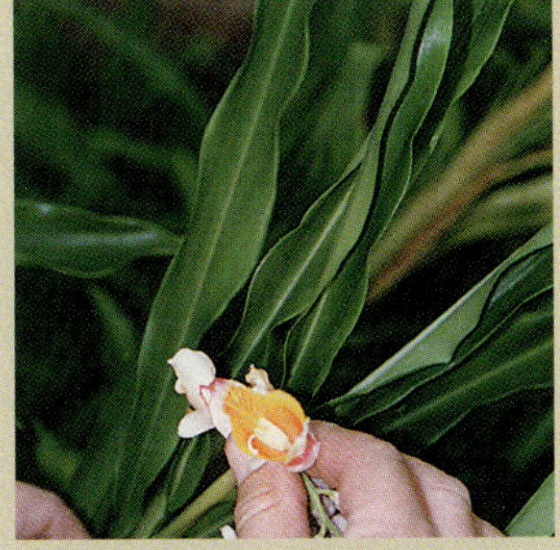

ALPINIA KATSUMADAI

A medium height species with very nice wavy leaves and upright yellow shell-like flowers; inflorescences are upright, not pendant. The plant grows to 4' in medium sun. Zone 7b and higher.

31150 Rhizome $12.95
31151 Growing Plant (6" pot)....$19.95

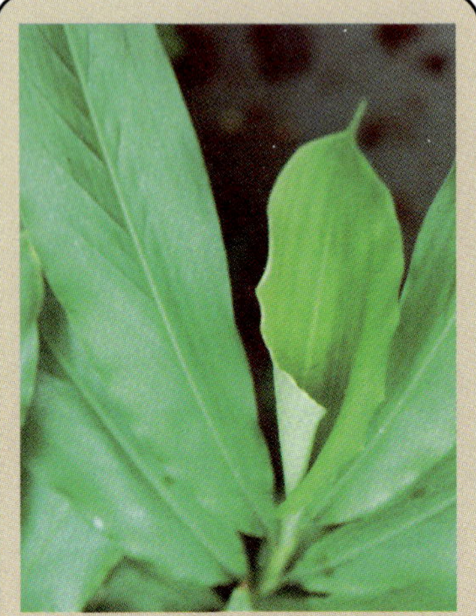

ALPINIA NUTANS

Has been incorrectly called Amomum cardamomum or 'Cardamon', but it is not true cardamon. Hardy foliage plant, often used as a shade groundcover. It rarely blooms, but the leaves smell of spice when rubbed. It grows to 3 feet (90cm) in shade. Zone 7 and higher. Great patio plant. Very hardy

31200 Rhizome.............................. $4.95
6($21.95) Save 26%
31201 Growing Plant (6" pot)......$8.95

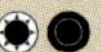

PHONE ORDERS:
1-800-624-9706
24 hours / 7days

FAX ORDERS:
1-337-365-6991
24 hours / 7days

FOR CUSTOMER SERVICE:
337-365-6998 - Mon.–Fri.,
8:30 am-4:00 pm C.T.

FOR INTERNET SERVICE:
http://www.stokestropicals.com
24 hours / 7 days

**E-MAIL
ORDERS/INQUIRIES:**
info@stokestropicals.com 24
hours / 7 days

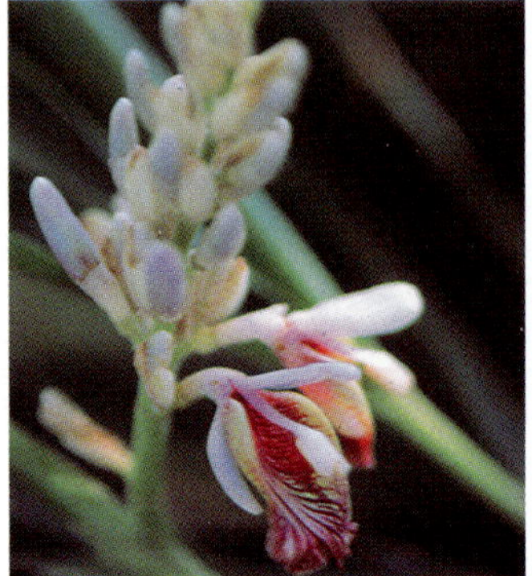

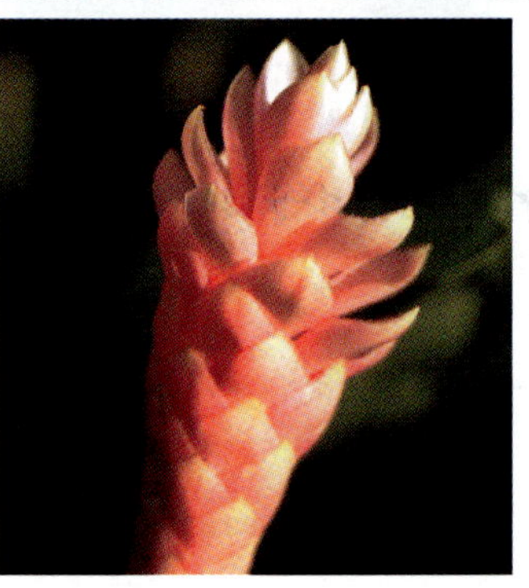

ALPINIA NUTANS 'Narrow Leaf'

A short cold-hardy Alpinia that flowers. Different from the regular nutans in having a much narrower leaf, it flowers easier and has the same wonderful spice fragrance. Nice deep-green leaves. Flowers on old growth are an added feature. Zone 7 and higher.
31210 Rhizomes $5.95
6($28.95) Save 19%
31211 Growing Plant (6" pot) $9.95

ALPINIA PURPURATA 'Kazu'

Called 'Kazu pink cone' ginger. Frequently used in cut flower industry. Blooms at 3' (90cm) to 4' (1.2m); can grow to 8' (2.4m) to 9' (2.7m). Grows well in full sun to medium shade. Zone 10 and higher. Must be greenhoused in colder areas.
31250 Rhizome $15.95
31251 Growing Plant (6" pot) $20.95

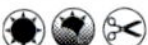

ALPINIA PURPURATA 'Kimi'

A very spectacular pink cone ginger cultivar that has a unique inflorescense. The top bracts that make up the pink cone are of lighter shade of pink. Very favored in the cutflower trade. Growing characteristics similar to regular *purpurata*. Zone 10 and higher. New.
31240 Rhizomes $14.95
31241 Growing Plant (6" pot) $19.95
31242 Growing Plant (4" pot) $7.95

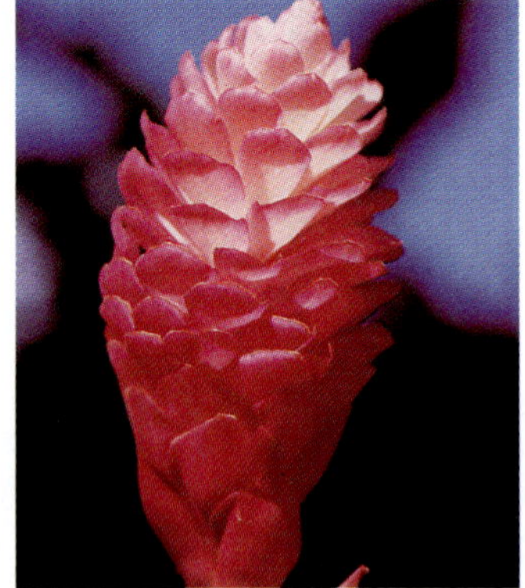

ALPINIA PURPURATA 'Pink'

Called "pink cone" ginger. Frequently used in cut flower industry. Blooms at 3' (90cm) to 4' (1.2m); can grow to 8' (2.4m) to 9' (2.7m). Grows well in full sun to medium shade. Zone 10 and higher. Must be greenhoused in colder areas.
31300 Rhizome $9.95
31301 Growing Plant(6" pot)..................$14.95
31302 Growing Plant(4" pot)....................$6.95

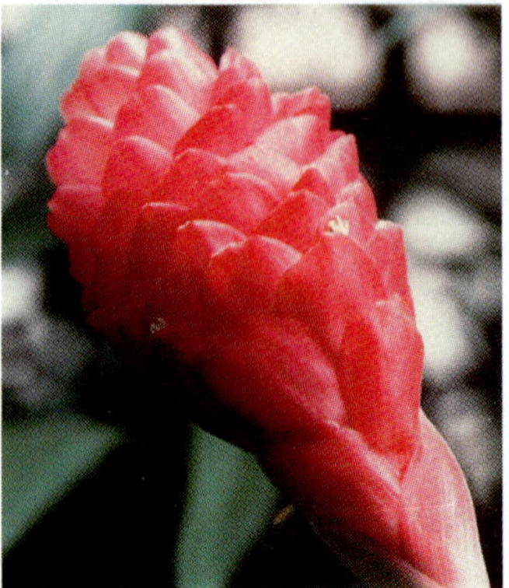

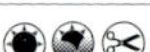

 Full Sun 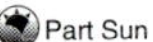 Part Sun 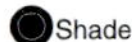 Shade Extra Water Fragrant Cut Flower 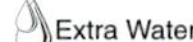 New 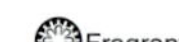

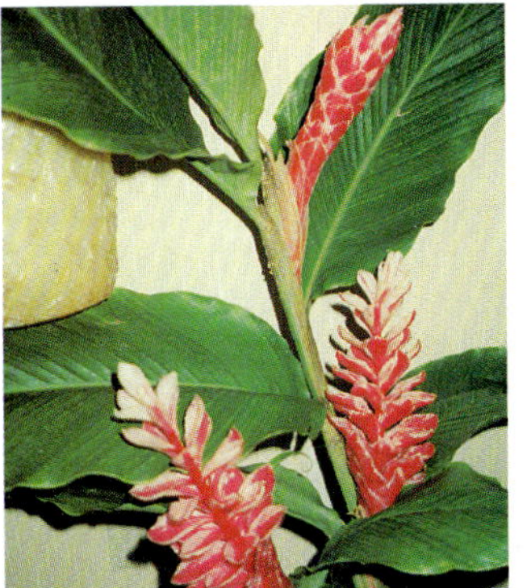

ALPINIA PURPURATA
'Polynesian Princess'

A dramatic looking new purpurata sport from the South Pacific. Has lovely variegated pink bracts that are less compact than other new cultivars of purpurata. Partial shade to full sun. Zone 10 and higher. Great cut flower. New.

31280 Rhizomes *$39.95*
31281 Growing Plant (6" pot) *$49.95*
31282 Growing Plant (4" pot) *$34.95*

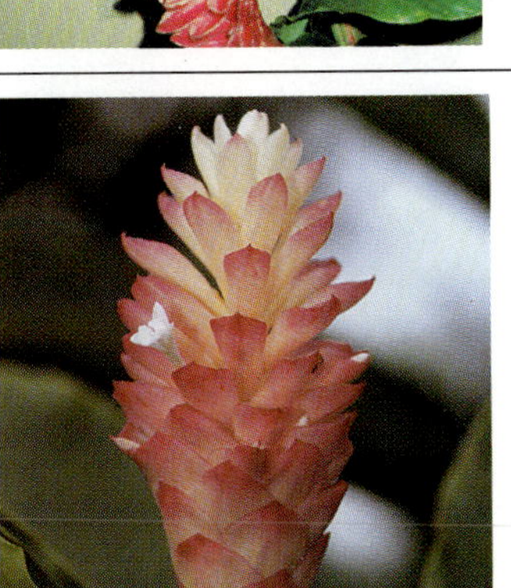

ALPINIA PURPURATA
'Strawberries & Cream'

A truly delightful cultivar of purpurata pink with white bracts that are frosted with pink edges. A great cut flower. Partial shade to full sun. Zone 10 and higher.

31360 Rhizomes *$21.95*
31361 Growing Plant (6" pot) *$26.95*

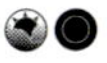

ALPINIA PURPURATA 'Tomi'

A great looking ginger with a rich dark pink inflorescence. Grows 6'-8'. Flowers year round. Zone 10 and higher. Makes great cut flower. New.

31340 Rhizomes *$15.95*
31341 Growing Plant (6" pot) *$22.95*

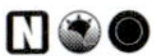

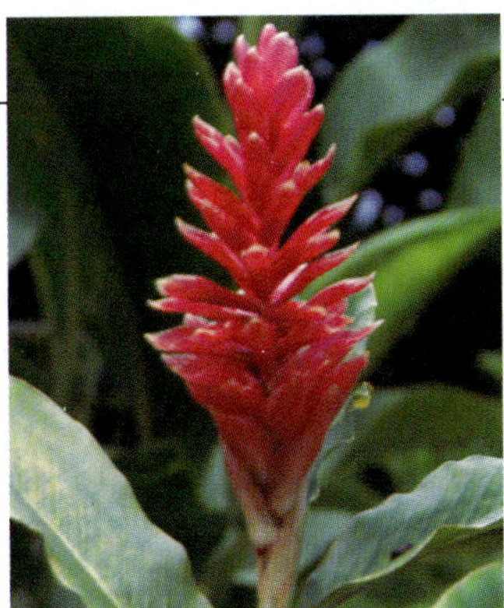

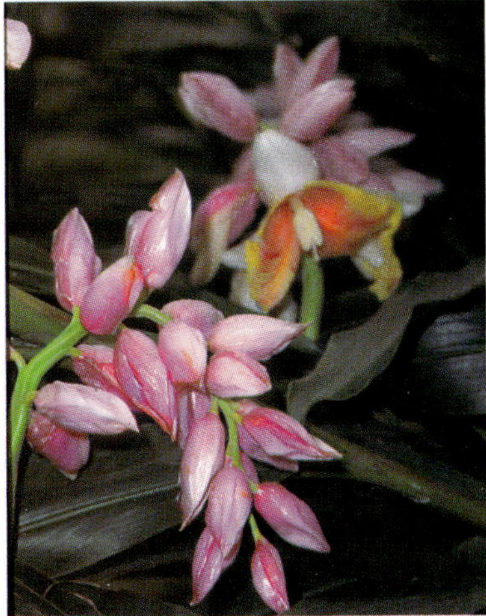

ALPINIA SP. 'Pink Perfection'

A spectacular new ginger with pink shell like flowers that individually open like snapdragons. Grows 5'-7'. Flowers freely in spring and summer on a slender elegant plant. Zone 10 and higher.

31060 Rhizome *$29.95*
31061 Growing Plant (6" pot) *$37.95*

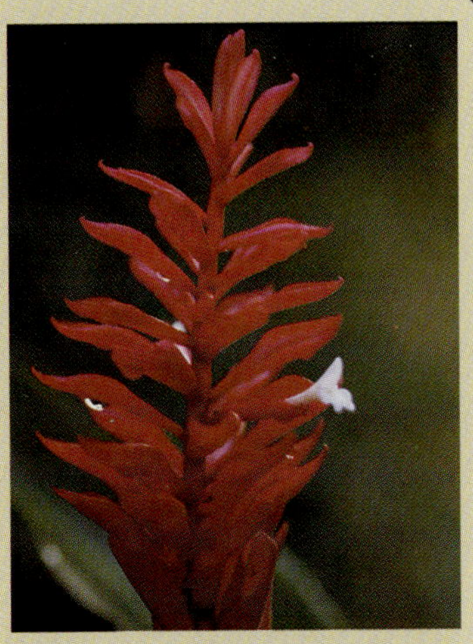

ALPINIA PURPURATA 'Red'

Called 'red cone' ginger. Frequently used in cut flower industry. Same growth and hardiness characteristics as 'pink cone' ginger.

31350 Rhizomes *$9.95*
31351 Growing Plant (6" pot) *$14.95*

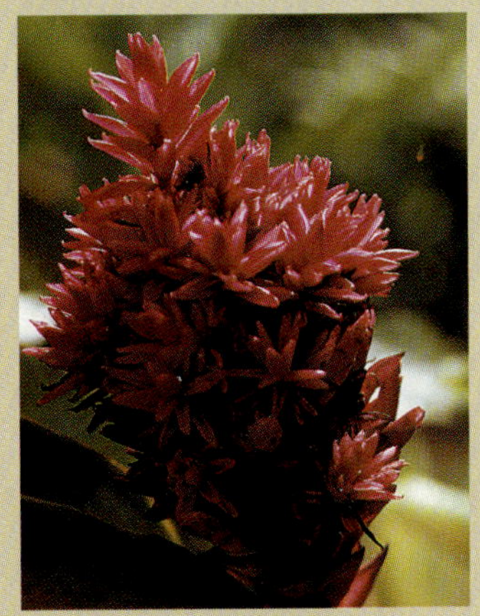

ALPINIA PURPURATA
'Tahitian'

The only double flowered purpurata known. A sensational double form of the red purpurata inflorescence; looks entirely different from other purpuratas but leaves and plant form are similar. Zone 10 and higher.

31390 Rhizomes *$9.95*
31391 Growing Plant (6" pot) *$14.95*

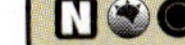

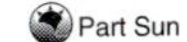 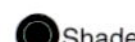 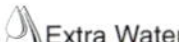

Full Sun   Part Sun   Shade   Extra Water   Fragrant   Cut Flower   New

33

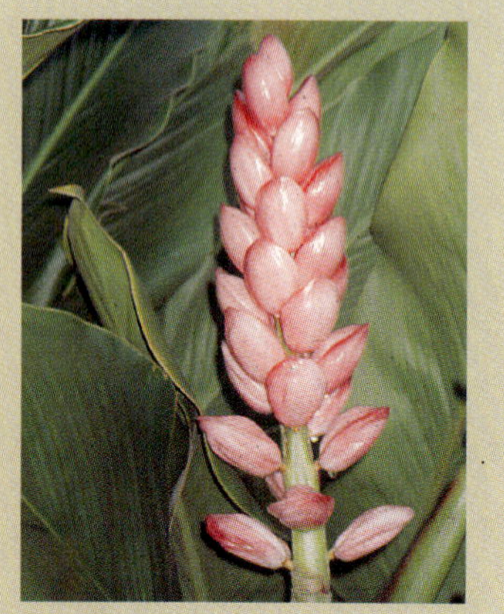

ALPINIA SP. 'Giant Pink'

An amazing ginger that has giant 12"-18" erect flower spikes. Flowers appear to be dipped in pink. Grows 6'-8' and flowers in spring and summer. From Northern Thailand. Zone 10 and higher. New.

31040 Rhizomes $29.95
31041 Growing Plant (6" pot)....$37.95

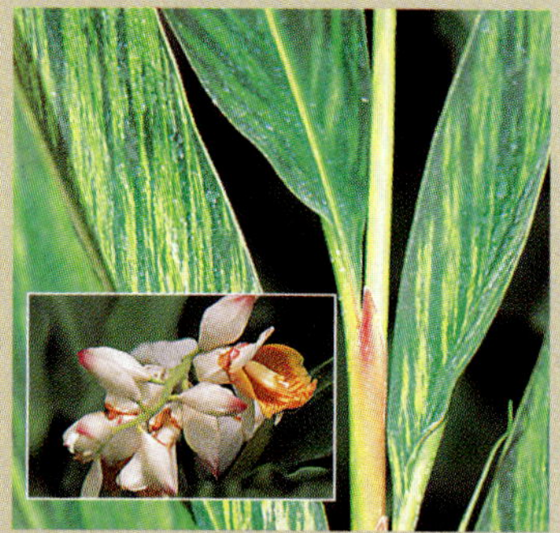

ALPINIA ZERUMBET VARIE-GATED 'Chinese Beauty'

Also called 'Yu Hwa,' this dramatic looking cultivar from China has a marbled variegation. Leaves are shiny dark green with light-green markings. Similar growth habit to the regular shell ginger (Alpinia zerumbet), growing to 7'-8' high. Beautiful pendant inflorescence with white and pink flowers. Medium to full sun. Zone 7b and higher.

31220 Rhizome...........................$18.95
31221 Growing Plant (6" pot)....$25.95

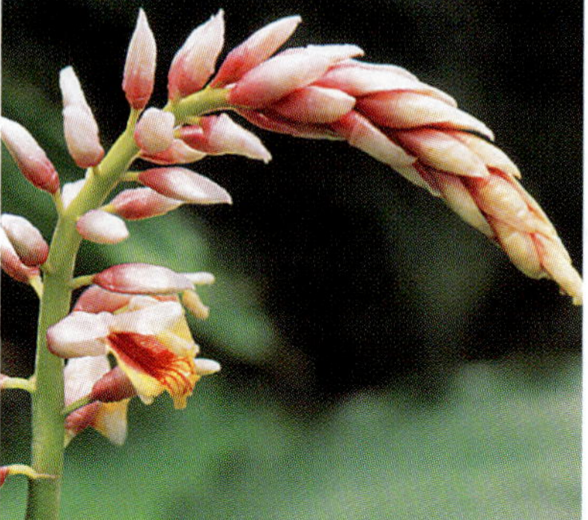

ALPINIA TONKINENSIS

Large plant 6' to 8' tall. Leaves linear, narrowed at base. Long panicle, 6" to 10". 3-5 flowers per bract almost sessile. Staminodes threadlike and curled at tip. Flower lip oval almost circular, with red veins 1/2" long and 3/8" wide. An outstanding large Alpinia. Probably Zone 9 and higher.

31380 Rhizome $14.95
31381 Growing Plant (6" pot) ..$21.95

ALPINIA VITTATA

Formerly called Alpinia sanderae. Commonly called the 'striped narrow leaf' ginger. The foliage is outstanding. Not as cold hardy as formosana; must be greenhoused in Zone 9 except in very warmest winters. Has white inflorescence with pink flowers. Grows to 5' (1.5m) in medium sun.

31400 Rhizome $14.95
31401 Growing Plant (6" pot) $19.95

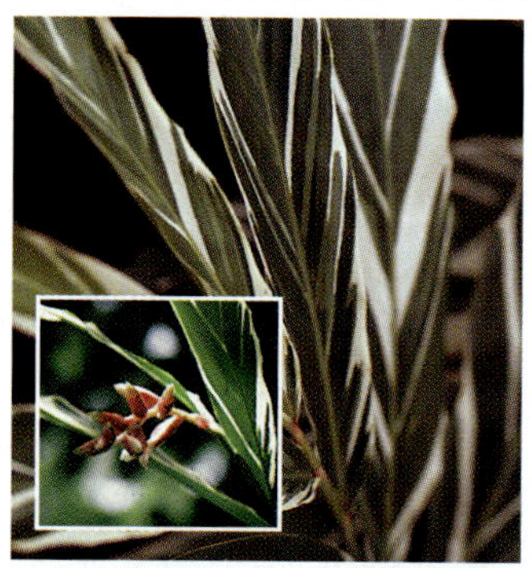

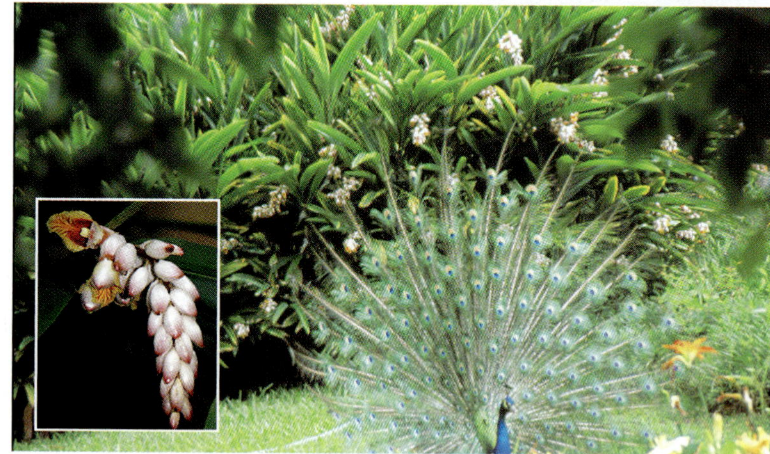

ALPINIA ZERUMBET

Called 'shell' ginger. Makes a good solid green foliage plant. Blooms in southern areas with mild winters. Large pendant inflorescence features white and pink flowers with red and yellow throats. Can be grown in full sun but will thrive in some shade. Can grow 7' (2.4m) to 9' (3m). Zone 7 and higher. One of the south's most common gingers.

31450 Rhizome $5.95

6($28.95) Save 19%

31451 Growing Plant (6" pot)...$9.95
31452 Growing Plant (4" pot)...$3.95

Full Sun   Part Sun   Shade   Extra Water   Fragrant   Cut Flower   New

TO ORDER CALL **1-800-624-9706**/24 HRS. OR VISIT OUR WEB SITE: www. stokestropicals.com

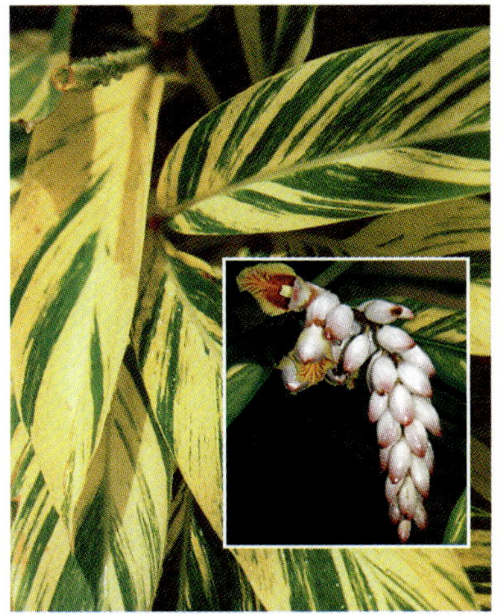

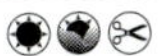

ALPINIA ZERUMBET VARIEGATED

Called 'variegated shell' ginger. Makes a beautiful foliage plant with outstanding yellow variegation. Following warm winters produces large pendant inflorescence with white and pink porcelain-like flowers. Can grow 5' to 6' and tolerates winter temperatures into the 20°F. Grows best in some shade but can tolerate full sun. Zone 7 and higher.

31500 Rhizome $6.95
6($34.95) Save 16%
31501 Growing Plant (6" pot) $11.95
31502 Growing Plant (4" pot) $4.95

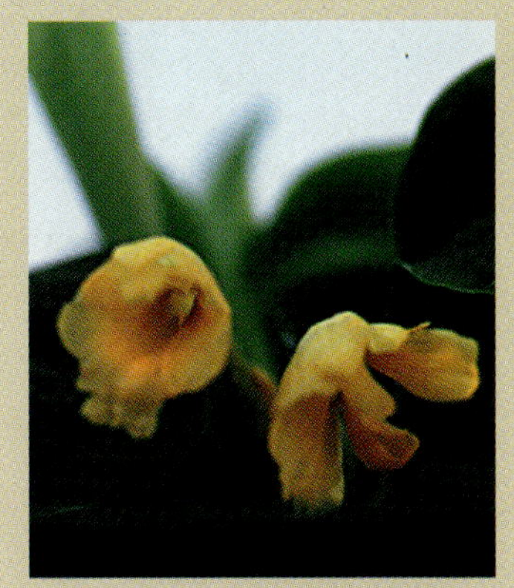

BOSENBERGIA AURANTIACA

The dark green fuzzy leaves with their gold stripe down the middle make this an attractive foliage plant. It produces many orange-gold flowers. Zone 10 and higher. Will grow to 5 inches (12.5cm) in shade.

31600 Rhizome............................ *$8.95*
31601 Growing Plant (6" pot) $15.95

BOESENBERGIA SP. 'Horn of Plenty'

A shade-loving plant that has broad, shiny, ribbed leaves and a red stem. Flower spikes appear mostly at ground level, but a few form between the leaves. The flower forms a 3" cream-colored tube with dark red on the inside. Zone 8 and higher.

31610 Rhizome $8.95
31611 Growing Plant (6" pot) $15.95

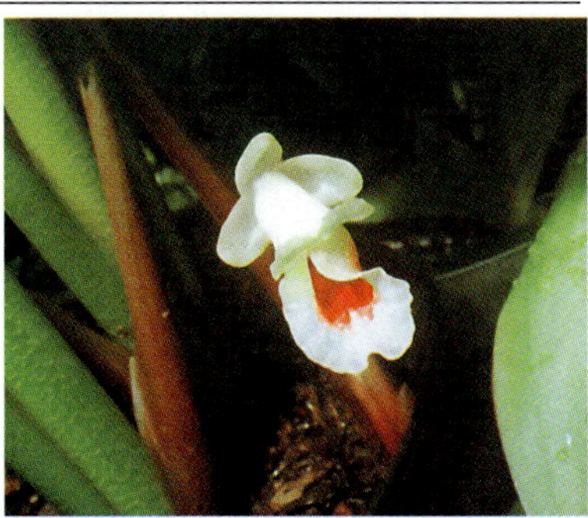

BURBIDGEA NITIDA 'Salmon Mousse'

A thin stemmed, foot tall plant that bears large flowers. Each flower lasts for three days and is gold for the first day and then turns salmon orange. Only grows well above 55°F (10.3° Celsius). Makes a lovely potted flowering plant for Halloween as it reaches maximum bloom at that time. Blooms at other times of the year in greenhouse. Probably Zone 10 and higher. A good houseplant.

31660 Rhizome ....$11.95   *31661 Growing Plant (6" pot)* $17.95

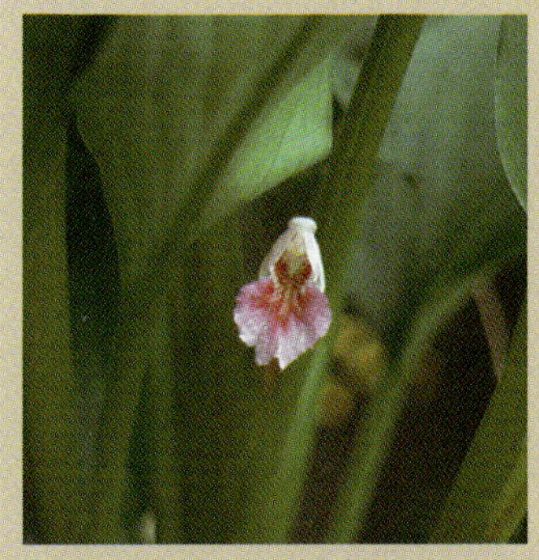

BOSENBERGIA ROTUNDA

Called 'Chinese keys'. An Asian spice plant valued for its roots. Small plant with dainty pink and blue flowers. Goes dormant in winter. The roots are used as a spice in the Orient. Height 2' (60cm) in shade to medium sun. Zone 8 and higher.

31650 Rhizome............................*$8.95*
31651 Growing Plant (6" pot)....$15.95

EDIBLE

BURBIDGEA SCHEIZOCHEILA 'Golden Brush'

A delightful small plant with waxy leaves that have bumpy texture. It grows to 1' in shade. Blooms in March or April and again in October. Many gold flowers are produced that open slowly. Plant is from Borneo. Good pot and houseplant. Zone 10 and higher.

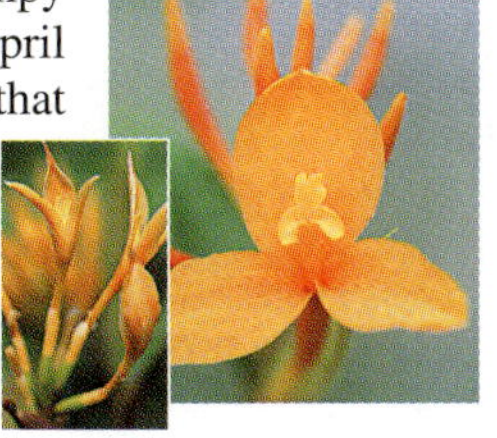

31670 Rhizome..$9.95
31671 Growing Plant (6" pot)............................$15.95
31672 Growing Plant (4" pot)................................$6.95

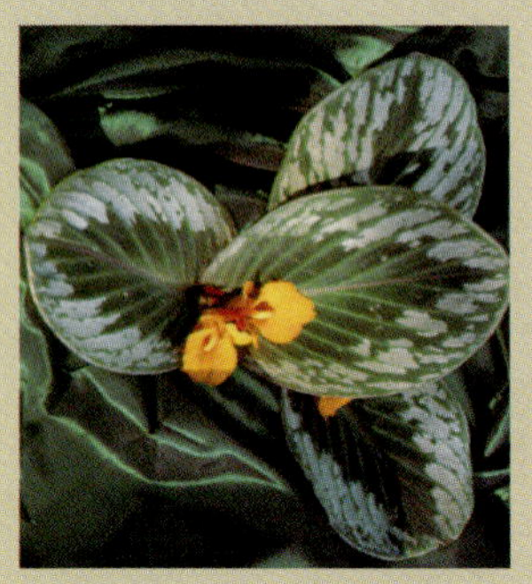

CORNUKAEMPFERIA AURAN-TIFLORA 'Jungle Gold'

This fantastic low-growing shade plant was previously classified as a Kaempferia. Recently it was named to a new genus: Cornukaempferia. It has an outstanding patterned leaf with dark maroon markings on a green leaf. Underside of leaves are lightly washed with maroon. And beautiful fiery orange/gold flowers emerge for weeks from the leaf axils. Collected from the jungle in Southeast Asia. Full shade. Like most Kaempferias goes dormant in winter. Probably zone 9 and higher.

35910 Rhizome.............................$9.95
35911 Growing Plant (6" pot) ...$13.95
35912 Growing Plant (4" pot).....$6.95

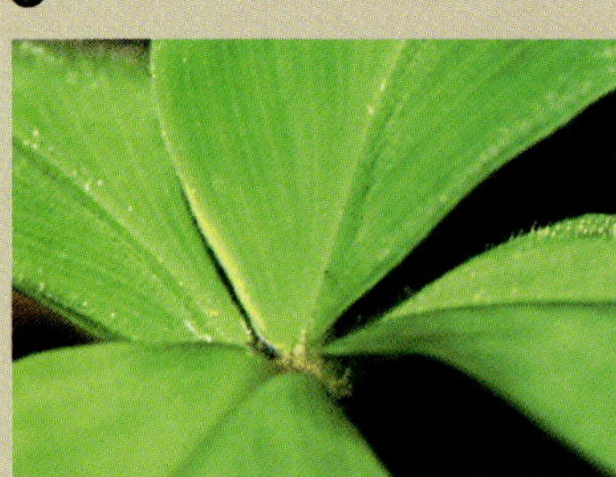

COSTUS ASAE 'Red Rose'

A beautiful native of Costa Rica is popular because of its attractive red inflorescences. The round fuzzy leaves help make this plant attractive as a foliage plant. A delight to touch. The plant will grow to 3' (1.8m) in shade. Zone 10 and higher.

31740 Rhizome.............................$9.95
31741 Growing Plant (6" pot) ...$16.95

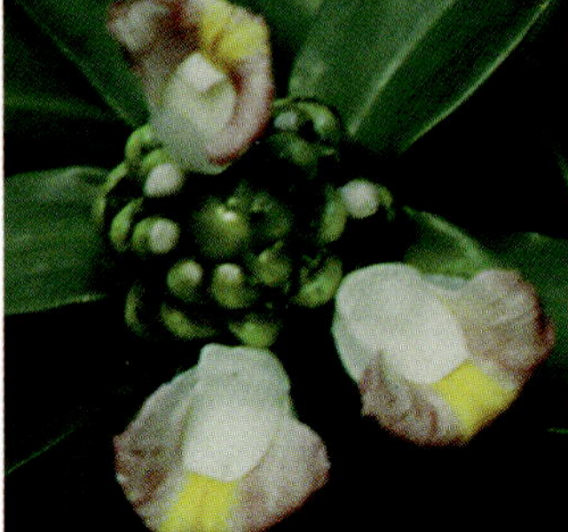
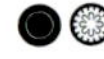

COSTUS ALLENII

Plant grows in deep shade in the jungles of Central America. The entire, spiral leafed plant is covered with long golden hairs. The short terminal bloom has tubular flowers with yellow and red stripes. Plant grows to 5' (1.5m). Zone 10 and higher.

31690 Rhizome $13.95
31691 Growing Plant (6" pot) $20.95

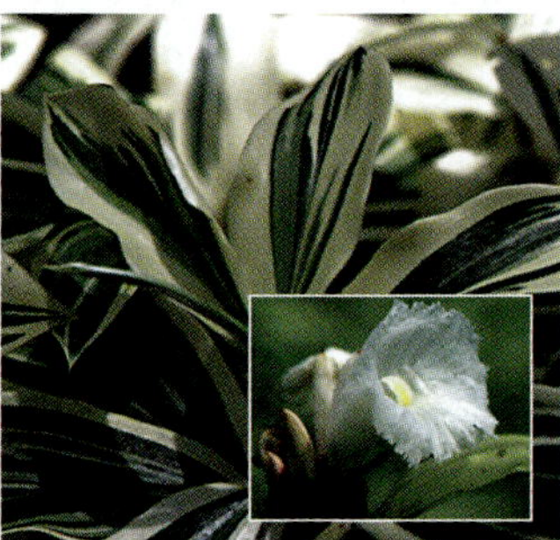
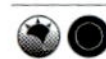

COSTUS CURVIBRACTEATUS

This vigorous grower produces many small reddish orange inflorescences that bloom until mid-winter. Plant is tender and needs to be greenhoused. Used for cut flowers and as pot plants. Native to Central America. Zone 10 and higher. Grows to 2' (60cm) in shade.

31800 Rhizome $12.95
31801 Growing Plant (6" pot) $18.95

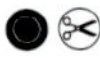

COSTUS AFER

Typical Costus with round spiraling stems and spindle shaped leaves. A rather large species that grows 7'-8' in medium shade. Has lovely pinkish flowers with yellow lip. One of the few Costus with fragrant flowers. Zone 9 and higher.

31680 Rhizome $13.95
31681 Growing Plant (6" pot) $20.95

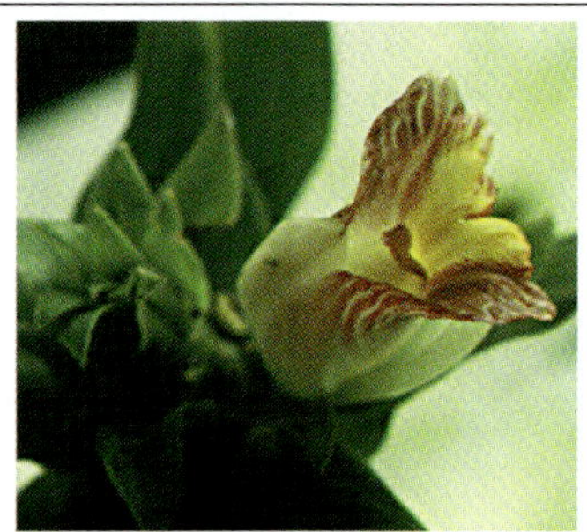

COSTUS AMAZONICUS VARIEGATED

A beautiful short (1'-3') growing plant with yellow and white flowers. Variegated leaves (more white than green) and spiraling stem are main attraction. Native to Brazil, Ecuador, and Peru. Zone 9 and higher. Full shade to medium sun.

31700 Rhizome $13.95
31701 Growing Plant (6" pot) $20.95

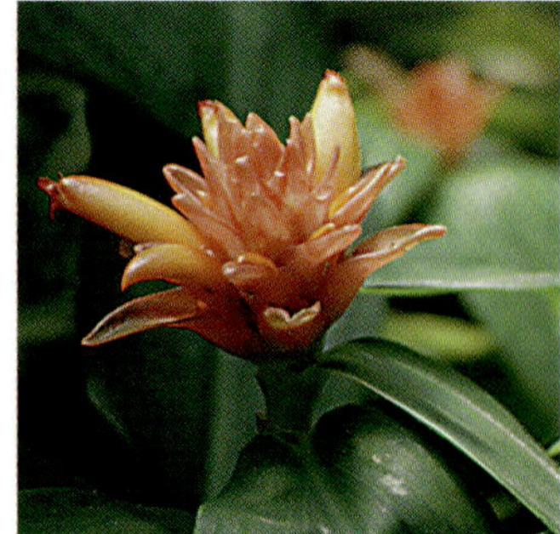

Ginger Collections
Save $5 (Rhizomes only) off listed prices by purchasing entire collection. See pages 66-68.

OUR MATCHLESS GUARANTEE

If for any reason you are not completely satisfied with your purchase, simply return it to us within 10 days of receipt for a prompt and friendly refund or exchange, whichever you prefer. If your purchase arrives in poor condition, please notify us as soon as possible so that we can take corrective action.

 Full Sun   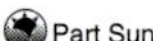 Part Sun   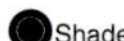 Shade   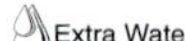 Extra Water   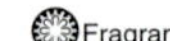 Fragrant   Cut Flower   New

TO ORDER CALL **1-800-624-9706**/24 HRS. OR VISIT OUR WEB SITE: www. stokestropicals.com

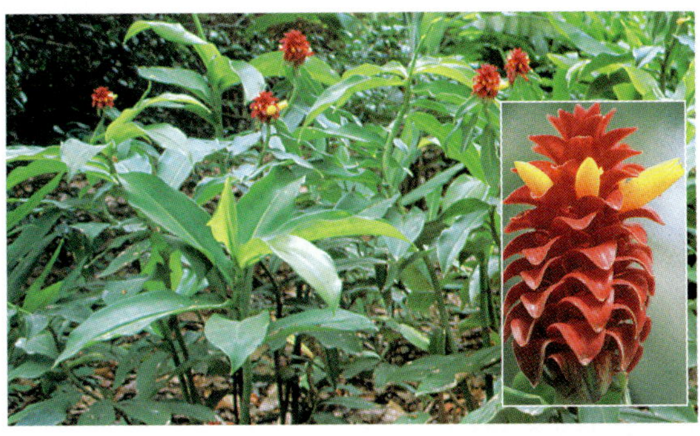

COSTUS BARBATUS

Called 'red tower' ginger. Fall in love with this wonderful plant by feeling the undersides of the leaves, which are as soft as down. The stems are slender and tend to spiral out of the ground and sway like charmed snakes. Like many tropical plants, they look best when among friends. Spiral leafed 6' to 8' tall with huge 7" (17.5cm) to 13" (32.5cm) tall deep-red inflorescence with large yellow flowers. Medium to full sun. Flowers April through November. Zone 9 and higher. Hummingbirds love them.

31750 Rhizome.................................*$10.95*   *31751 Growing Plant (6" pot)*.......*$18.95*

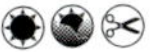

COSTUS CURVIBRACTEATUS HYBRID 'Green Mountain'

This vigorous grower produces many delightful terminal inflorescences all summer and fall. Reddish orange bracts of inflorescence have beautiful green tips. Flowers over a long period: spring to winter. Native to Central America. Grows to 4' in shade. We are very excited about the potential for this new hybrid. Zone 10 and higher. Great pot plant and can be greenhoused.

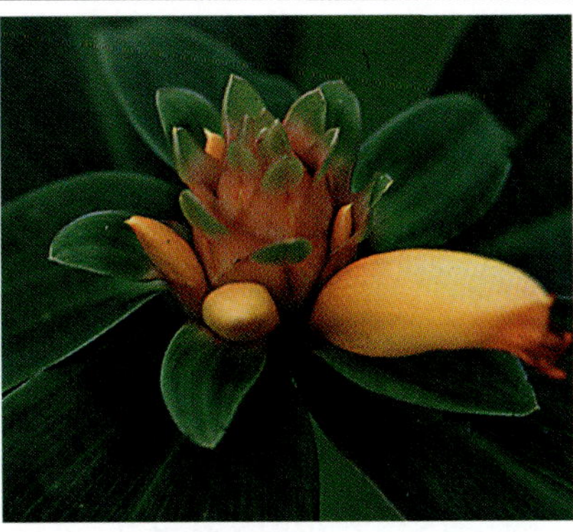

31810 Rhizome.................................*$9.95*   *6($45.95) Save 17%*
31811 Growing Plant (6" pot).........*$16.95*   *31812 Growing Plant (4" pot)* *$6.95*

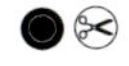

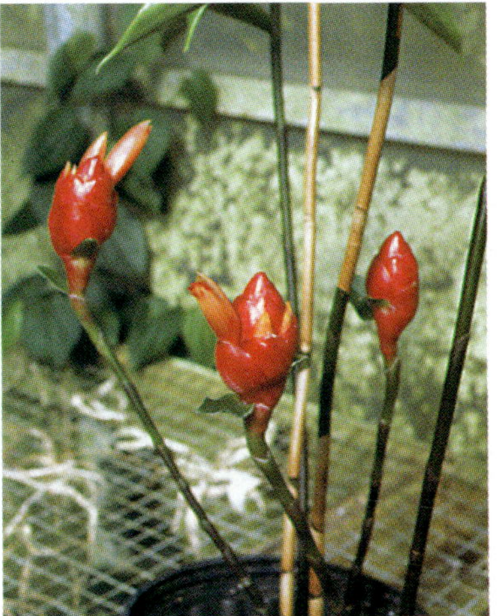

COSTUS ERYTHROTHYRSUS 'Red Lollipop'

A fantastic new Costus that is compact (24"-30") that has numerous shiny-red 3" spikes on separate 1' basal stems. Sometimes cones are produced terminally on spiral stems. Plant blooms profusely at any time of year. Spikes retain color long after small orange flowers are gone. Prefers part shade. Probably zone 9 and higher.

31860 Rhizome *$11.95*
31861 Growing Plant (6" pot) *$18.95*

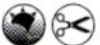

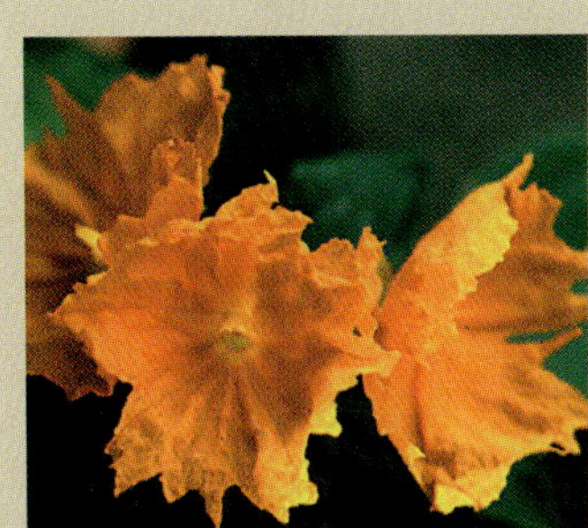

COSTUS CUSPIDATUS

Called 'Fiery Costus' and Costus igneus (incorrectly). A fantastic plant that is medium size 2' (60cm) and flowers continuously almost year round. It's inflorescence is a brilliant fiery crepe orange that is distinct from any other ginger. Frequently 2 or 3 terminal flowers are produced at one time. Plant has nice clumping growth habit. Native of Brazil. Medium shade. Good container plant. Zone 8 and higher.

31900 Rhizome...............................*$6.95*
6($34.95) Save 16%
31901 Growing Plant (6" pot) ...*$12.95*
31902 Growing Plant (4" pot) *$4.95*

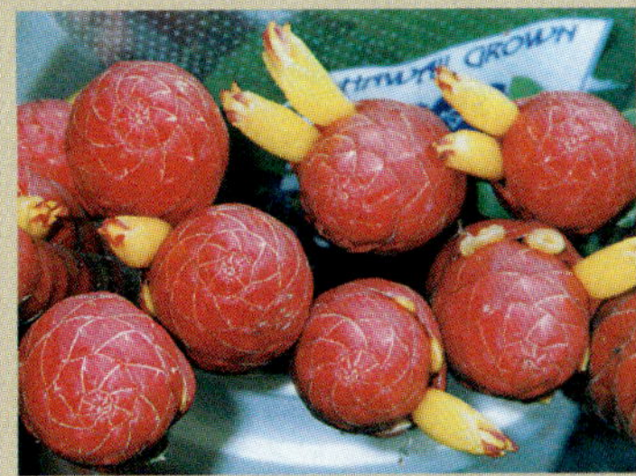

COSTUS ERYTHROCRINUS 'Eskimo Kiss'

One of the most spectacular of all Costus flowers. Inflorescence is bright shiny red round balls with tight bracts from which canary yellow flowers appear in a spiral. Plant has spiraling stem and grows 3'–4'. Makes great cut flower. Flowers attract hummingbirds. Probably Zone 9 and higher.

31730 Rhizome *$11.95*
31731 Growing Plant (6" pot) ...*$18.95*

❋ Full Sun   ◐ Part Sun   ● Shade   💧Extra Water   ✺Fragrant   ✂ Cut Flower   N New

37

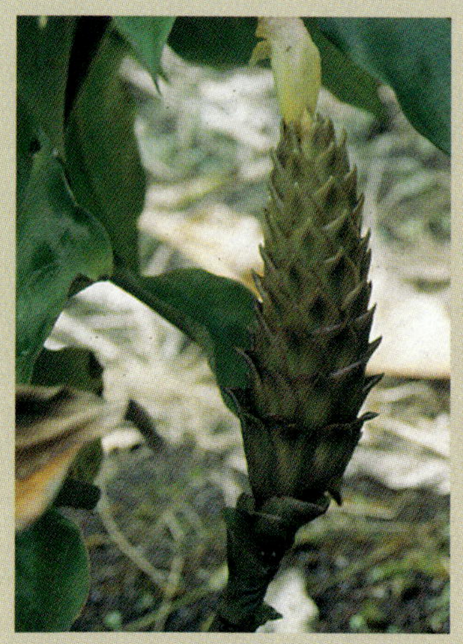

COSTUS LONGIBRACTEATUS
'Long Kiss'

A great looking ginger from Ecuador with a 10"-12" floral cone. Grows 6'-8'. Great plant for Costus collectors. Probably zone 9 and higher. New. Medium to full sun.
31870 Rhizome............................$27.95
31871 Growing Plant (6" pot) ...$34.95

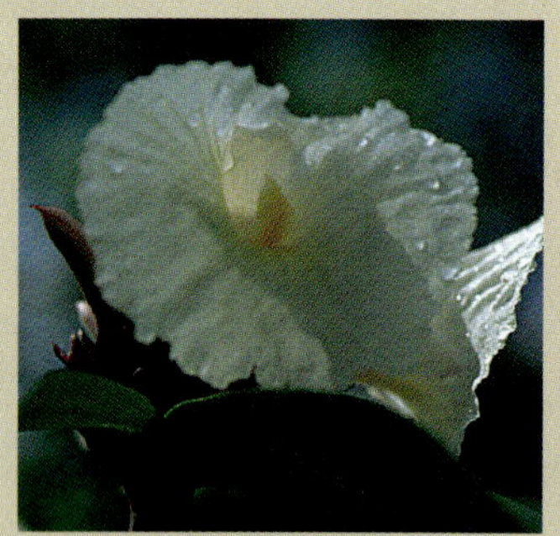

COSTUS SPECIOSUS

Called 'crepe' ginger. Rhizomes are used to make medicines in India. Produces red cones terminally with white translucent flowers resembling crepe paper. Blooms during summer and fall. Medium to full sun. Grows 6' (1.8m) to 9' (2.7m) in height. Zone 8 and higher.
32450 Rhizome.............................$6.95
6($34.95) Save 16%
32451 Growing Plant (6" pot)....$13.95

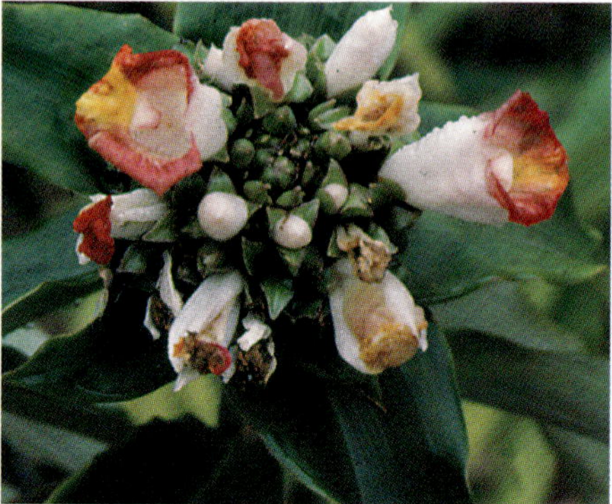

COSTUS MALORTIEANUS

Known as the 'Stepladder Ginger', this popular shade-loving foliage plant has large round fuzzy leaves and red and yellow striped flowers. Height is 2' (60cm). Zone 8 (if well protected) and higher. Medium shade.
31950 Rhizome $7.95
6($39.95) Save 16%
31951 Growing Plant (6" pot) $13.95

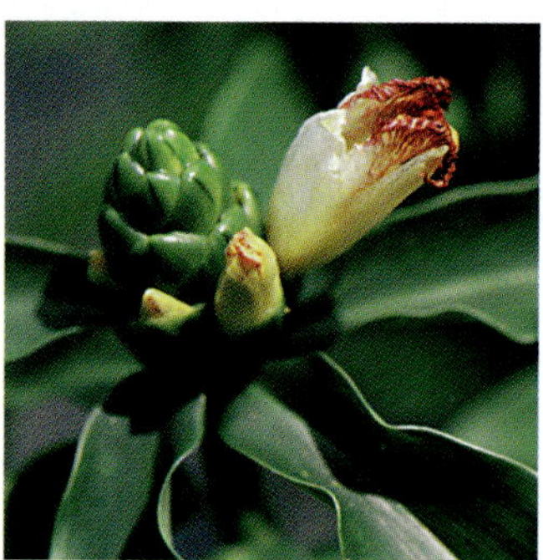

COSTUS PULVERULENTUS

Native to Central and South America. Flowers range from bright red, to yellow-orange. Species used for cut flowers and grows to 5' (1.5m) in medium sun. Zone 9 and higher.
32100 Rhizome.....................$11.95
*32101 Growing Plant
(6" pot) $18.95*

COSTUS LUCANUSIANUS
'Sweet African'

A wonder ginger from West Africa (Cameroon), with beautiful flowers that are fragrant. Medium sun. Grows 6'-8'. Zone 10 and higher. New.
32120 Rhizome.................$14.95
*32121 Growing Plant
(6" pot) $21.95*

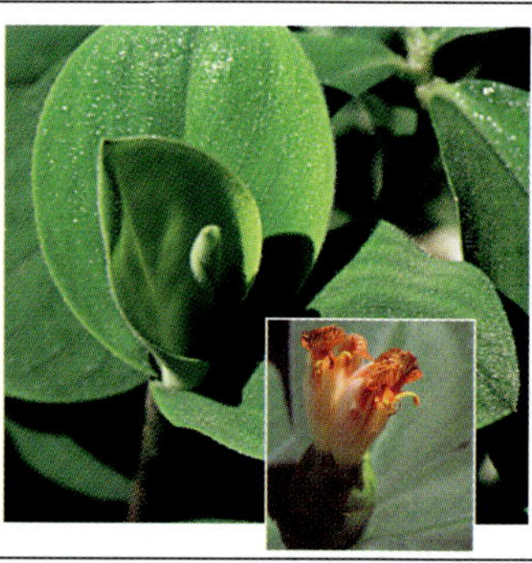

COSTUS PICTUS

A tall species with red spotted stems that can be used as cut foliage. It has thin stems and narrow leaves and blooms basally in spring and terminally in summer. Grows 6' (1.8m) to 7' (2.1m) in medium sun. Easy to grow Costus. Produces outstanding spiraling effect when grown in pot. Zone 8 and higher.
32050 Rhizome $6.95
6($34.95) Save 16%
32051 Growing Plant (6" pot) $10.95

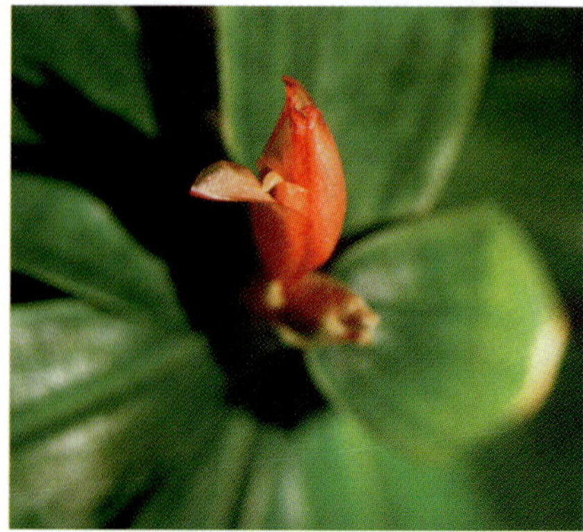

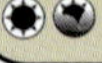 Full Sun 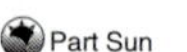 Part Sun 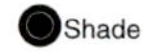 Shade 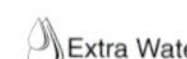 Extra Water 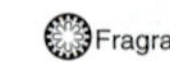 Fragrant 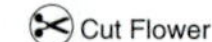 Cut Flower 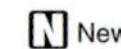 New

TO ORDER CALL **1-800-624-9706**/24 HRS. OR VISIT OUR WEB SITE: www. stokestropicals.com

Gingers

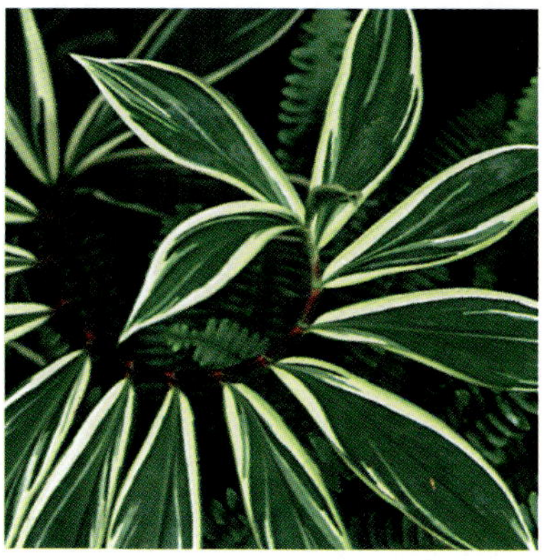

COSTUS SPECIOSUS VARIEGATED

Called 'variegated crepe ginger'. Great reddish spiral stems with sharply variegated foliage make it a standout in the garden landscape. Underside of leaves hairy. Dark maroon terminal cones from which white "crepe" flowers emerge. Medium to full sun. Grows from 5' (1.5m) to 7' (2.1m). Not as hardy as non-variegated form. Zone 9 and higher. Great container plant.

32500 Rhizome *$11.95*
32501 Growing Plant (6" pot) $18.95

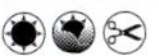

COSTUS SPECIOSUS 'Tetraploid'

A fantastic new cultivar of Costus speciosus that grows shorter (3'- 4') and flowers more freely. White crepe flowers emerge from a burgundy-red terminal cone from summer to fall. Easy to grow, easy to flower, short, and relatively cold hardy. Zone 8 and higher.

32460 Rhizome *$10.95*
32461 Growing Plant (6"pot) *$17.95*

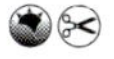

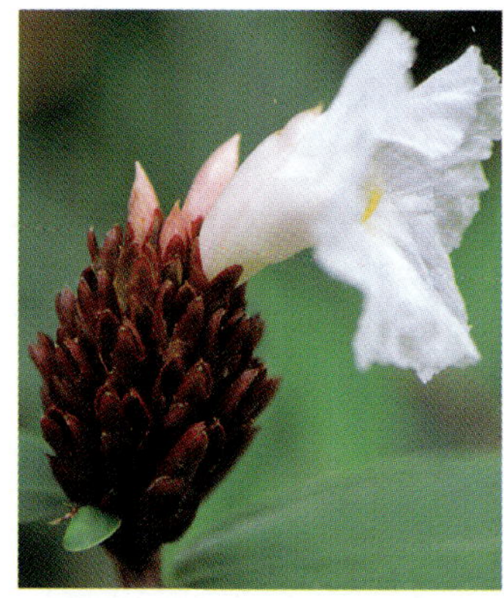

COSTUS SPICATUS

Called the 'Indianhead' ginger. It is a rather common species that is easy to grow. Produces red cones in summer with orange flowers; can be used as a cut flower. Grows 6' (1.8m) to 7' (2.1m) in medium sun. Outstanding spiralling stems. Makes great container plant. Zone 8 and higher.

32550 Rhizome *$6.95*
6($34.95) Save 16%
32551 Growing Plant (6" pot)$ *$12.95*

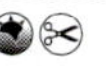

A WONDERFUL CENTERPIECE PLANT FOR YOUR PATIO OR GARDEN

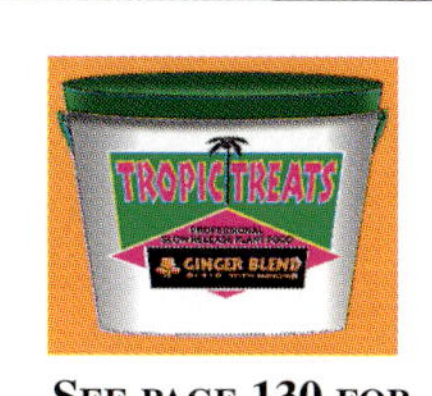

SEE PAGE 130 FOR GINGER FERTILIZER.

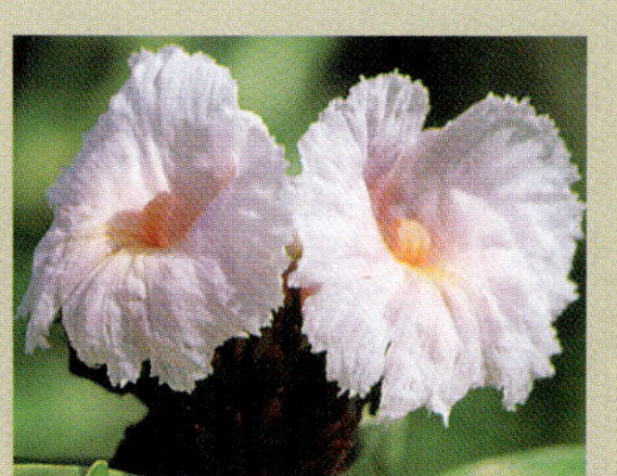

COSTUS SPECIOSUS 'Pink Shadow'

A variation of Costus speciosus with white flowers blushed with pink. Flowers emerge from terminal red cones. Blooms during summer and fall. Medium to full sun. Grows 6' (1.8m) to 9' (2.7m) in height. Zone 8 and higher.

32540 Rhizome...........................*$10.95*
32541 Growing Plant (6" pot)....*$17.95*

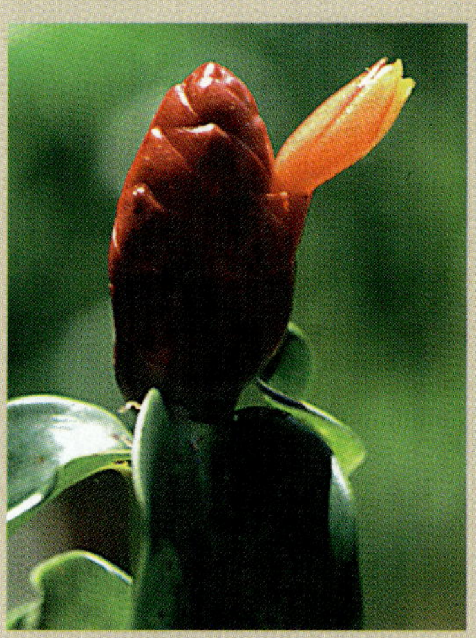

COSTUS SP. 'French Kiss'

Called 'French Kiss' because of its brilliant red conical terminal inflorescence. General form of the plant is similar to *Costus spicatus*. Grows 5' to 6' in medium shade to full sun. Nice addition for the *Costus* enthusiast. Zone 9 and higher.

32200 Rhizome............................*$7.95*
32201 Growing Plant (6" pot)....*$13.95*

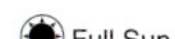 Full Sun 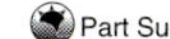 Part Sun 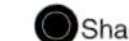 Shade 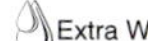 Extra Water 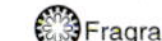 Fragrant 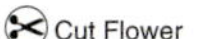 Cut Flower 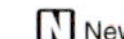 New

39

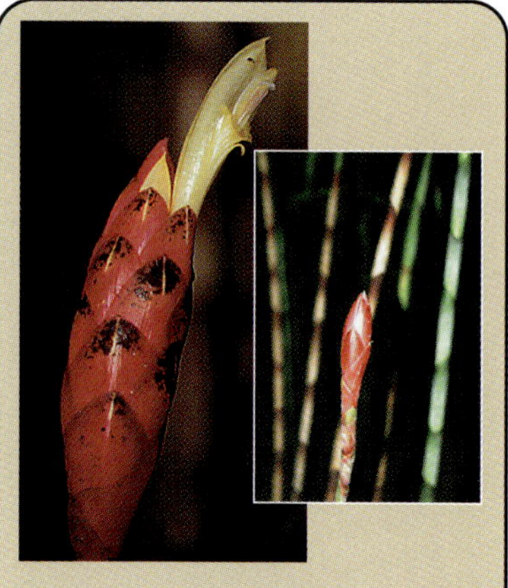

COSTUS STENOPHYLLUS

Known as 'Bamboo Ginger'. Stems and inflorescences are used in the cutflower trade. This attractive foliage plant has stems that are colored with alternating bands of brown and light brown. This Costa Rican native is endangered in the wild. Basal inflorescences are bright red. Plant grows 4' to 6' in the shade. Zone 10 and higher.

32650 Rhizome.............................$12.95
32651 Growing Plant (6" pot) ...$19.95

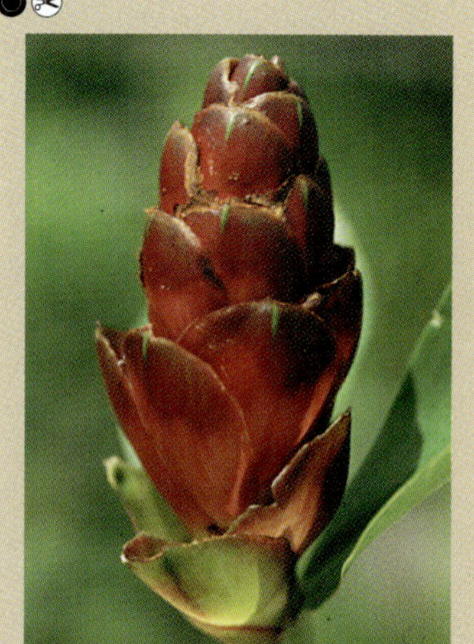

COSTUS SPIRALIS

Short plant with red cone and pink flowers. This South American native grows to 4' (1.2m) in medium sun. Zone 9 and higher.

32600 Rhizome...........................$11.95
32601 Growing Plant..................$18.95

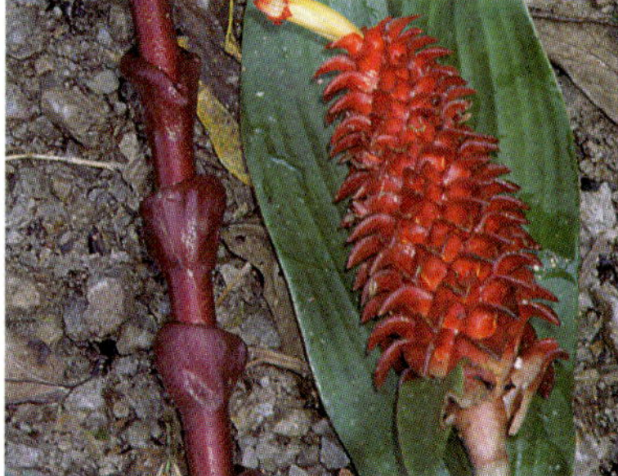

COSTUS SP 'Maroon Chalise'

A startling ginger with a maroon stem with overcupping ligules, solid green leaves and a brilliant red inflorescence—all in one package. Grows 3'-4' tall. Flowers year round. From Peru. Zone 10 and higher. New.

32110 Rhizome $23.95
32111 Growing Plant (6" pot) $30.95

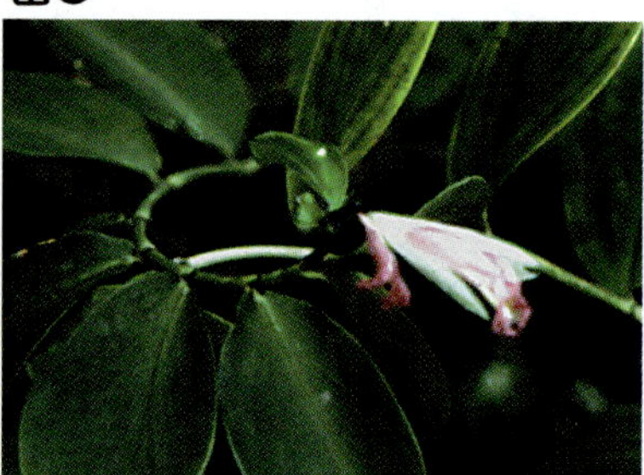

COSTUS TAPPENBECKIANUS

Small purple flowers are produced by this small attractive foliage plant. The plant blooms terminally and basally, with small inflorescences that usually produce only a few flowers. It grows to 3' (1.8m) in shade. Zone 10 and higher.

32700 Rhizome $13.95
32701 Growing Plant (6" pot) $20.95

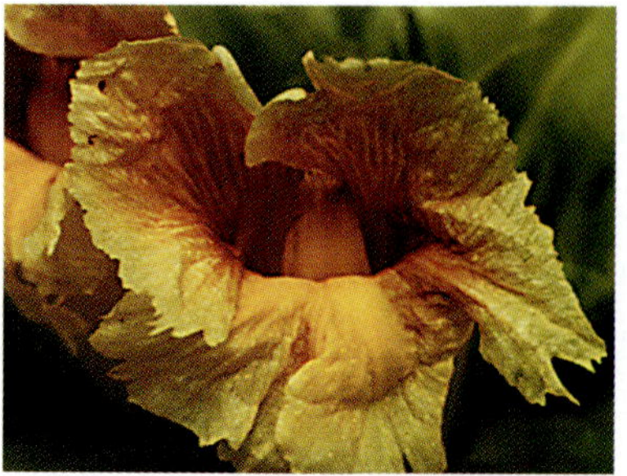

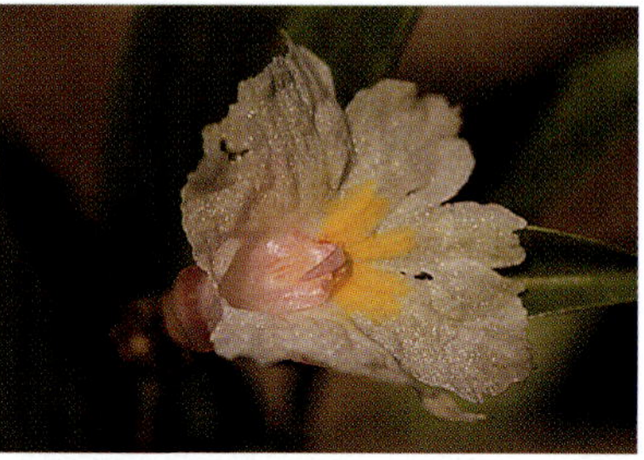

COSTUS TALBOTII 'Blushing Spiral'

A thin spiral ginger with narrow leaves. White tipped flowers backed by 3 pink petals with a splash of yellow. Flowers are produced both terminally on stems and on basal spikes. Blooms easily in 6' pot in any season in greenhouse. Probably Zone 10 and higher. Grows in medium shade to 3' tall.

32640 Rhizome $13.95
32641 Growing Plant (6" pot) $20.95

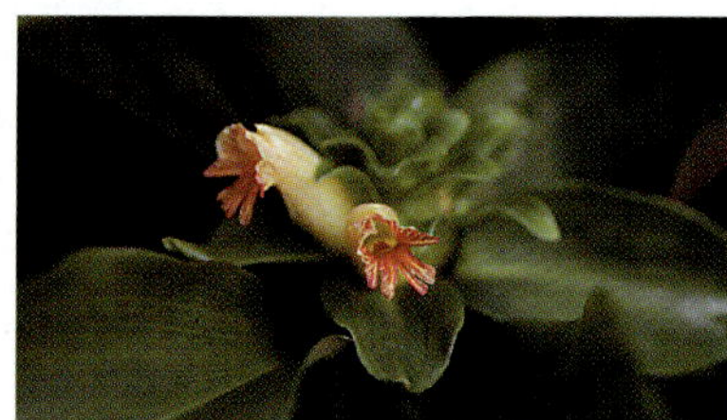

COSTUS VARZEARUM

A great looking medium-size ginger growing to 3'-4' in medium sun. Native of Brazil. A very nice looking foliage plant with dark green leaves with maroon undersides. Produces small attractive tubular flowers that have red and yellow throats. Probably Zone 9 and higher.

32730 Rhizome $13.95
32731 Growing Plant (6" pot) $20.95

COSTUS VILLOSISSIMUS

Dubbed the 'Porcupine Costus' because of the stiff fuzzy hairs covering its leaves and stems. Grows in medium to full sun 6' (1.8m) to 12' (3.6m). Beautiful yellow flowers. Zone 10 and higher.

32710 Rhizome $13.95
32711 Growing Plant (6" pot) $20.95

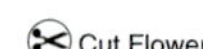

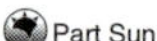

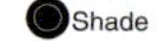

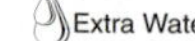

⬤ Full Sun   ✦ Part Sun   ⬤ Shade   Extra Water   Fragrant   ✂ Cut Flower   N New

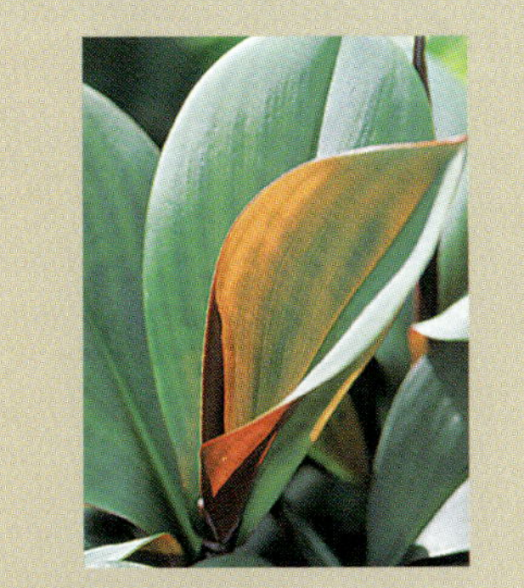

COSTUS VINOSUS

A very striking costus from Panama. Extremely showy vegetation; tends to be shy bloomer. Undersides of leaves and entire stems are oxblood colored. Grows to 3'. Full shade plant. Leaf sheaths (ligules) completely inside stems are cupped which allows them to trap water, which may serve as a defensive mechanism against certain pests. Zone 10 and higher.

32720 Rhizome..............................$14.95
32721 Growing Plant (6" pot) ...$21.95
32722 Growing Plant (4" pot) $7.95

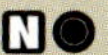

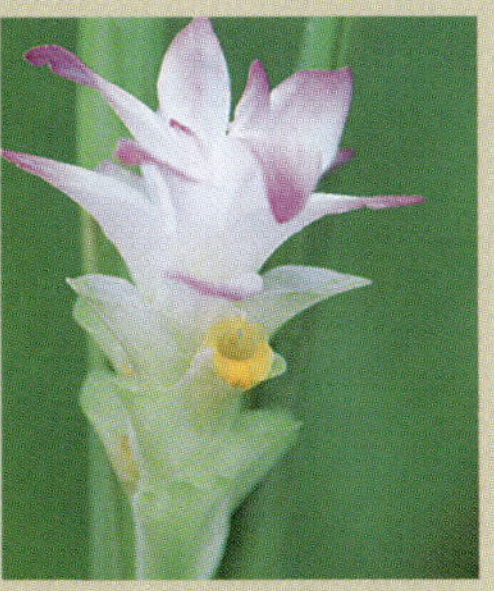

CURCUMA AMADA
'Emperess'

A fantastic new Curcuma similar in size and leaf to Curcuma cordata. Leaves 48"-51" long. Huge inflorescence 4" wide x 6" tall nestled in plant leaf axils. Wonderfully colored bracts are fuzzy to the touch. True flowers are yellow with dark yellow center stripe on lower lip. Probably Zone 9 and higher.

32930 Rhizome..............................$9.95
32931 Growing Plant (6" pot) ...$13.95

CURCUMA AERUGINOSA

Known as the 'Pink and Blue' ginger which refers to its blue rhizome and pink inflorescence. The plant is a spring bloomer, that occasionally blooms in summer. The deep maroon stripe on the leaf makes this an attractive foliage plant. Rhizomes have a blue center. The plant grows to 3' (1.8m) in medium sun. Zone 7b and higher.

32750 Rhizome $10.95
32751 Growing Plant (6" pot) $14.95

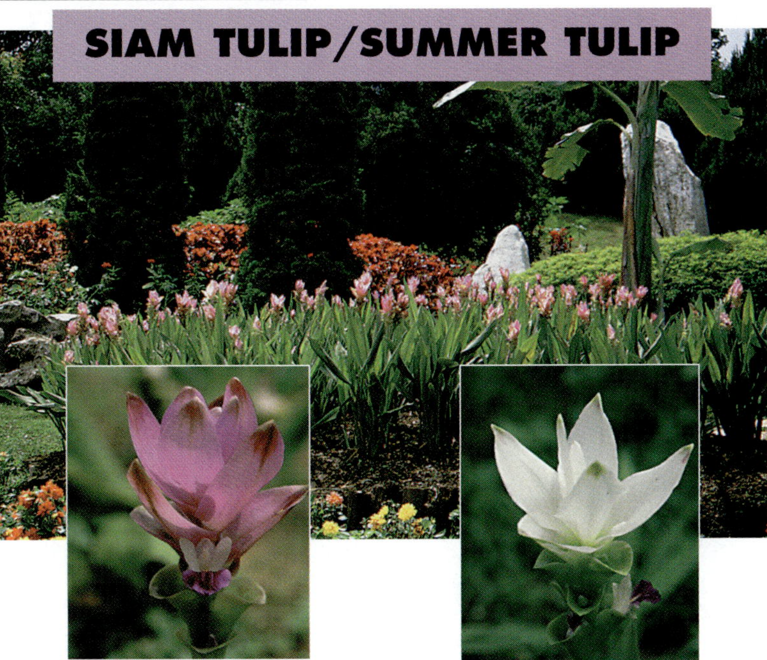

CURCUMA ALISMATIFOLIA
'Pink'

A strikingly beautiful ginger that superficially resembles a tulip. Introduced from Thailand. Produces a beautiful dark, rose-pink inflorescence that makes a great cut flower. Has long narrow stiff leaves that resemble tulip leaves. Grows to 2' in medium to full sun. Blooms all summer. Probably Zone 8 and higher. Dormant November to May/June.

32850 Rhizome $4.95
6($21.95) Save 26%
32851 Growing Plant (6" pot) $7.95
32852 Growing Plant (4" pot) $2.95

CURCUMA ALISMATIFOLIA
'White'

A sport from the 'Pink'. Not as big a plant or as large flowered as "Pink". Probably Zone 8 and higher.

32800 Rhizome $8.95
6($45.95) Save 15%;
32801 Growing Plant (6" pot) $12.95
32802 Growing Plant (4" pot) $5.95

RARE

CALL 24 HRS. / 7 DAYS

TO PLACE AN ORDER:
1-800-624-9706

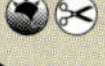 Full Sun   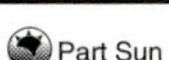 Part Sun   Shade   Extra Water   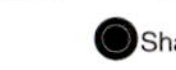 Fragrant    Cut Flower   New

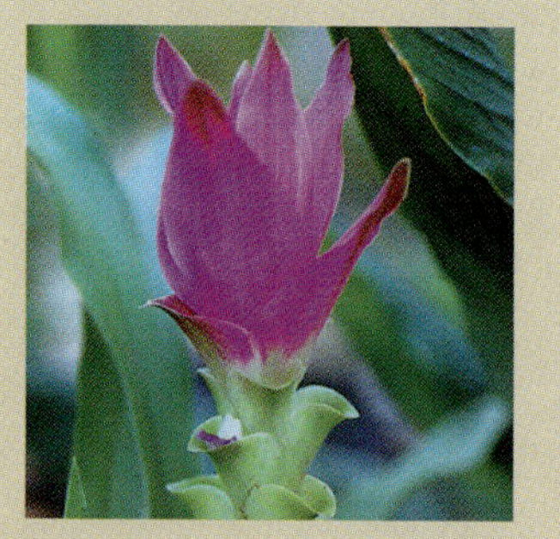

CURCUMA ALISMATIFOLIA 'Rose'

A sport from the 'Pink'. Not as big a plant or as large flowered as pink. Probably Zone 8 and higher.

32900 Rhizome............................. $8.95
6($45.95) Save 17%
32901 Growing Plant (6" pot)....$12.95
32902 Growing Plant (4" pot)......$5.95

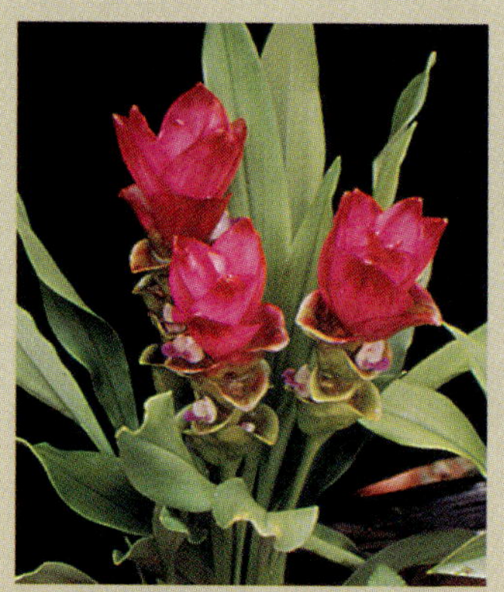

CURCUMA ALISMATIFOLIA 'Thai Supreme'™

Another remarkable cultivar that is like a blush version of 'Thai Beauty'. The reduced magenta pigment results in the bracts taking on a vertical lined appearance. Bracts are not quite as cupped and are longer with more pointed tips. Overall a very unique alismatifolia cultivar. Similar in all other respects to 'Thai Beauty'. New.

32920 Rhizome.......................... $11.95
32921 Growing Plant (6" pot)....$16.95

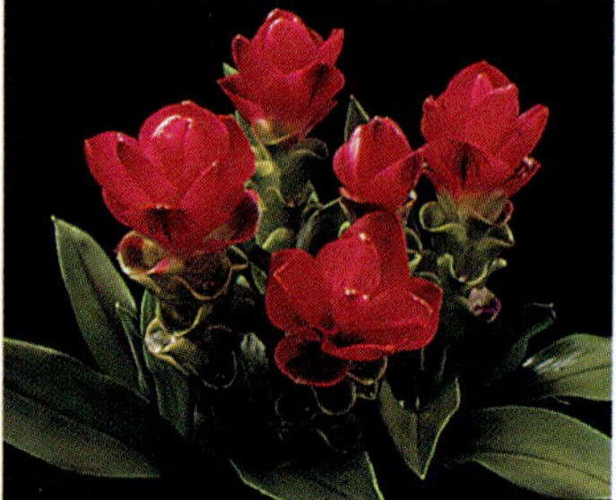

CURCUMA ALISMATIFOLIA 'Thai Beauty'™

A wonderful new hybrid form of the wild 'pink' *alismatifolia* that has exquisite hot magenta bracts. Terminal colored bracts are large and cupped. Leaves are outstanding; upright and broad and frequently having a faint maroon midstripe. Makes great cut flower. Probably Zone 8 and higher. Dormant November to May/June. Same growing characteristics and requirements as other *alismatifolias*. New.

32910 Rhizome............................... $11.95   32911 Growing Plant (6" pot) $16.95

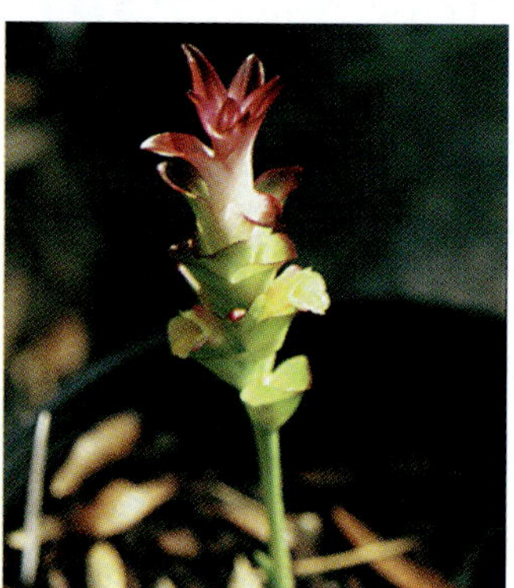

CURCUMA ATTENUATA

Plant has inflorescence that is white with maroon top. This species blooms in spring and summer and is slow growing with thin, slightly fuzzy leaves. Plant grows to 3' (1.8m) in medium sun. Probably Zone 8 and higher.

32950 Rhizome $7.95
32951 Growing Plant (6" pot) $12.95
32952 Growing Plant (4" pot) $4.95

CURCUMA AURANTIACA

Called 'Rainbow Curcuma' because of striking range of colors in inflorescence. Inflorescence is 10"-12" high and 4" in diameter on 3'- 3½' plant. Leaves are corrugated like Curcuma cordata (Jewel of Thailand). One of our best-looking Curcumas. Probably Zone 9 and higher. Medium shade. Blooms until first frost.

32760 Rhizome $9.95
6($45.95) Save 17%
32761 Growing Plant (6" pot) $16.95
32762 Growing Plant (4" pot)...........................$6.95

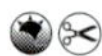

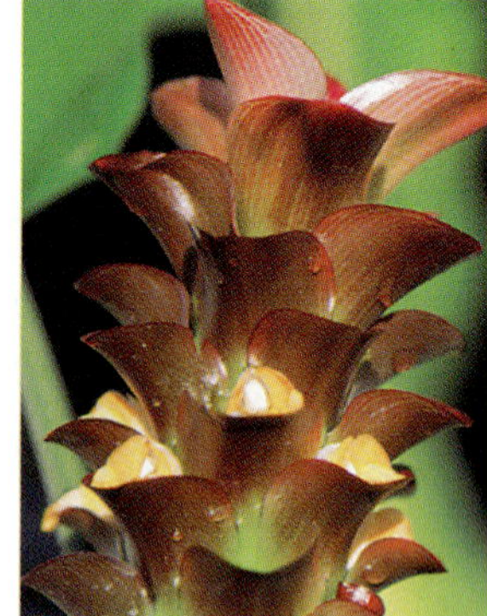

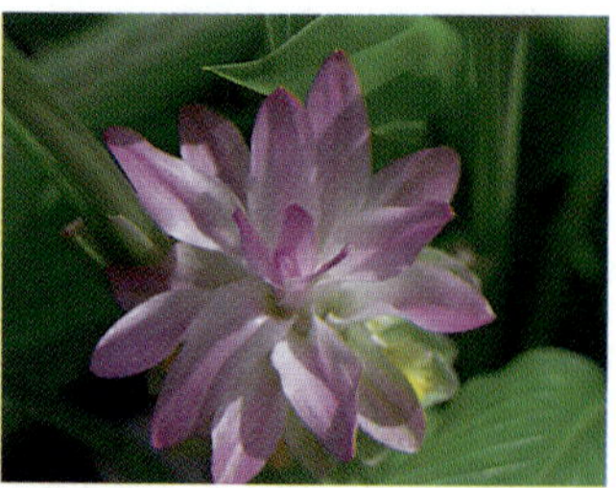

CURCUMA AUSTRALASICA

Called 'Aussie Plume'. Wonderful large ginger with central dark rose inflorescence. Full sun. Height to 5' (1.5m). Goes dormant in November but returns in May. Zone 8 and higher. One of our most popular gingers.

33000 Rhizome $7.95
6($39.95) Save 16%
33001 Growing Plant (6" pot) $12.95
33002 Growing Plant (4" pot) $4.95

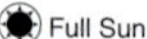 Full Sun 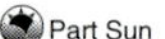 Part Sun 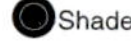 Shade   Extra Water   Fragrant   Cut Flower   N New

CURCUMA CORDATA 'Jewel of Thailand'

Rare ginger from Thailand. Very beautiful with tall 8" to 12" waxy pink inflorescence. Excellent cut flower. Grows to 3'-4' in medium sun. Blooms July through October. Zone 9 and higher. Dormant November to May.

33050 Rhizome......................................*$7.95*
6($39.95) Save 16%
33051 Growing Plant (6" pot)..........................*$12.95*
33052 Growing Plant (4" pot)..........................*$4.95*

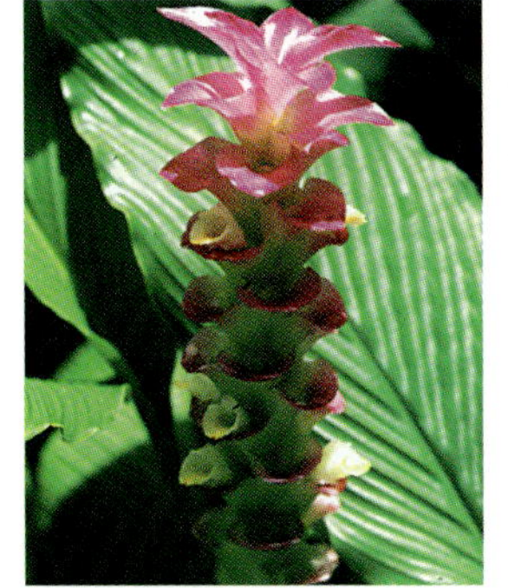

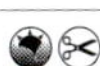

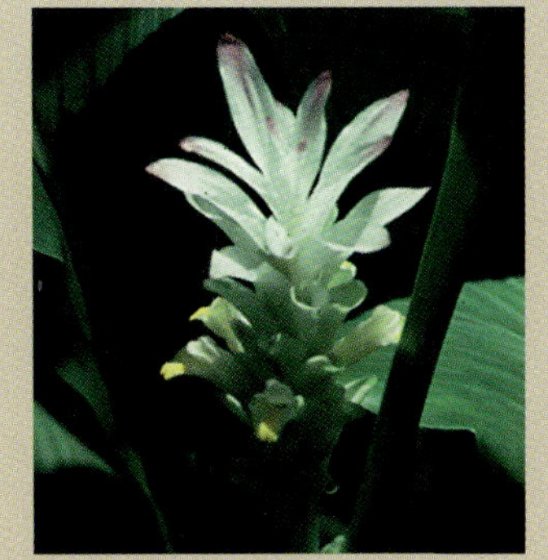

CURCUMA ELATA

Called 'Giant Plume' ginger. This is one of the first gingers to bloom in spring. Large pink inflorescence is produced before leaves appear. Plants can reach 6' to 7' in height. Grows well in medium to full sun. Zone 7 and higher. Goes dormant in November but returns in April or May.

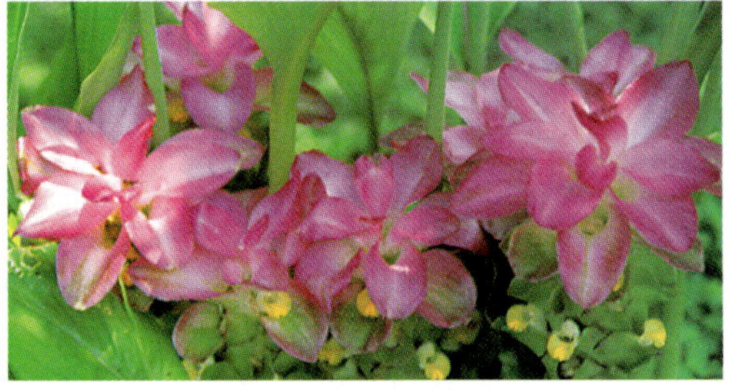

33150 Rhizome ....*$12.95*   *33151 Growing Plant (6" pot)*.....*$19.95*

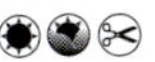

CURCUMA DOMESTICA

Also known as Curcuma longa, this ginger is the source of the spice turmeric used in Oriental and Asian cooking. The coloring agent, flavoring, and dye are made from its rhizomes. Grows to 4' (1.2m) in medium to full sun. Zone 7b and higher. Goes dormant in November but returns in May.

33100 Rhizome............................*$9.95*
33101 Growing Plant (6" pot)....*$14.95*

CURCUMA FLAVIFLORA

This rare species has been given the common name 'Fiery Curcuma' because of its red bracts and orange flowers. A new introduction from Thailand that grows to 3 feet (1.8m) in shade. Zone 8 and higher. This summer and fall bloomer has a unique bloom that remains at ground level.

33200 Rhizome *$14.95*
33201 Growing Plant (6" pot) *$21.95*

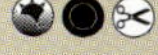

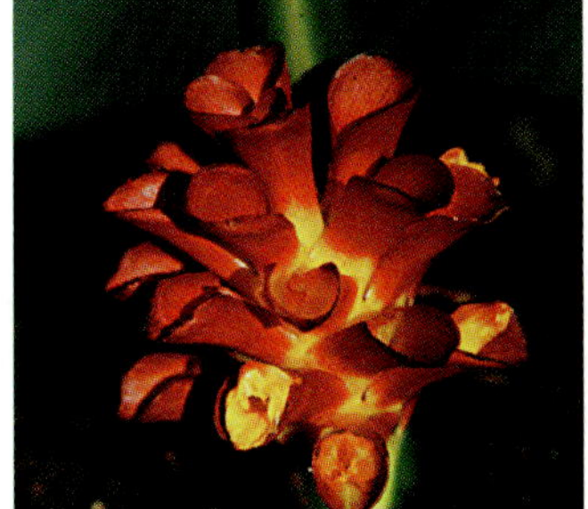

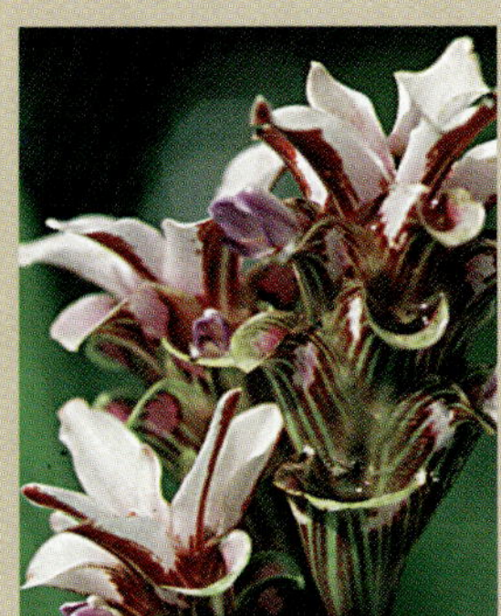

CURCUMA GRACILLIMA 'Burnt Burgundy'

A beautiful small delicate ginger from Thailand with burgundy colored inflorescence with darker (burnt) streaks in bracts. Inflorescence is held above long narrow, dark- green leaves. Grows 1½' (45cm) to 2' (60cm) high in medium sun. An absolute must for collectors. Blooms appear in summer. Zone 9 and higher. Goes dormant in November but returns in May.

33250 Rhizome.....................................*$9.95*
33251 Growing Plant (6" pot).........................*$14.95*

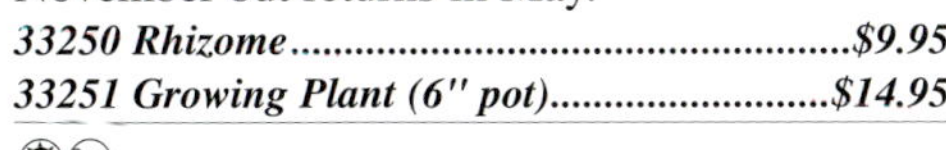

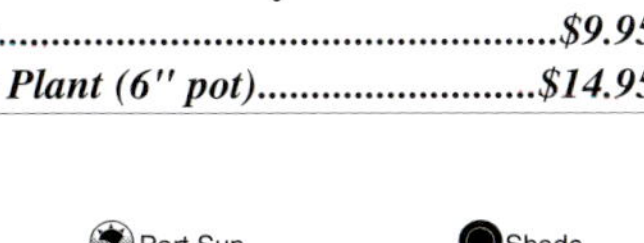

CURCUMA GRACILLIMA 'Candy Cane'

A rare, small delicate ginger, introduced from Thailand. Striking inflorescence (white stripped with maroon) is proudly held above plant. Grows to 2' in medium sun. Blooms appear in summer. Goes dormant November to May. Zone 9 and higher.

33300 Rhizome............................*$6.95*
6($34.95) Save 16%
33301 Growing Plant (6" pot)....*$11.95*
33302 Growing Plant (4" pot)......*$3.95*

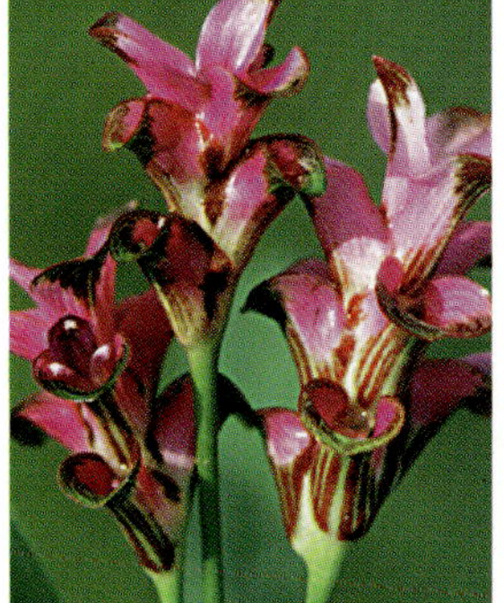

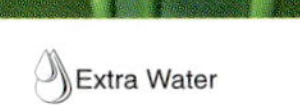

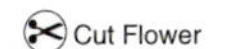

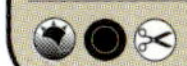

☀ Full Sun   🌤 Part Sun   ● Shade   💧 Extra Water   ✻ Fragrant   ✂ Cut Flower   Ⓝ New

TO ORDER CALL **1-800-624-9706**/24 HRS. OR VISIT OUR WEB SITE: www. stokestropicals.com

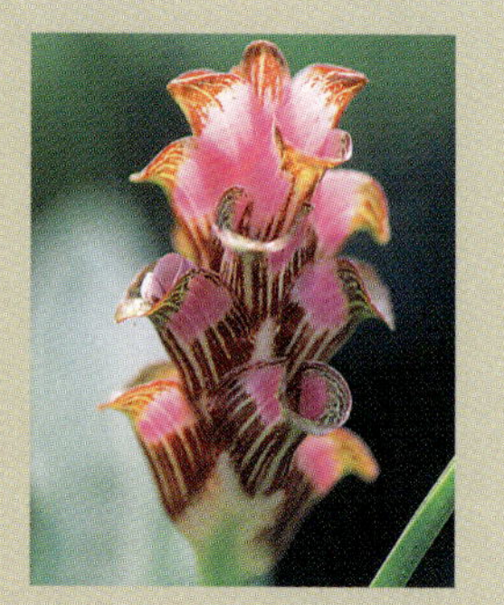

CURCUMA GRACILLIMA 'Lavender Stripe'

A beautifully patterned inflorescence produced on (12"-16") stalk. Inflorescence is lighter lavender color as opposed to dark maroon pattern of Curcuma gracillima 'Burnt Burgundy.' Part shade to almost full sun. Blooms from summer to late fall. Goes dormant in November and returns in May. Probably Zone 8 and higher. Good cut flower.

33350 Rhizome...........................$10.95
33351 Growing Plant (6" pot)....$15.95

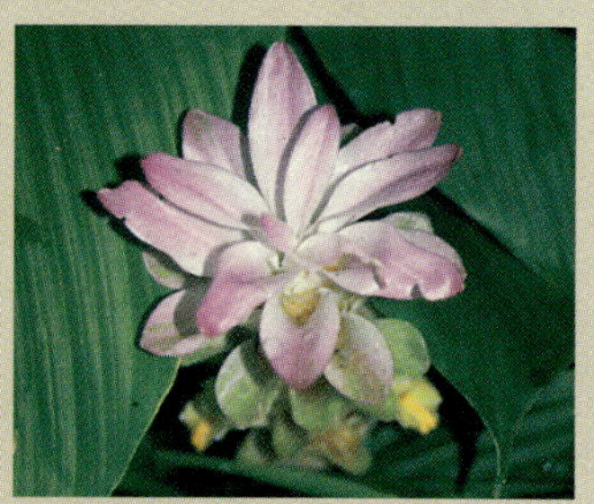

CURCUMA PETIOLATA 'Hidden Lily'

Probably the most cold hardy of the Curcumas. A fast growing plant that produces whitish pink inflorescence "hidden" down in plant in summer through fall. Hence the name. Grows to 3' in medium to full sun. Zone 7 and higher. Goes dormant in November but returns in May.

33550 Rhizome.......................... $8.95
6($39.95) Save 16%
33551 Bareroot Plant.................$13.95

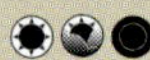

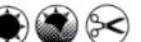

CURCUMA HARMANDII 'Emerald Pagoda'

New introduction from Thailand that we like a lot and have named 'Emerald Pagoda' because of its "tiered" inflorescence: an emerald green colored stalk of bracts with small orchidlike light-bluish white flowers. Medium to full sun. Probably Zone 9 and higher. A different looking Curcuma.

33360 Rhizome $11.95
33361 Growing Plant (6" pot) $16.95

CURCUMA INODORA

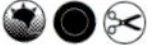

This attractive spring bloomer has a large pink inflorescence and grows to 4' (1.2m) in medium sun. Probably Zone 8 and higher. From India. Goes dormant in November but returns in May. Leaves have red center stripe or "feather" (see inset).

33400 Rhizome................................ $6.95
33401 Growing Plant (6" pot) $11.95

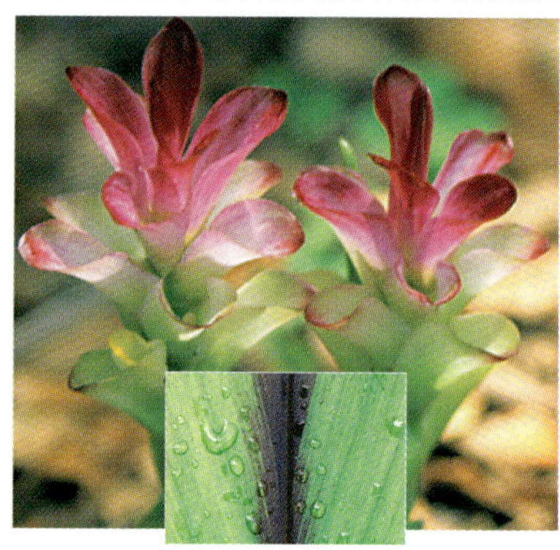

CURCUMA ORNATA

Differs from *elata* in that leaves have a red central stripe and flowers appear later in spring after the leaves. Inflorescence is short and has broad white bracts with purple tips. Plant grows 4' to 5' in medium sun. Zone 8 and higher. Other Curcumas with a red midstripe are: inodora, zedoaria, aeruginosa and yunnanensis. Dormant November to May.

33450 Rhizome..$10.95
33451 Growing Plant (6" pot)....................$16.95

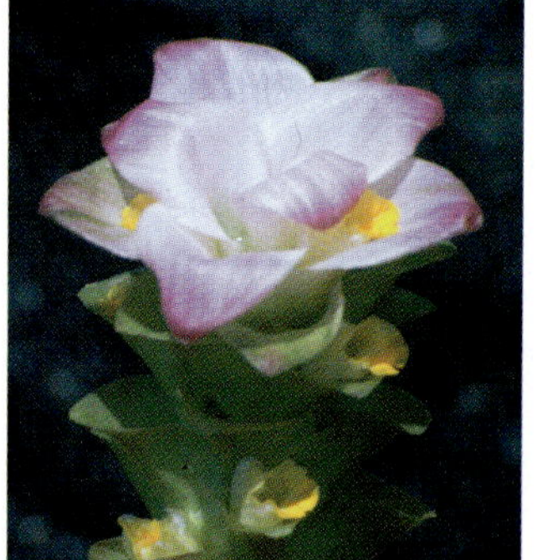

CURCUMA PARVIFLORA

'White Angel' is a new introduction that is very attractive for a small species. Inflorescence is made up of a stack of bracts with deep forest green basal bracts and pure white terminal bracts. This plant grows to 1' (30cm) and blooms freely in a 6" (15cm) pot. Will take medium sun. Zone 8 and higher. Goes dormant in November but returns in May.

33500 Rhizome $14.95
33501 Growing Plant (6" pot) $21.95

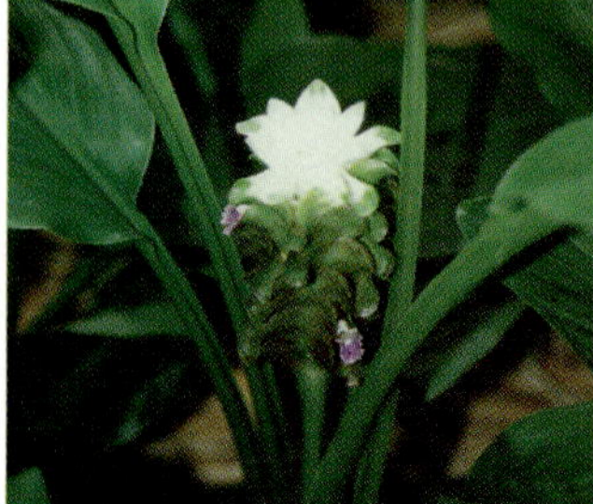

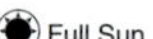 Full Sun 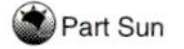 Part Sun 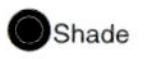 Shade 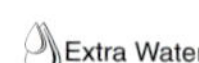 Extra Water 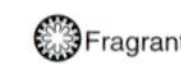 Fragrant 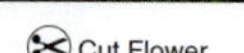 Cut Flower  New

TO ORDER CALL **1-800-624-9706**/24 HRS. OR VISIT OUR WEB SITE: www. stokestropicals.com

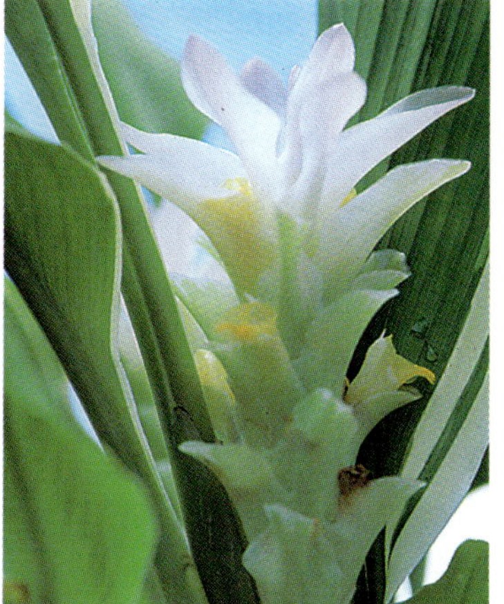

CURCUMA PETIOLATA VARIEGATED 'Emperor'

Similar to the common "hidden lily" except that leaves are beautifully variegated. Prefers medium sun. Plant is worth having because of foliage alone. Central blooms are an extra. Zone 7 and higher. A very popular ginger that is difficult to keep in stock. Goes dormant in November but returns in May.

33600 Rhizome $8.95
6($45.95) Save 17%
33601 Growing Plant (6" pot)..........$13.95
33602 Growing Plant (4" pot)............$5.95

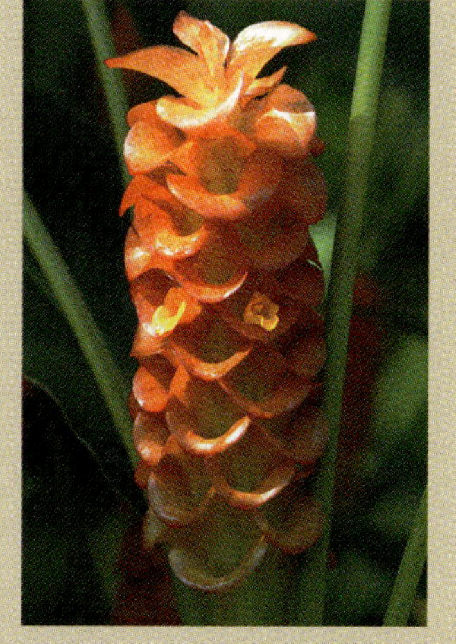

CURCUMA PIERRIANA 'Sleeping Princess'

An amazing Curcuma species from Thailand. Short plant that grows to 2' in medium to full sun. Broad thick textured glossy green leaves. Multiple inflorescences arise from short basal stalks near leaf bases. Inflorescence starts off as insignificant maroonish cream pointed bracts. Stalks of inflorescence slowly extend and "sleeping" flowers emerge from inside bracts. Flowers are a beautiful white with deep maroon tipped petals, and golden yellow stripe on lower petal. Several (4-6) flowers appear at once. Probably Zone 9 and higher.
33850 Rhizome $8.95
33851 Growing Plant (6" pot) $13.95

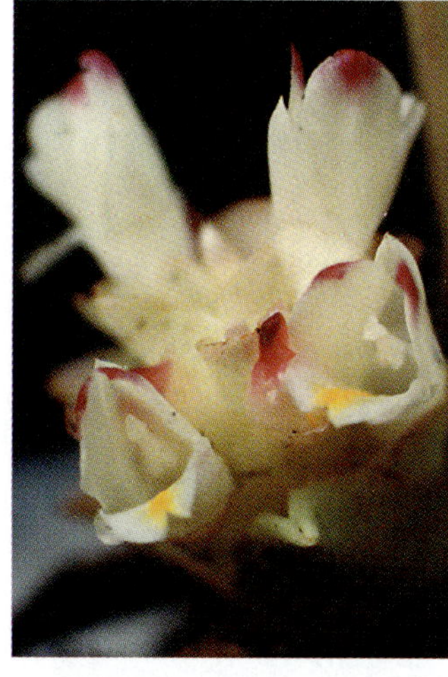

CURCUMA ROSCOEANA

Called the 'Jewel of Burma'. Medium plant to 24" high. Does well in shade to medium sun. Striking pure orange inflorescence appears in center of graceful cluster of foliage. Excellent pot plant. Keep dry in winter. Makes good cut flower. Without a doubt one of the most beautiful of all the gingers. A must for the serious collector. Zone 9 and higher.
33650 Rhizome............................ $9.95
6($39.95) Save 16%
33651 Growing Plant (6" pot)... $14.95
33652 Growing Plant (4" pot)..... $6.95

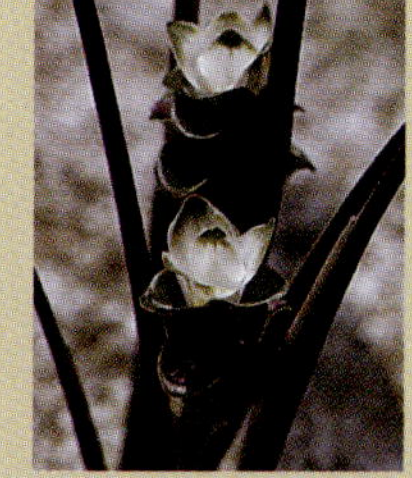

CURCUMA SP. 'Candy Corn'

What a splash of color! Bunches of basal inflorescences appear in spring and summer. Plant has typical Curcuma leaves to 24" tall. Like other Cucumas goes dormant in late fall and winter. Zone 10 and higher. New.
33310 Rhizome $19.95
33311 Growing Plant (6" pot) $26.95

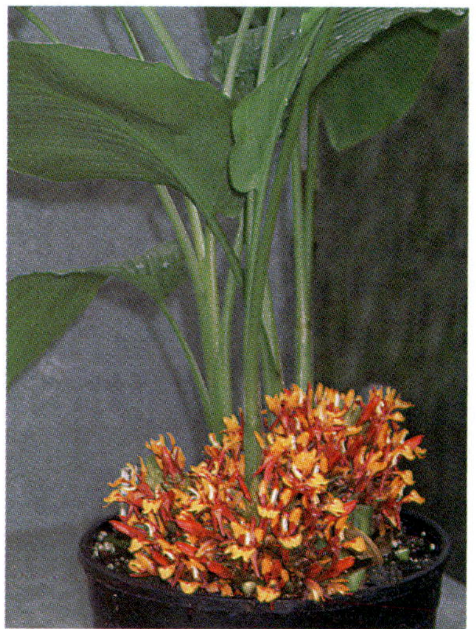

CALL 24 HRS. / 7 DAYS
TO PLACE AN ORDER:
1-800-624-9706
FOR INFORMATION:
1-337-365-6998

CURCUMA SP. 'Green & White'

A truly spectacular Curcuma with reddish stems and inflorescence with emerald green bracts topped with snow white bracts with green tips. Medium shade. Collected from Thailand. Probably Zone 9 and higher. *Call about availability.*
33430 Rhizome............................$29.95

Available in 2001

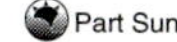 Full Sun   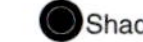 Part Sun   Shade   Extra Water   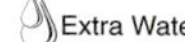 Fragrant   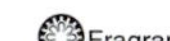 Cut Flower   New

Gingers

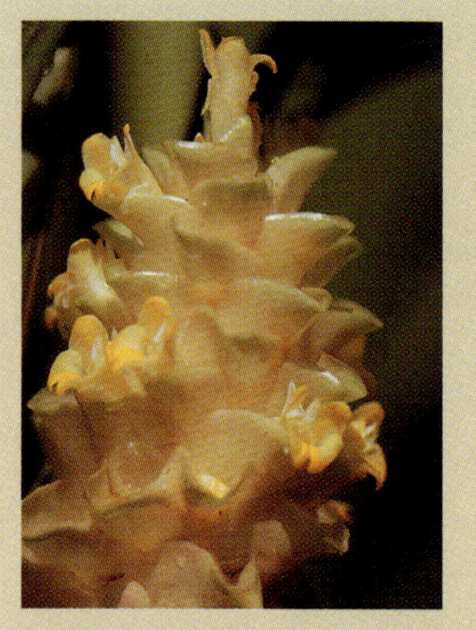

CURCUMA SP. 'Ivory Ice'

A special looking new Curcuma from Thailand with ivory-colored bracts holding orange, yellow flowers. Plant grows 2'-3' in medium shade. Probably Zone 9 and higher.
33880 Rhizome.............................$15.95
33881 Growing Plant (6" pot) ...$20.95

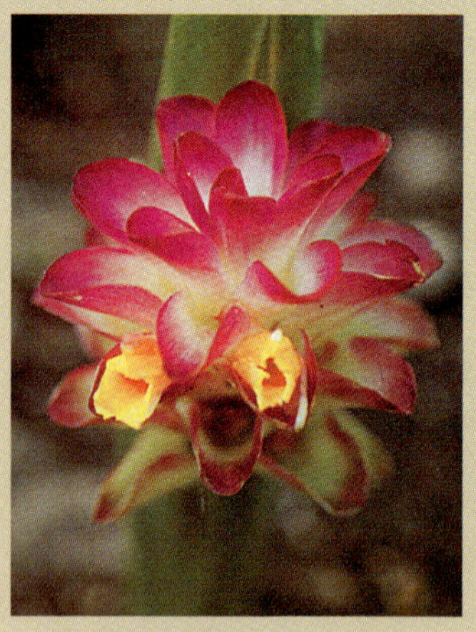

CURCUMA SP. 'Ribbon'

A magnificient new curcuma from Thailand with narrow leaves and a hot pink tipped inflorescence holding golden yellow flowers. Medium shade. Probably Zone 9 and higher.
33680 Rhizome $9.95
33681 Growing Plant (6" pot) ...$15.95
33682 Growing Plant (4" pot) $6.95

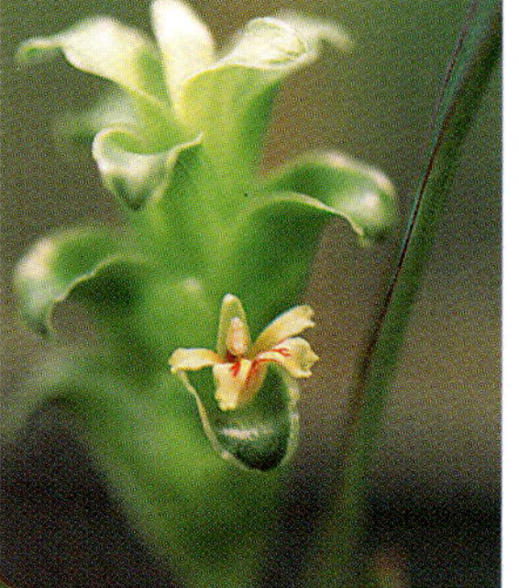

CURCUMA SP. 'Green Goddess'

A tiny Curcuma species that comes from Cambodia. Short 8" plant with a small inflorescence composed of green bracts that bear tiny cream-colored flowers with maroon stripes. Narrow leaves are 8" long with a slight maroon mid-stripe. Makes a good pot plant. Can take almost full sun. Probably Zone 9 and higher.
33660 Rhizomes $10.95
33661 Growing Plant (6" pot)........................$15.95

CURCUMA SP. 'Khymer Orange'

A strikingly beautiful new ginger from Cambodia with a beautiful burnt-orange inflorescence with delightful orange flowers. May be related to Curcuma *aurantiaca* but is distinct in size and inflorescence shape. Plant is smaller than *aurantiaca*, growing 1½'-2' high and with a lamp globe-shaped inflorescence. Late-summer to late-fall bloomer. Likes medium shade. Probably Zone 9 and higher.
33410 Rhizome $13.95
33411 Growing Plant (6" pot) $19.95

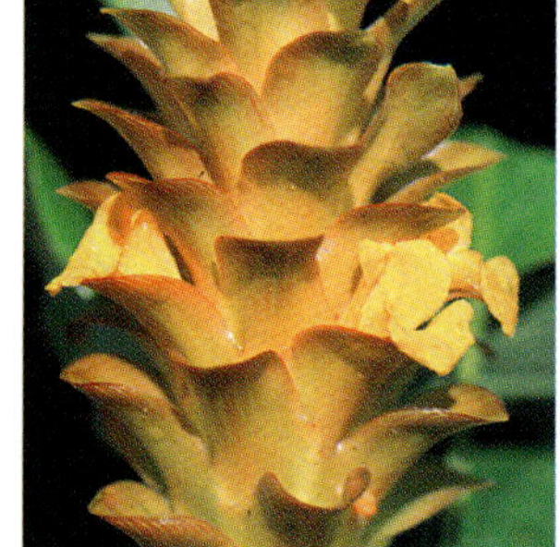

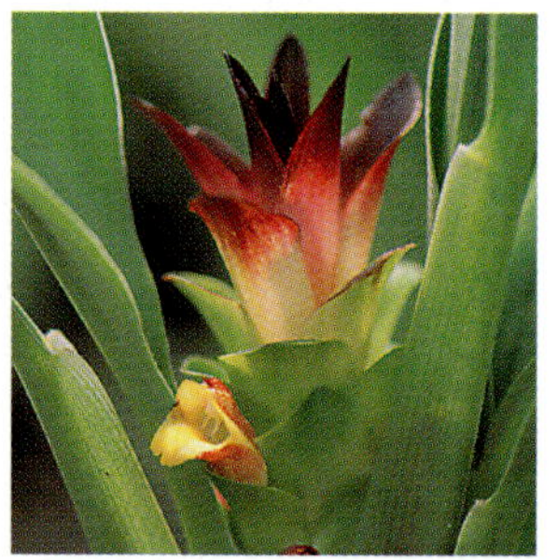

CURCUMA SP. 'Maroon Beauty'

Another wonderful Curcuma from Thailand. Plant has tough dark-green leaves with fuzzy undersides. Leaves grow to 2' high in medium sun. From late summer to early fall, produces a deep maroon inflorescence. A wonderful, tough little plant. Probably Zone 9 and higher.
33860 Rhizome $12.95
33861 Growing Plant (6" pot) $17.95

CURCUMA SP. 'Pink Pearl'

A new introduction from Cambodia. Species not known for certain, may be *sparganifolia*. A strikingly different *Curcuma* with rose-colored cupped bracts that have white "diamond" tips. Comes in 3 different colors and shapes as pictured here. Tall stem extends high above long narrow leaves. Small white flowers deep within bracts. Medium to full sun. Makes outstanding cut flower lasting for more than a week. Probably Zone 9 and higher. Dormant November to May. Makes great pot plant in well lit areas as well as great plant for mass plantings in beds.

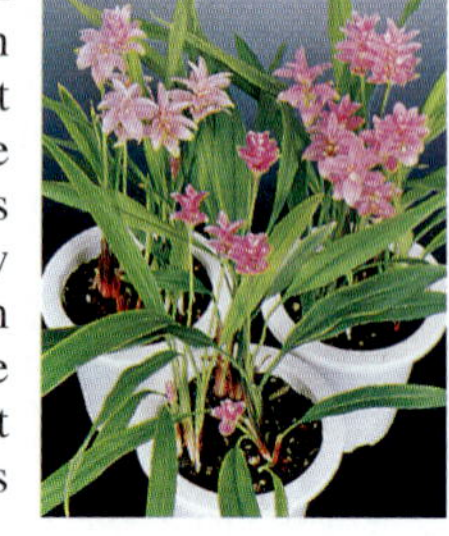

*33750 Rhizome ....$9.95**   *6($45.95) Save 17%*
33751 Growing Plant (6" pot) $14.95
33752 Growing Plant (4" pot) $6.95

**Note: If you order rhizomes you could get any one, or all three, of the flower types.*

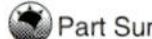 Full Sun   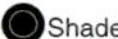 Part Sun   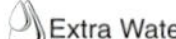 Shade   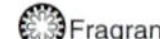 Extra Water   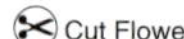 Fragrant   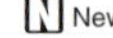 Cut Flower   N New

TO ORDER CALL **1-800-624-9706**/24 HRS. OR VISIT OUR WEB SITE: www. stokestropicals.com

Gingers

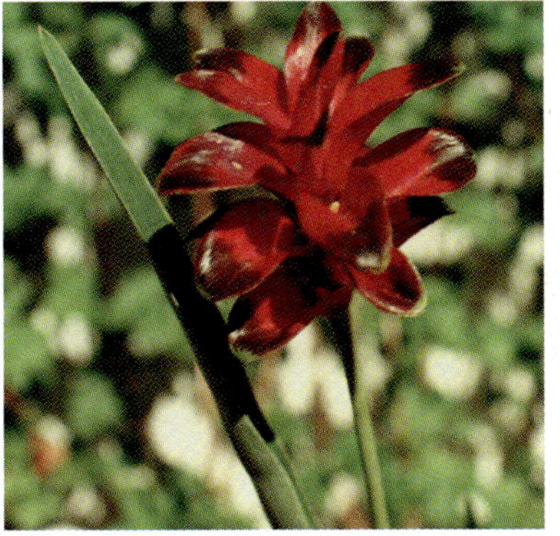

CURCUMA SP. 'Siam Ruby'

Similar to 'Pink Pearl' except tips of rose pink bracts are tipped in brilliant dark emerald green. May be same species but different color variation. Dormant November to May. Probably Zone 9 and higher.

33800 Rhizome $15.95
33801 Growing Plant (6″ pot) $20.95

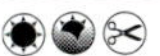

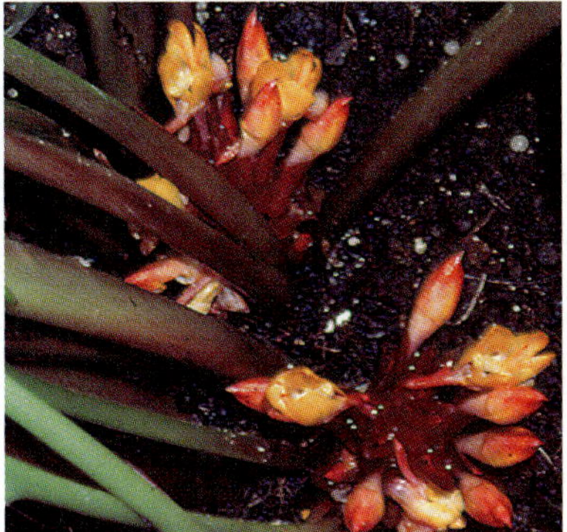

CURCUMA SP. 'Sri Pak'

A rare beauty from Vietnam. Grows to 24″. Extremely colorful flowers arising from soil at base of leaves in summer. Like all Curcumas, goes dormant in fall and returns in late spring. Probably Zone 9 and higher. New.

33820 Rhizome $9.95
33821 Growing Plant (6″ pot) $15.95

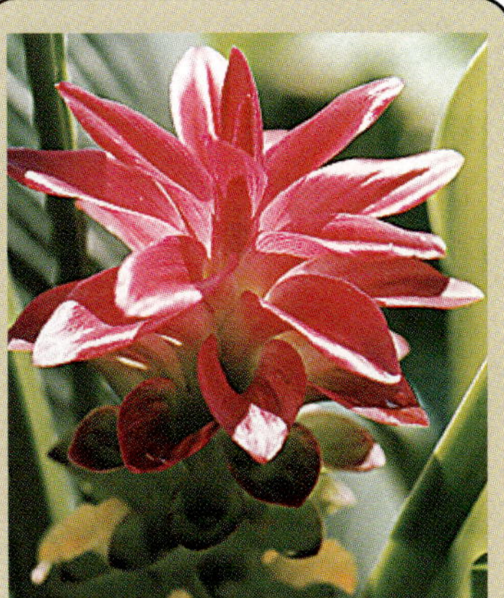

CURCUMA SUMATRANA

Also called 'Olena'. A knockout. Short plant with large bright pink central inflorescence. Height to 24″. Medium sun. Flowers summer to fall. Dormant November to April. One of our most popular gingers. Zone 8 and higher.

33900 Rhizome..............................$7.95
6($39.95) Save 16%
33901 Growing Plant (6″ pot) ...$12.95

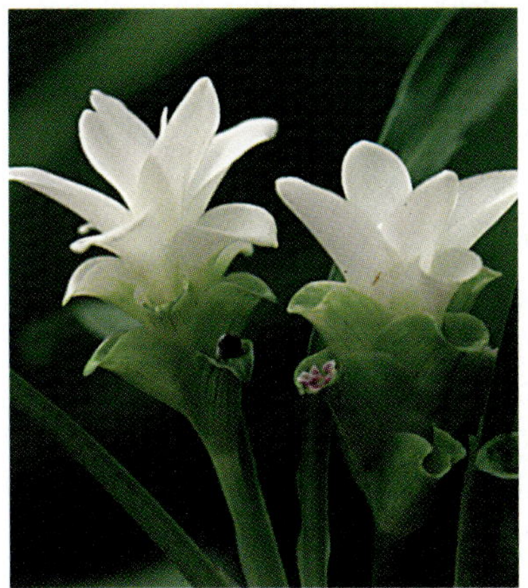

CURCUMA THORELII
'Chiang Mai Snow'

A beautiful species introduced from Thailand. Has a large snow white inflorescence. Plant grows 1$\frac{1}{2}$'-2' (60cm) high. Prefers medium sun. Blooms early summer to fall. Goes dormant in November but returns in May. A must for the collector. Zone 9 and higher.

34000 Rhizome $11.95
34001 Growing Plant (6″ pot) $17.95

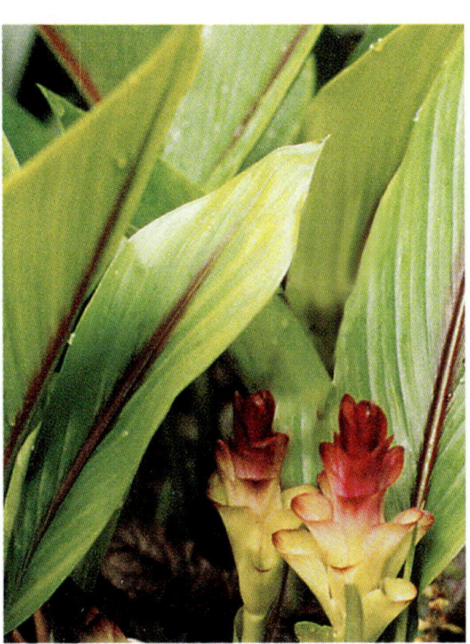

CURCUMA ZEDOARIA

This spring bloomer has large maroon inflorescence with a maroon stripe in the middle of the leaves. It grows to 3 feet. Goes dormant in November but returns in May. Likes medium shade. Zone 8 and higher.

34050 Rhizome $13.95
34051 Growing Plant (6″ pot) $18.95

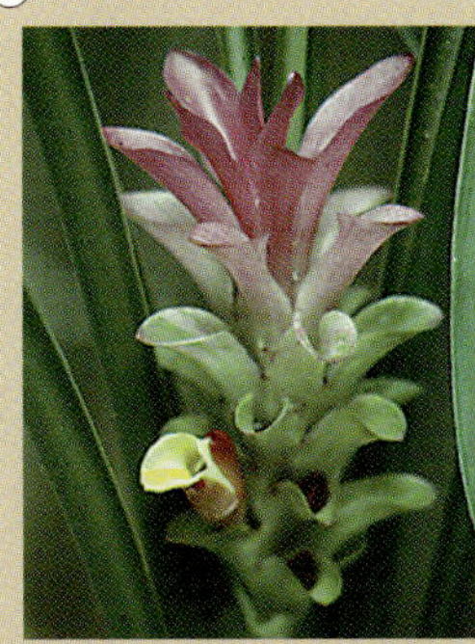

CURCUMA YUNNANENSIS
'Yunnan Plume'

A tall plant with lance shaped leaves having a purplish stripe down the middle. It has blooms featuring many narrow upright bracts that are bright plum colored. Has a long blooming season (July to Oct.) and prefers lightly filtered sun. Zone 8 and higher.

34010 Rhizome..........................$14.95
34011 Growing Plant (6″ pot)....$19.95

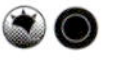

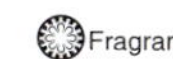

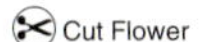

Full Sun   Part Sun   Shade   Extra Water   Fragrant   Cut Flower   New

47

Gingers

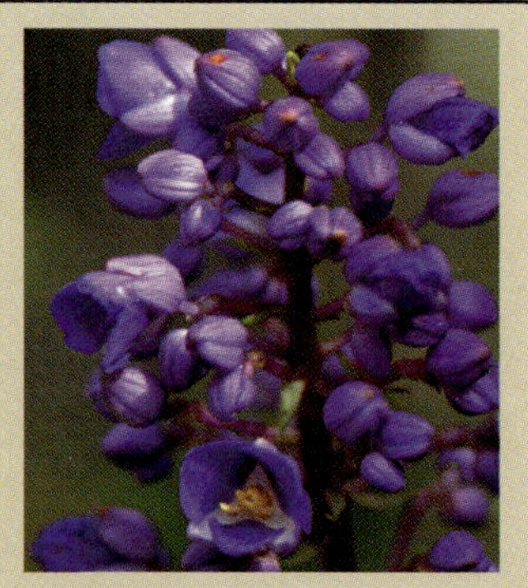

DICHORISANDRA THYRSIFLORA

Called 'blue ginger', however it is not a true ginger (is in the spiderwort family). Superficially resembles a *Costus* with spirally arranged dark green leaves and strong stems that terminate in large heads of rich blue flowers with white and yellow interiors. Prefers medium shade and moist soil. Grows 5' to 6'. Blooms in late summer to late fall. Zone 8 and higher. A very popular seller.
34100 Rhizome...............................$8.95
6($45.95) Save 15%
34101 Growing Plant (6" pot)....$16.95
34102 Growing Plant (4" pot)......$6.95

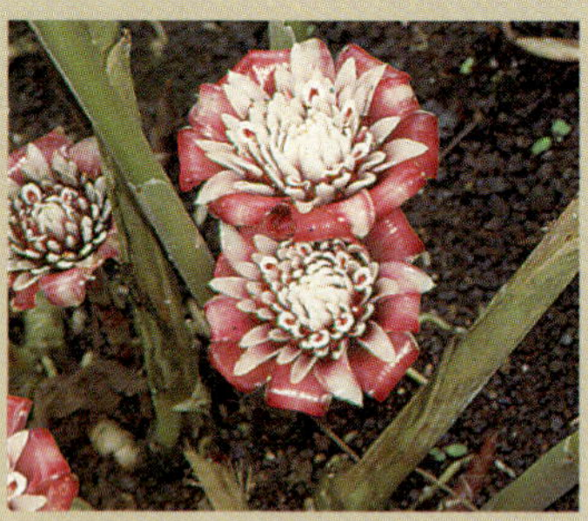

ETLINGERA VENUSTA
'Malay Rose'

What a ginger! An absolutely beautiful plant with short basal inflorescence. Plant grows 6'-8'. Flowers in spring and summer. Flowers make good cuts. Zone 10 and higher. New.
34210 Rhizome $19.95
34211 Growing Plant (6" pot) ...$26.95

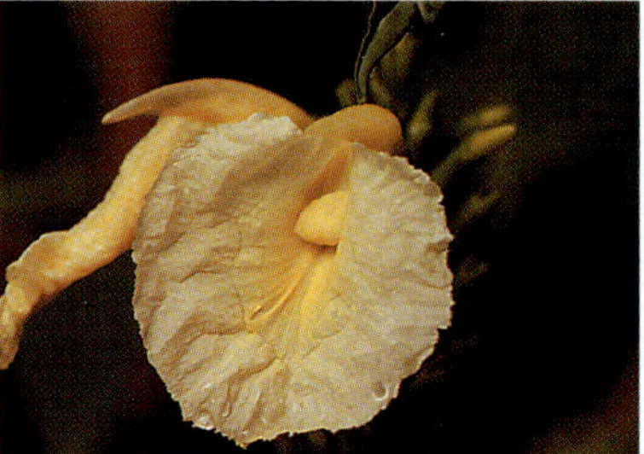

DIMEROCOSTUS STROBILA-CEOUS GUITTERREZII

A dramatic tall 7'-10' Costus-like plant with a spiraling stem and Costus-like flower. Flowers are creamy colored with yellow center borne on stem terminals. Does well in containers. Full sun. Zone 10 and higher.
34120 Rhizome $17.95
34121 Growing Plant (6" pot) $23.95

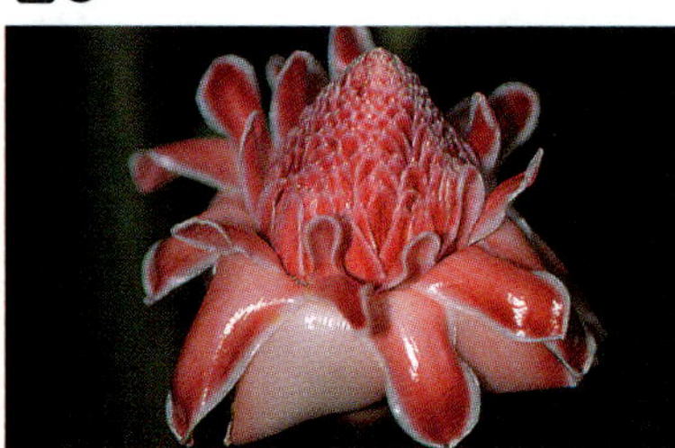

ETLINGERA ELATIOR
'Pink Torch Ginger'

Its basal inflorescences are used for cut flowers. This Southeast Asia native is grown as an ornamental around the world. The basal inflorescences are tall and spread at the top like a torch. Young inflorescences are eaten in some Asian countries. Needs 2 years growth in a warm climate before blooming. Plant grows 6' (1.8m) to 20' (6m) in full sun. Zone 10 and higher. The inflorescence is glossy pink.
34150 Rhizome $20.95
34151 Growing Plant (6" pot) $25.95

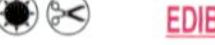
EDIBLE

OUR MATCHLESS GUARANTEE

If for any reason you are not completely satisfied with your purchase, simply return it to us within 10 days of receipt for a prompt and friendly refund or exchange, whichever you prefer. If your purchase arrives in poor condition, please notify us as soon as possible so that we can take corrective action.

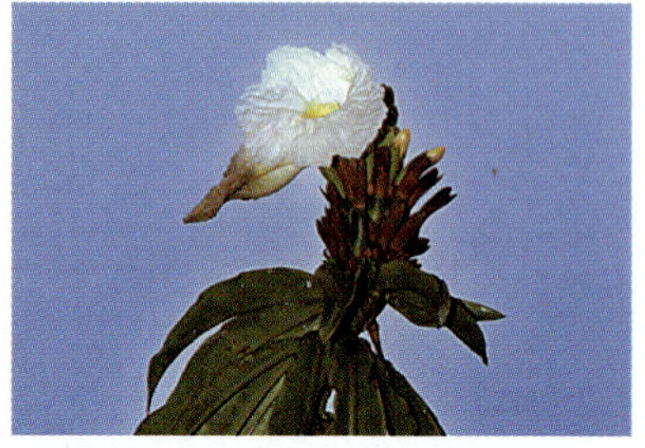

DIMEROCOSTUS STROBILA-CEOUS STROBILACEOUS

The original species type with white crepe flowers with small yellow centers borne on a terminal cone. Flower closely resembles that of Costus speciosus. Plant is tall reaching 7-10" and more. Full sun. Zone 10 and higher.
34110 Rhizome $17.95
34111 Growing Plant (6" pot) $23.95

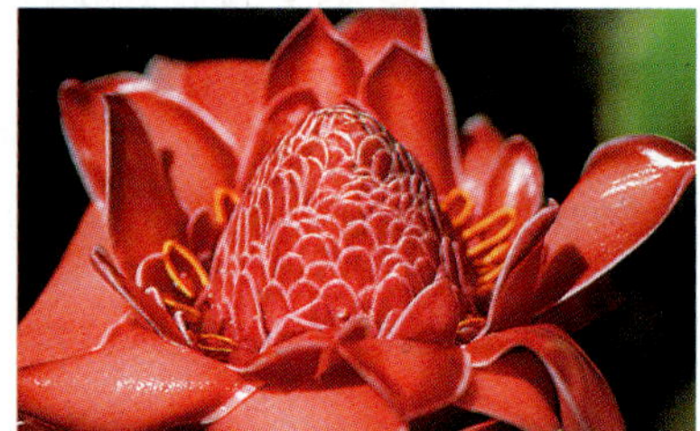

ETLINGERA ELATIOR
'Red Torch Ginger'

Its basal inflorescences are used for cut flowers. This Southeast Asia native is grown as an ornamental around the world. The basal inflorescences are tall and spread at the top like a torch. Young inflorescences are eaten in some Asian countries. This plant has attractive foliage and stems because of the maroon coloring of the stem and undersides of leaves. Needs 2 years growth in a warm climate before blooming. The plant grows 6' (1.8m) to 20' (6m) in full sun. Zone 10 and higher. The inflorescence is glossy red with red flowers that have yellow margins.
34200 Rhizome $20.95
34201 Growing Plant (6" pot) $25.95

EDIBLE

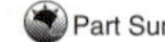 Full Sun   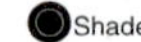 Part Sun   Shade   Extra Water   Fragrant   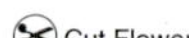 Cut Flower   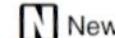 New

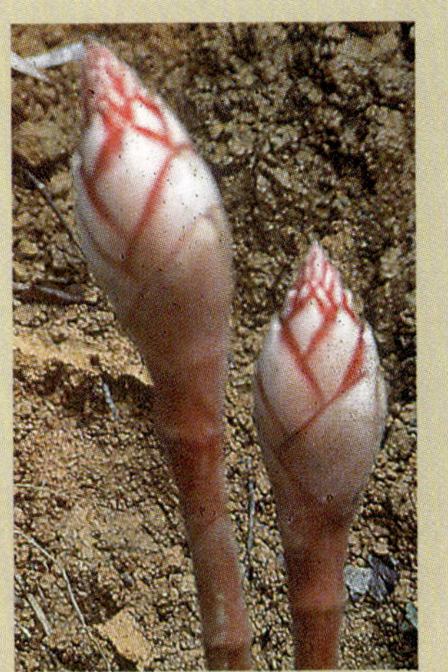

ETLINGERA MAINGAYI
'Sultan's Bud'

A wonderful new ginger from Malaysia that grows to 6'-8'. Flowers in spring and summer. Makes good cut flower. Zone 10 and higher. New.

34140 Rhizome...........................$21.95
34141 Growing Plant (6" pot) ...$28.95

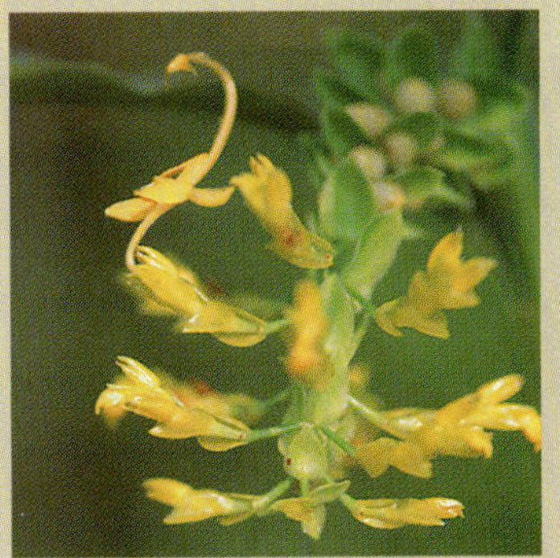

GLOBBA OBSCURA

A nice *Globba* species that grows to 2' (60cm) in full shade. Both bracts and flowers are yellow so once bracts appear plant looks like it is in full bloom. From a distance, because of overall yellow color, superficially resembles *Globba schomburgkii*. Probably Zone 8 and higher.

34260 Rhizome.............................$6.95
34261 Growing Plant (6" pot)....$11.95

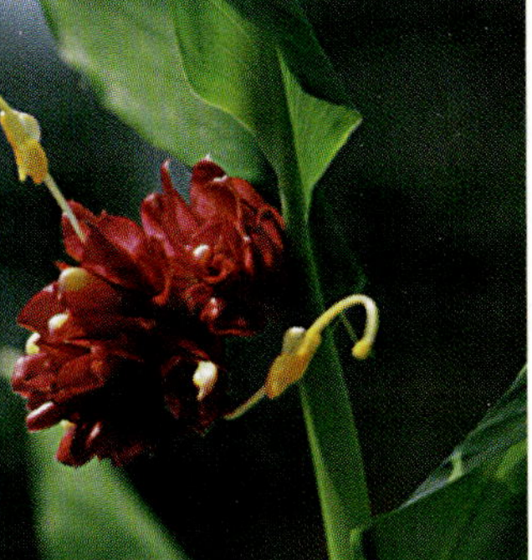

GLOBBA GLOBULIFERA
'Purple Globe'

Attractive shade plant with a purplish maroon globe-shaped inflorescence. This plant makes bulbils; grows to 2' in shade. Bulbils are small plants that grow from the seeds while still held in the inflorescence. Zone 8 and higher. Goes dormant in winter.

34250 Rhizome........................... $4.95
34251 Growing Plant (6" pot)....................$7.95

GLOBBA SCHOMBURGKII
'Yellow Dancing Girl'

Delicate, beautiful yellow inflorescence is produced under terminal leaf of each stem. Flowers start in the summer and continue into fall. Plant is cold hardy and naturalizes in Zone 9. Grows to 2' high in shade. Spreads by bulbils making large colonies. Goes dormant in winter. Zone 7b and higher.

34350 Rhizome $2.95
34351 Growing Plant (6" pot) $5.95

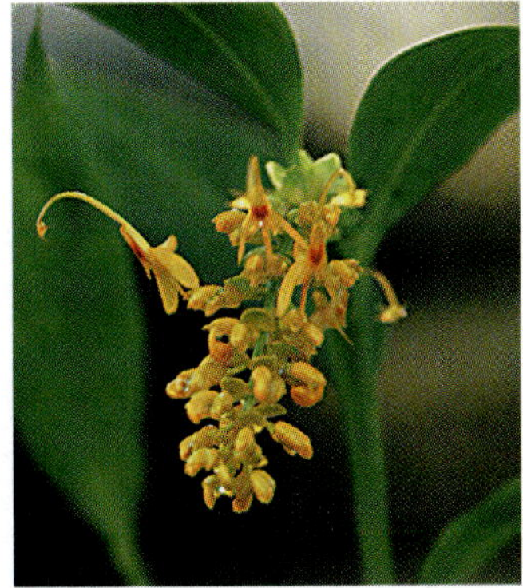

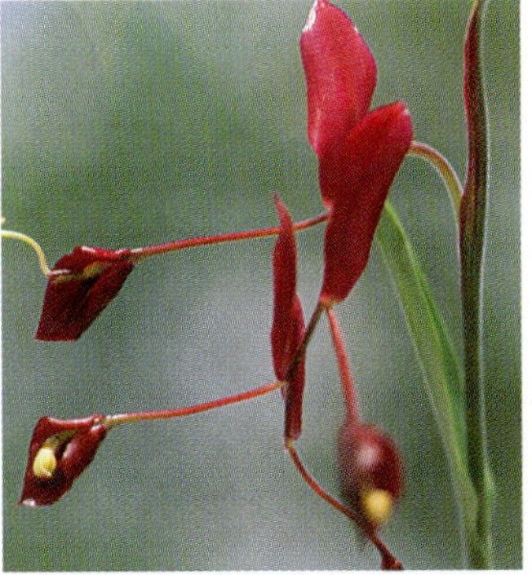

GLOBBA SP. 'Bamboo Leaf'

A beautiful little Globba that has thin stems and small narrow leaves that resemble bamboo. A tough shade loving plant that produces a typical dancing girl flower with shiny deep-maroon bracts. Makes a good ground cover or pot plant, growing 12"-18" high. Probably Zone 8 and higher. An elegant small plant. Goes dormant in winter.

33870 Rhizome $7.95
33871 Growing Plant (6" pot) $12.95

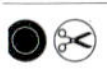

GLOBBA WINITII
'Mauve Dancing Girl'

Elegant small plant with purple bracts and yellow flowers. Grows to 2' (60cm). Likes shade. Makes excellent cut flower that lasts for weeks. The most beautiful of the Globbas. A good windowsill plant. A must for collectors. Goes dormant in winter. Zone 9 and higher. One of our most popular Globbas.

34400 Rhizome......................... $5.95
6($28.95) Save 19%;
34401 Growing Plant (6" pot) $10.95
34402 Growing Plant (4" pot) $3.95

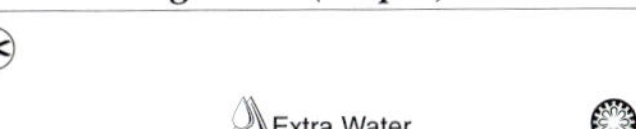

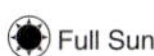 Full Sun　　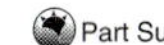 Part Sun　　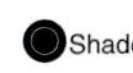 Shade　　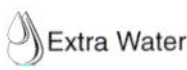 Extra Water　　Fragrant　　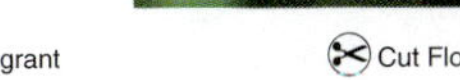 Cut Flower　　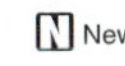 New

49

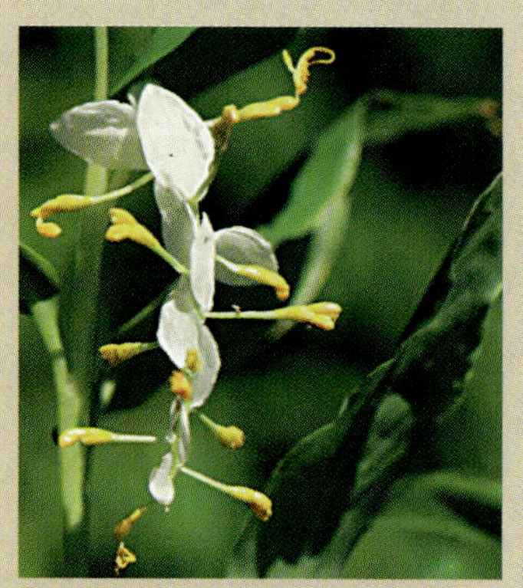

GLOBBA WINITII 'White Dragon'

One of the wonderful "dancing girls". An unbelievably beautiful new variety from Thailand with pure white bracts and small yellow flowers. Grows to 2' (60cm). Likes shade. Makes excellent cut flower that lasts for weeks. A good windowsill plant. Goes dormant in winter. Zone 9 and higher.

34500 Rhizome $6.95
6($28.95) Save 19%;
34501 Growing Plant (6" pot) ..$11.95
34502 Growing Plant (4" pot) $4.95

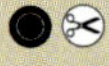

HEDYCHIUM COCCINEUM 'Disney'

Available but not pictured. Same as Hedychium coccineum except dark maroon coloring on stems and leaf undersides. In very limited supply. Grows to 6' (1.8m) in medium sun. Attracts butterflies. Very different looking from regular coccineum.

35360 Rhizome $15.95
*35361 Growing Plant
(6" pot)* $21.95
*35362 Growing Plant
(4" pot)* $10.95

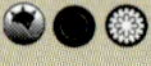

GLOBBA WINITII 'Red Leaf'

New from Thailand. Delicate small plant with purple bracts and yellow flowers. Grows to 2' (60cm). Likes shade. Makes excellent cut flower that lasts for weeks. This plant has beautiful leaves that are maroon underneath. A good windowsill plant. A must for collectors. Zone 9 and higher.

34450 Rhizome $7.95
34451 Growing Plant (6" pot) $12.95

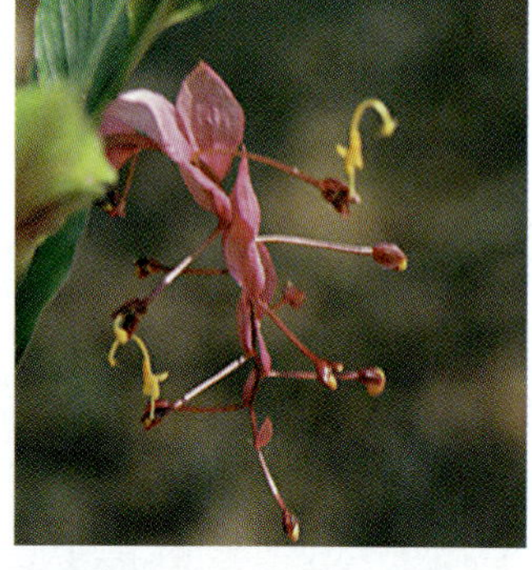

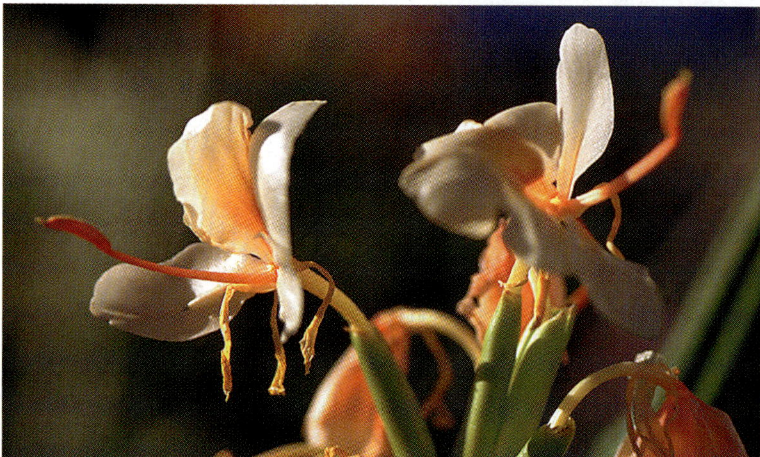

HEDYCHIUM ANGUSTIFOLIUM 'Peach'

Called 'Narrowleaf' ginger. Grows 6' (1.8m) to 7' (2.1m) in medium shade. Large terminal inflorescence of yellow (aging to peach) flowers borne on elegant dark green, narrow leaves. Zone 8 and higher.

34700 Rhizome ....$7.95   *6($39.95) Save 16%*
34701 Growing Plant (6" pot) $13.95

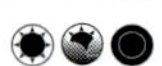

HEDYCHIUM COCCINEUM

Called 'Orange Bottlebrush' ginger. Tall thin species with a long spike of delicate orange flowers. The spike blooms simultaneously and is unusually showy. Grows to 6' (1.8m) in medium sun. A knockout plant. Zone 8 and higher. Attracts butterflies.

34800 Rhizome $13.95
34801 Growing Plant (6" pot) $19.95

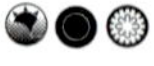

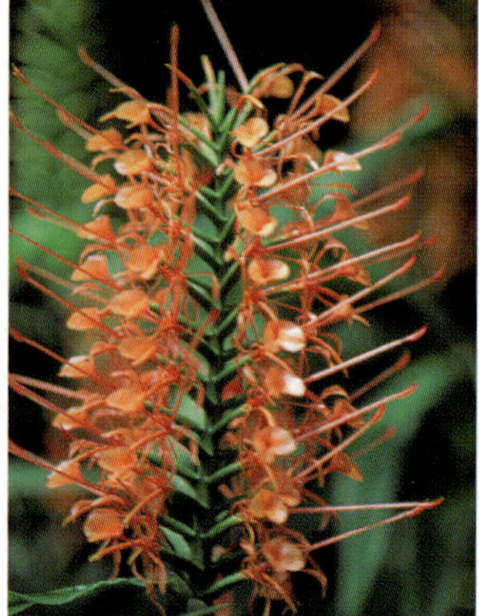

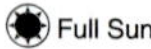 Full Sun   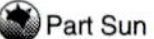 Part Sun   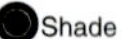 Shade   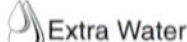 Extra Water   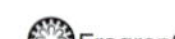 Fragrant   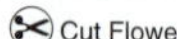 Cut Flower   N New

HEDYCHIUM COCCINEUM CV. 'Tara'

This lovely variety of the well known coccineum ginger is superior to it in every way. Brought back from the Himalayas by Tony Schilling of Kew Gardens; it is the hardiest Hedychium in Britain. It is a large plant (6'-8' tall) with blue waxy stem and leaves that are topped with a foot-long spike sporting a mass of flaming orange flowers-often two at a time from the bracts. Has the typical gardenia fragrance of the species but flowers much earlier and longer (June-September). Zone 7 and higher. Attracts butterflies.

35730 Rhizome $19.95
35731 Growing Plant (6" pot) $25.95
35132 Growing Plant (4" pot) $15.95

HEDYCHIUM CORONARIUM X COCCINEUM 'Shooting Star'

A majestic new hybrid with wonderful inflorescence that is half coronarium and half coccineum. Has nice fragrance. Leaves are slightly variegated with "shooting stars" of creamy color on the medium green pointed leaves. Grows 4'-5' in medium to full sun. Probably Zone 7 and higher.

35620 Rhizome $19.95
35621 Growing Plant (6" pot) $25.95

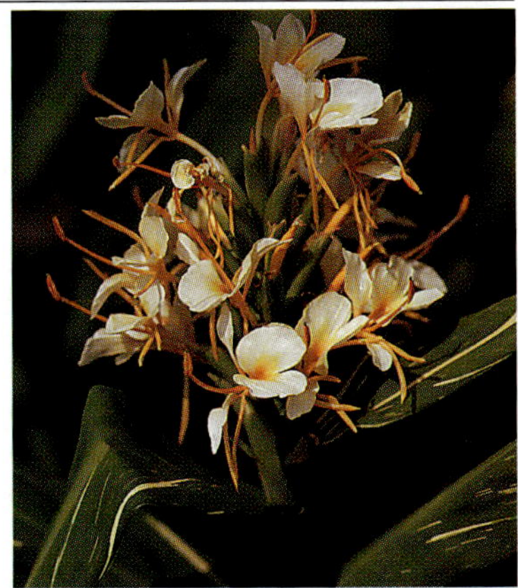

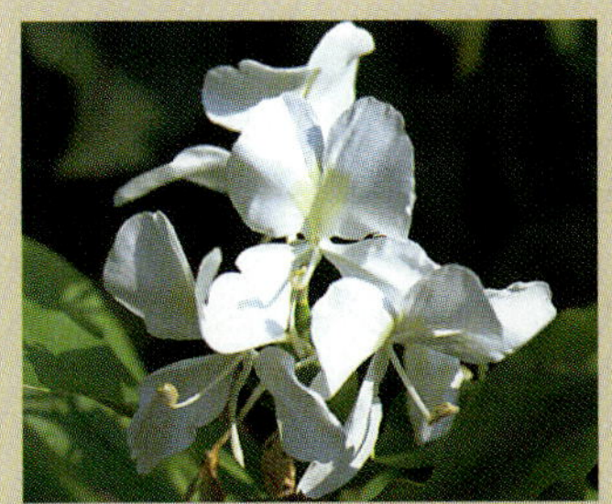

HEDYCHIUM CORONARIUM

Called 'White Butterfly' ginger. Few other plants are as redolent as this mariposa. Originally from India and Indonesia, it traveled to Hawaii, where it remains popular for use in leis. The most fragrant of the Hedychiums, the largest flower, and the hardiest. Flowers from late summer into the fall. Prefers partial shade but will grow in full sun. Grows 4' (90cm) to 5' (1.2m). Zone 7 and higher. Will grow in water.

34900 Rhizome..............................$3.95
6($18.95) Save 20%;
34901 Growing Plant (6" pot)......$7.95
34902 Growing Plant (4" pot)......$2.95

HEDYCHIUM DENSIFLORUM

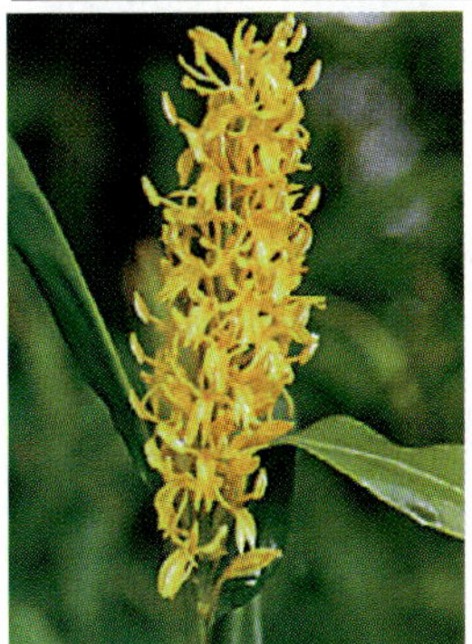

A magnificent Hedychium with a very dense (hence species name, densiflorum) flower head of rich golden-yellow flowers. The Plant grows to 5'-7' in partial shade. One of our most beautiful Hedychiums when in bloom. Zone 7 and higher. Supplies limited.

34970 Rhizome..$12.95
34971 Growing Plant (6" pot) $17.95

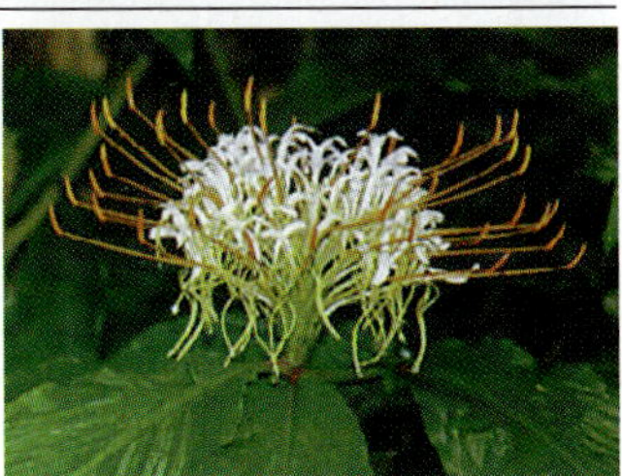

HEDYCHIUM ELLIPTICUM

A great looking Hedychium growing to 6'-7'. Flower head is striking with a bouquet of fragrant white flowers with very long yellow stamens sticking out like porcupine quills. Prefers some shade. Probably Zone 7 and higher. Supplies limited.

34980 Rhizome.....................$11.95
34981 Growing Plant (6" pot) $16.95

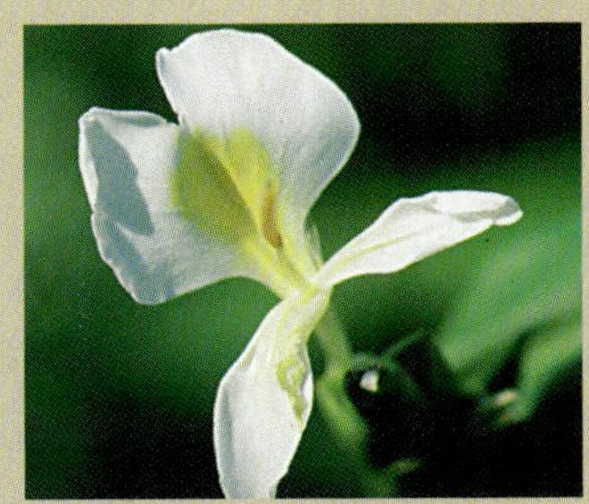

HEDYCHIUM CORONARIUM CHRYSOLEUCUM

Like the 'White Butterfly' ginger, except has a yellow center. Same outstanding attributes: fragrant, large flower, and hardy. Flowers from late summer well into the fall. Prefers partial shade but will grow in full sun. Grows 3' to 4' high. Zone 7 and higher.

34950 Rhizome............................ $9.95
34951 Growing Plant (6" pot)....$15.95

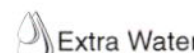
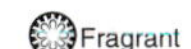
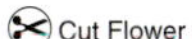

Full Sun   Part Sun   Shade   Extra Water   Fragrant   Cut Flower   New

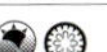

Gingers

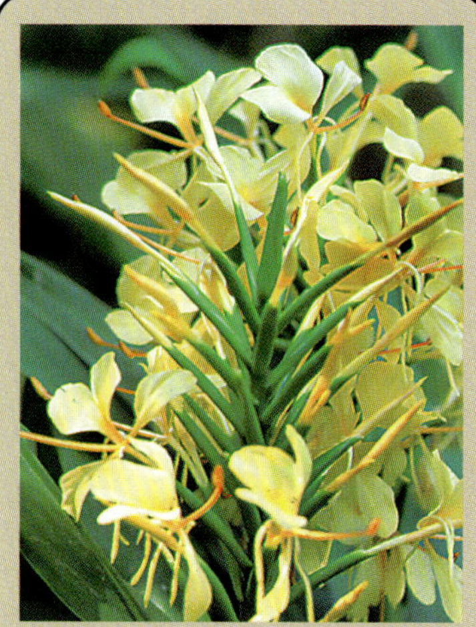

HEDYCHIUM GARDNERI-ANUM 'Fiesta Kahili'

Often called 'Kahili' ginger. Has sturdy stems with large leathery leaves. Inflorescence is outstanding with many fragrant yellow flowers with red stamens. Medium to full sun. Grows 4' to 6'. Zone 8 and higher.

35100 Rhizome..............................$7.95
6($39.95) Save 16%
35101 Growing Plant (6" pot)....$12.95
35102 Growing Plant (4" pot)......$4.95

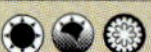

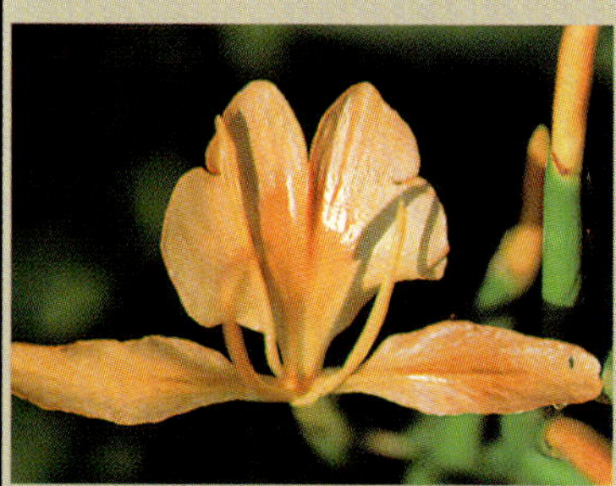

HEDYCHIUM HYBRID 'Double Eagle'

This *Hedychium* is 5' (1.5m) to 6' (1.8m) topped with a 6" (15cm) spike of large coppery gold flowers. Zone 7 and higher. Blooms from July to September. Medium shade. Nice fragrance.

35320 Rhizome...........................$16.95
35321 Growing Plant (6" pot)....$21.95

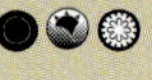

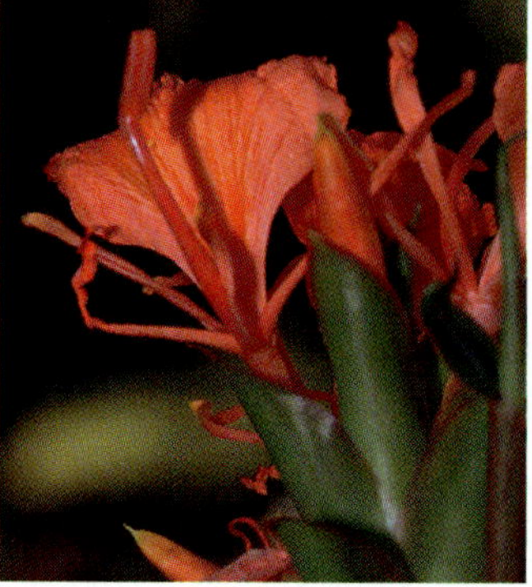

HEDYCHIUM GREENII 'Red Leaf Ginger'

In summer and fall produces large reddish-orange flowers on a maroon colored stem with leaves that are tinged in red underneath. Can be used as foliage plant. Grows 5' (1.5m) to 6' (1.8m) in medium shade. Unique among Hedychiums in producing plantlets on old inflorescence. Zone 7 and higher. Not fragrant.

35250 Rhizome $10.95
35251 Growing Plant (6" pot) $15.95

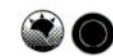

HEDYCHIUM HYBRID 'Anne Bishop'

A great new addition to our butterfly ginger line. Obtained from Hawaii in 1996, it grows 5' (1.5m) to 6' (1.8m) in medium to full sun. It has large terminal inflorescence with mass of orange, fragrant flowers. Probably Zone 8 and higher.

35310 Rhizome $15.95
35311 Growing Plant (6" pot) $20.95

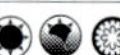

Rhizomes are available only from December 15st to May 1st. This is their period of dormancy. Rhizomes should be planted when soil temperatures warm up.

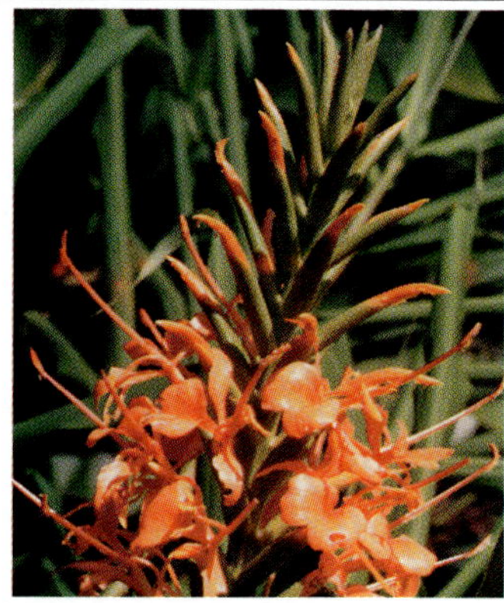

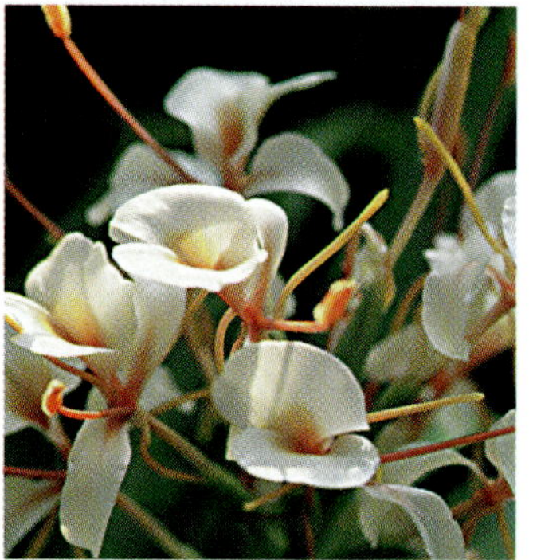

HEDYCHIUM HYBRID 'Ayo'

A very nice butterfly ginger that we obtained from Mr. Ayo in Louisiana in the Spring of 1996. We have dubbed it "Ayo" in his honor. It is similar to *angustifolium* in general appearances however flowers and fragrance are distinctly different. Medium shade. Zone 9 and higher.

34650 Rhizome $7.95
6($39.95) Save 16%
34651 Growing Plant (6" pot) $12.95

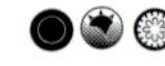

HEDYCHIUM HYBRID 'Carnival'

A very special (3'-4') butterfly ginger with huge 12"-14" flower spikes of yellow and orange flowers. Each spike flowers continuously for 5-7 weeks. Zones 8 and higher. One of our best ever flowering Hedychiums.

35130 Rhizome $18.95
35131 Growing Plant (6" pot) $23.95

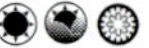

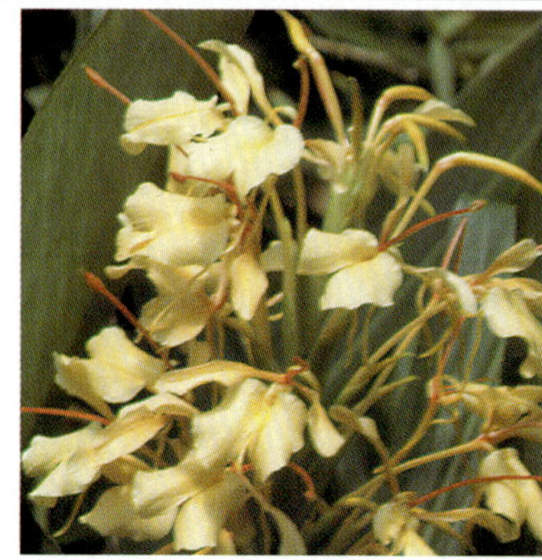

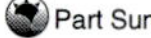 Full Sun   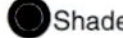 Part Sun   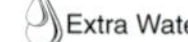 Shade   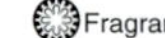 Extra Water   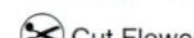 Fragrant   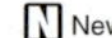 Cut Flower   N New

TO ORDER CALL **1-800-624-9706**/24 HRS. OR VISIT OUR WEB SITE: www. stokestropicals.com

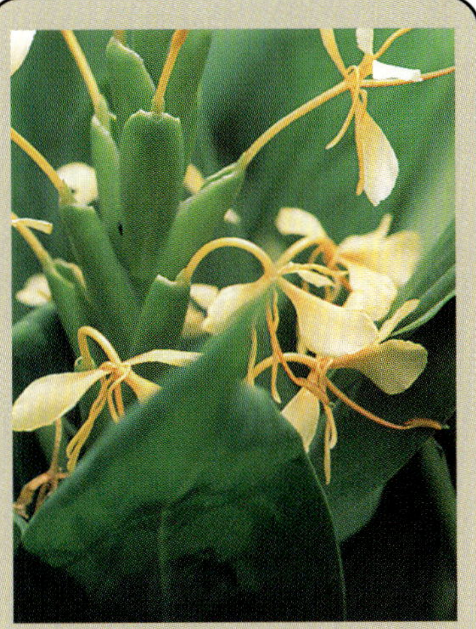

HEDYCHIUM HYBRID 'Filagree'

A very nice medium-size butterfly ginger with very fragrant slim or "filagree" flowers. Plant only grows to 3'-5'. Free blooming from July to November. Zone 7 and higher.
35670 Rhizome..............................$7.95
6($39.95) Save 16%
35672 Growing Plant (6" pot)....$12.95

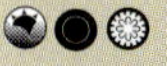

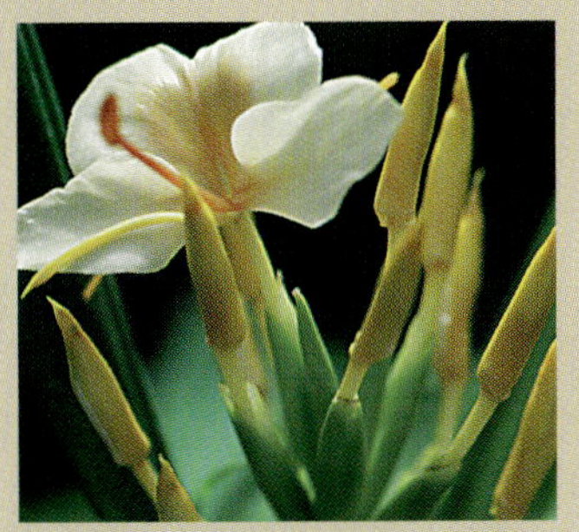

HEDYCHIUM HYBRID 'Gold Flame'

Vigorous plant with erect white flowers with a burnt gold center, fragrant. Height to 5'. An outstanding hybrid rapidly gaining popularity. Medium shade. Zone 8 and higher.
34550 Rhizome..............................$14.95
34551 Growing Plant (6" pot)....$19.95

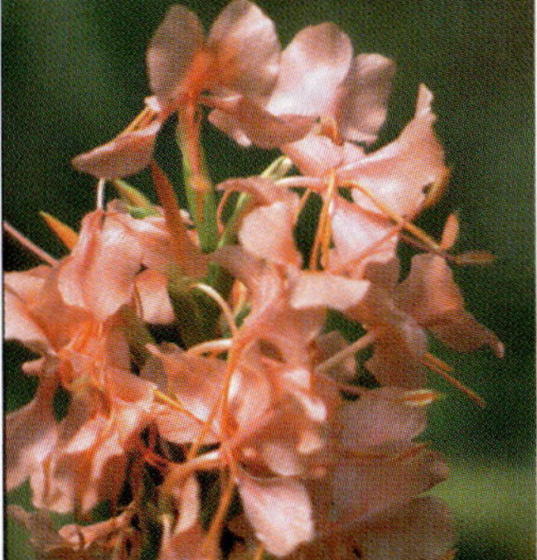

HEDYCHIUM HYBRID 'Elizabeth'

Lovely butterfly ginger with raspberry-colored flowers with wavy edges. Height 6'–8' (1.8m to 2.4m). Medium sun. Dormant after first freeze but returns in March. A truly spectacular plant. Zone 7 and higher. One of our most popular tall Hedychiums.
35350 Rhizome $16.95
35351 Growing Plant (6" pot) $21.95
35352 Growing Plant (4" pot) $10.95

HEDYCHIUM HYBRID 'Fireworks'

A strong upright plant (to 4') with waxy leaves that are reddish underneath. The flowers have an unearthly appearance, since each is a bundle of orange-red fibers with yellow tips, giving the 6" inflorescence the appearance of exploding fireworks. Grows well in full sun. Zone 8 and higher. Flowers June through October. Zone 7 and higher.
35560 Rhizome $17.95
35561 Growing Plant (6"pot)..................$22.95

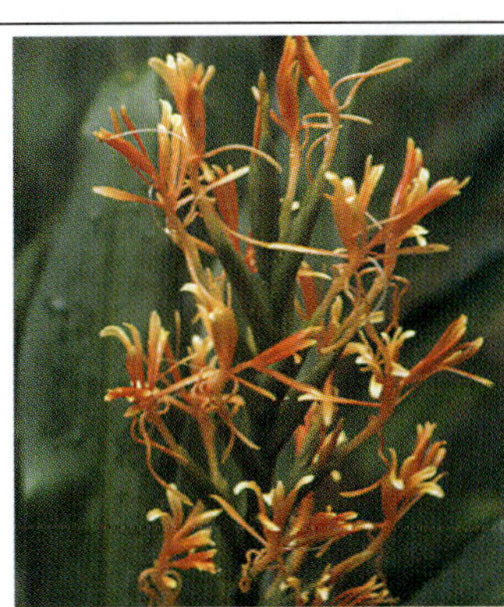

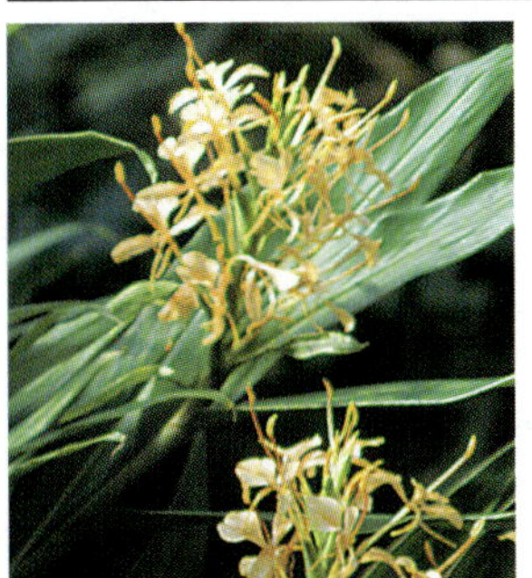

HEDYCHIUM HYBRID 'Golden Glow'

Magnificent 4' butterfly ginger; prolific bloomer from May to midwinter or first freeze. Flower spikes put on a resplendent show with large numbers of clear, golden-orange flowers. Zones 8 and higher. In very limited supply.
35460 Rhizome $18.95
35461 Growing Plant (6"pot) $23.95

HEDYCHIUM HORSFIELDII

Was classified as Brachychilum horsfieldii. Now correctly placed in genus Hedychium. A short 2'-3' plant with unusual looking small yellow flowers on long pedicels. Very fragrant. Flowers in winter if protected from cold. Seed pods split open revealing orange interior with beads of dark red seeds. Probably Zone 9 and higher. Medium shade.
35160 Rhizome $13.95
35161 Growing Plant (6" pot) ..$18.95

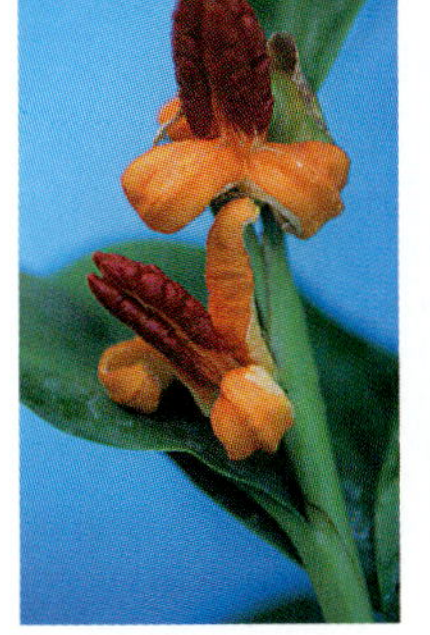

Seed pod

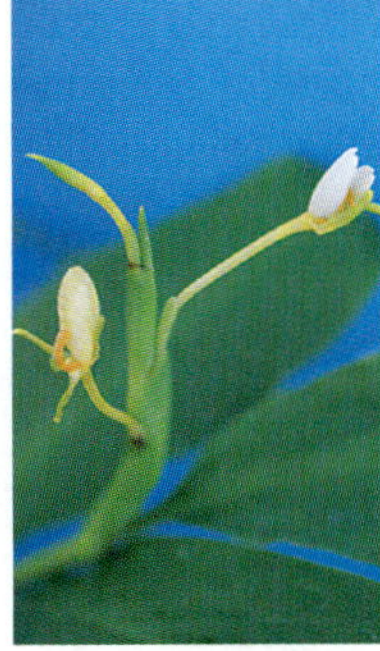

Flower

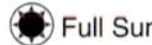 Full Sun 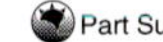 Part Sun 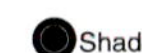 Shade  Extra Water 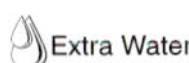 Fragrant 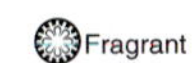 Cut Flower 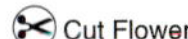 New

53

Gingers

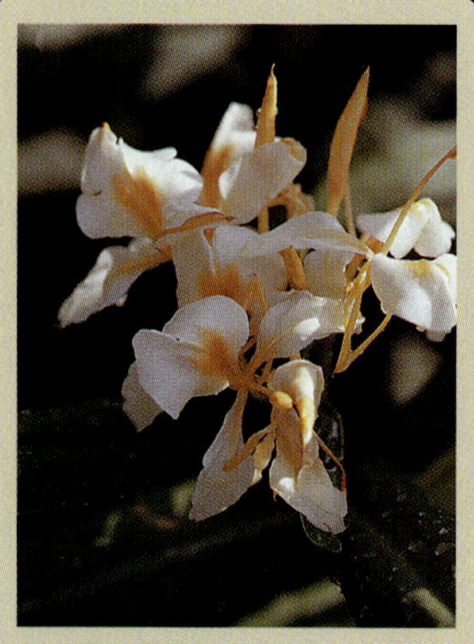

HEDYCHIUM HYBRID 'Kinkaku'

A great looking medium size butterfly ginger with large shiny peach flowers atop dark greenleaved stems. Grows to 6' (1.8m). Medium sun. Zone 7 and higher.

35500 Rhizome...........................*$13.95*
35501 Growing Plant (6" pot) ...*$18.95*

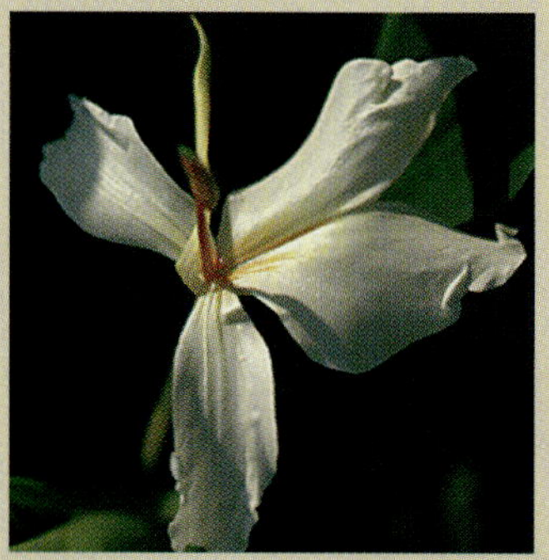

HEDYCHIUM HYBRID 'Luna Moth'

A real dazzler, the 'Luna Moth' has giant white flowers resembling a moth in flight. Flowers are fragrant. Plant grows in medium shade to 4' (1.2m). Zone 8 and higher.

35530 Rhizome...........................*$10.95*
35531 Growing Plant (6" pot) ...*$15.95*
35532 Growing Plant (4" pot) *$6.95*

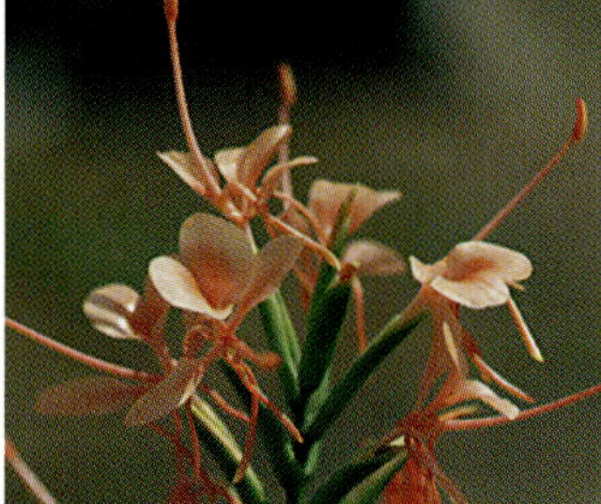

HEDYCHIUM HYBRID 'Lemon Beauty'

One of our tall Hedychiums with spikes that have many bright yellow, large fragrant flowers with pink stamens. Blooms from August through October. Grows 6' tall in medium sun. Zone 7 and higher.

35520 Rhizome *$15.95*
35521 Growing Plant (6" pot) *$20.95*

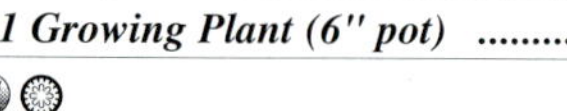

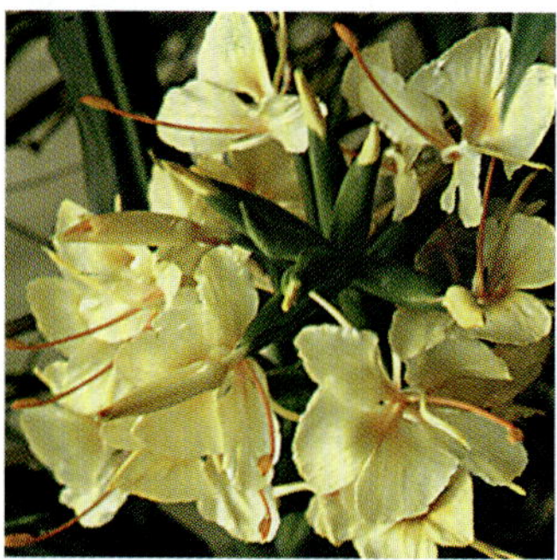

HEDYCHIUM HYBRID 'Mutant'

A very different looking thin, white stringy flower on a medium size 4' (1.2m) plant makes this a collector's item. Flowers are quite fragrant. Grows in medium sun. Zone 8 and higher.

35600 Rhizome *$10.95*
35601 Growing Plant (6" pot) *$15.95*

HEDYCHIUM HYBRID 'Kewense'

A knockout. Probably named after the world famous Kew Gardens in England. This outstanding tall 6' to 7' butterfly ginger has a mass of pink raspberry flowers that are slightly fragrant. Medium sun. Narrow bluish green leaves. Zone 7 and higher.

35450 Rhizome *$17.95*
35451 Growing Plant (6" pot) *$22.95*

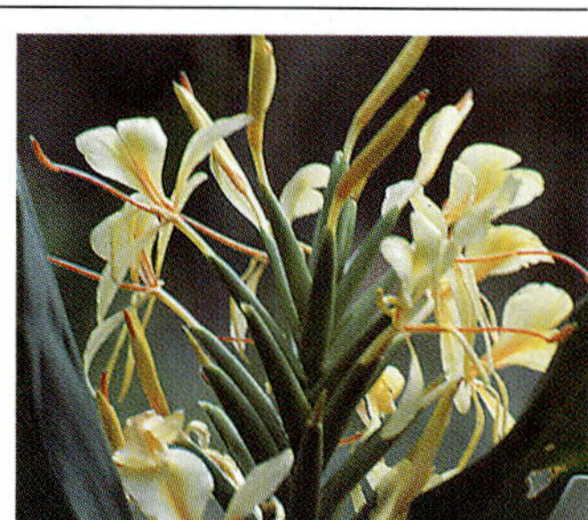

HEDYCHIUM HYBRID 'Lemon Sherbet'

A tall 6'-8' (2.4m) robust plant with a 12" (30cm) long spike with up to fifty 3" (7.5cm) yellow ruffled flowers with pink stamens. Blooms from June through September. Zone 8 and higher.

35510 Rhizome *$16.95*
35511 Growing Plant (6" pot) *$21.95*

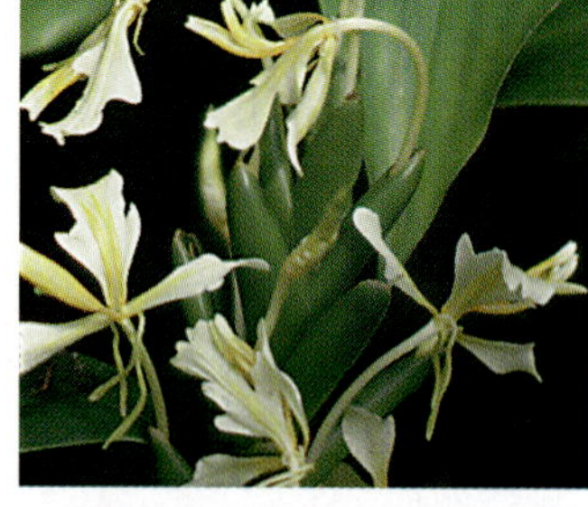

HEDYCHIUM HYBRID 'Kai Yang'   COCONUT FRAGRANCE

(Not Pictured) An unusual butterfly ginger hybrid that has cream colored flowers and a wonderful coconut fragrance. Flower and plant similar to Hedychium 'Kinkaku' . Grows 5' (1.5m) to 6' (1.8m) in medium sun. Zone 8 and higher.

35400 Rhizome...*$7.95*   *6($39.95) Save 16%*
35401 Growing Plant (6" pot) *$12.95*
Note: last offered for $17.95 and $27.95!

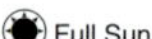 Full Sun   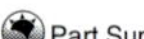 Part Sun    Shade    Extra Water   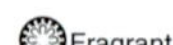 Fragrant   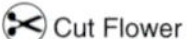 Cut Flower   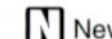 New

TO ORDER CALL **1-800-624-9706**/24 HRS. OR VISIT OUR WEB SITE: www. stokestropicals.com

HEDYCHIUM HYBRID 'Pink Flame'

This *Hedychium* is 5' (1.5m) tall with a short spike that has many large, white flowers with a pink flame-like spot in the middle of the lip. Medium shade. The flowers are fragrant and bloom from July through October. Zones 7 and higher.

35610 Rhizome $16.95
35611 Growing Plant (6" pot) $21.95

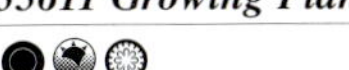

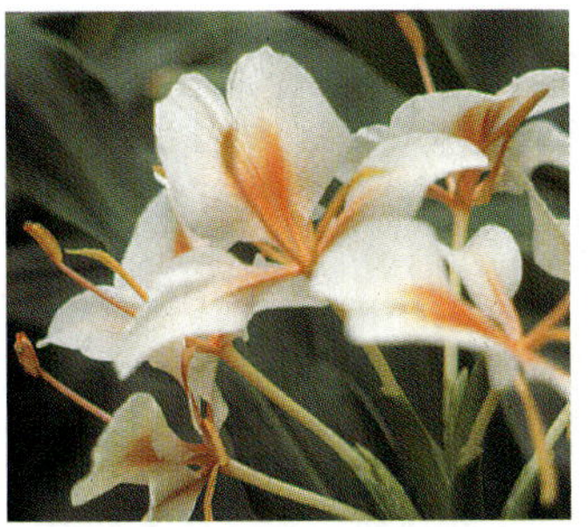

HEDYCHIUM HYBRID 'Pink V'

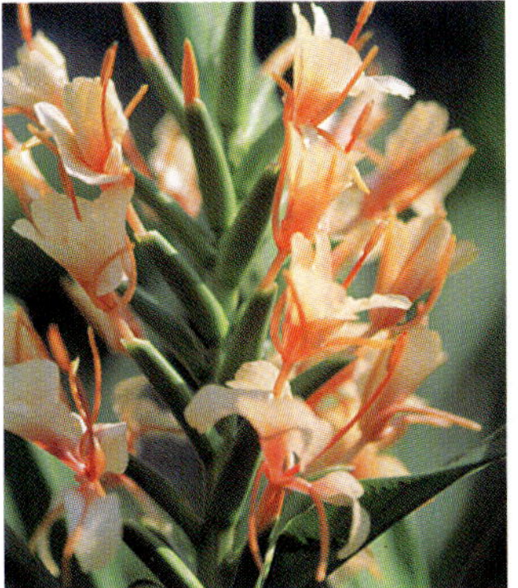

Sensational new hybrid. Very showy, lovely cream colored flowers with salmon throats; large flowers with citrus fragrance. Blooms from June to frost. Grows 6' (1.8m) to 7' (2.1m). Medium sun. Zone 7 and higher.

35540 Rhizome $14.95
35541 Growing Plant (6" pot) $19.95
35542 Growing Plant (4" pot) $9.95

Orders Placed Through Our Web Site Receive a 15% Discount

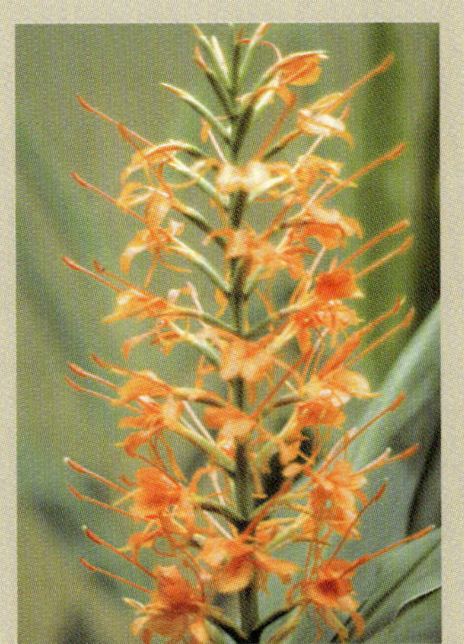

HEDYCHIUM HYBRID 'Raffilii'

A new Hedychium with a blazing orange inflorescence. Inflorescence can be 7"-9" tall on a 6'-7' plant. Blooms in fall of the year. Zone 7 and higher.

35550 Rhizome...........................$13.95
35551 Growing Plant (6" pot)....$18.95

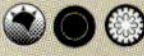

HEDYCHIUM HYBRID 'Tropic Bird'

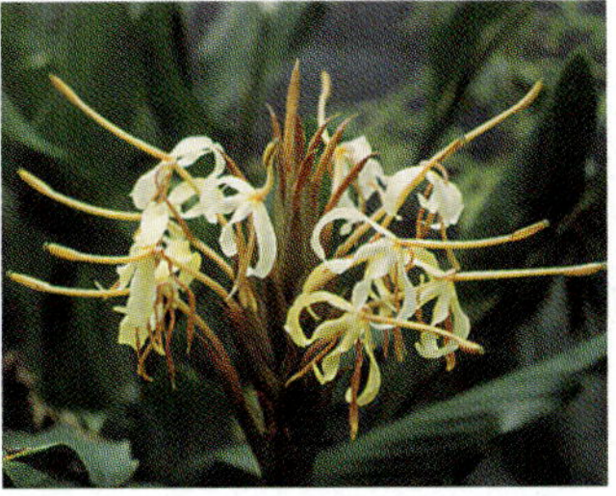

A very strong growing plant only 1 ¹/₂' high but with 1'-long waxy leaves. The free-blooming flower spikes have bracts covered with golden hair and waxy flowers that curve backwards and have the amazing property of lasting for 4-5 days. Color changes from white to cream to gold. The flowers have a strong, spicy, clove-like scent and bloom in flushes. Peak flowering from September to February makes them an ideal greenhouse crop. They maintain good blooming and foliage even when minimum temperatures are 45-50 degrees F. Zone 8 and higher.

35680 Rhizome $17.95
35681 Growing Plant (6" pot) $22.95

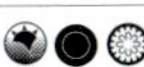

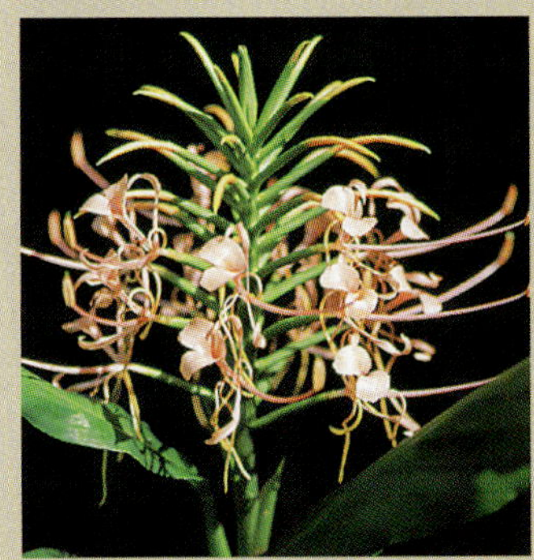

HEDYCHIUM HYBRID 'Pink Sparks'

Another wonderful and different butterfly hybrid that stands out in the garden landscape. Grows 5' (1.5m) to 6' (1.8m) in medium sun. Young shoots are bronze. Slightly fragrant small pinkish flowers with long pink stamens that are densely clumped on tips of tall strong stems. Flowers August - October. Zone 7 and higher.

35650 Rhizome...........................$14.95
35651 Growing Plant (6" pot) ...$21.95

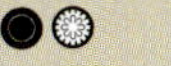

HEDYCHIUM HYBRID 'White Starburst'

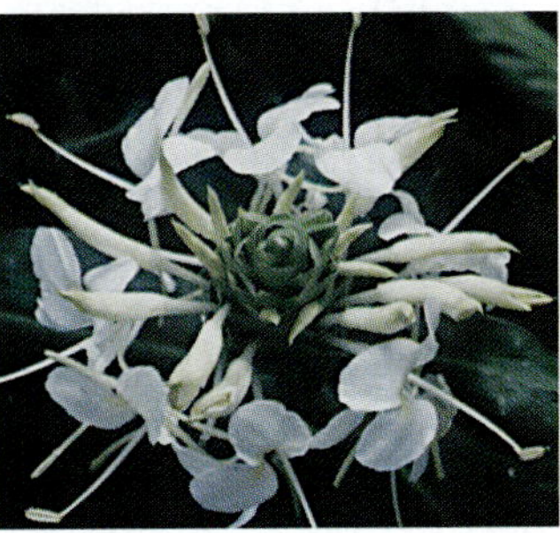

Plant is 6' (1.8m) tall and has a ring of ten medium sized white, fragrant flowers in a pinwheel like ring. Blooms September through November. Zone 7 and higher.

35660 Rhizome $16.95
35661 Growing Plant (6"pot)..................$21.95

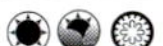

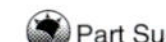 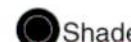 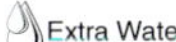

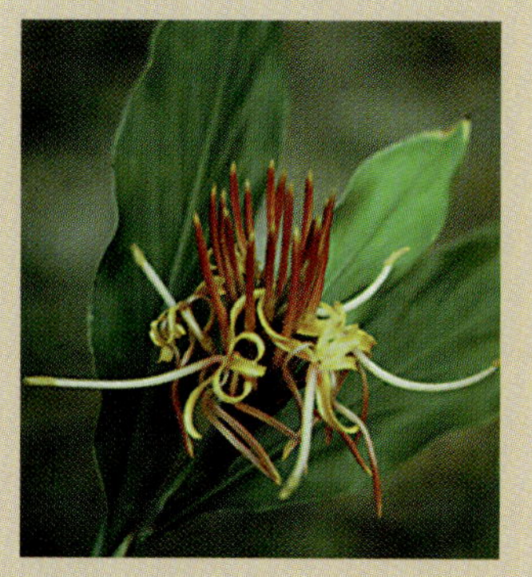

HEDYCHIUM LONGICORNUTUM

Outstanding epiphytic species that has a wonderful bloom that is bright yellow and orange. Grows 2' (60cm) in full sun. Native to Malaysia. Zone 9 and higher. Blooms February –April. Good house plant.

35685 Rhizome............................$15.95
35686 Growing Plant (6" pot) ...$21.95

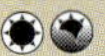

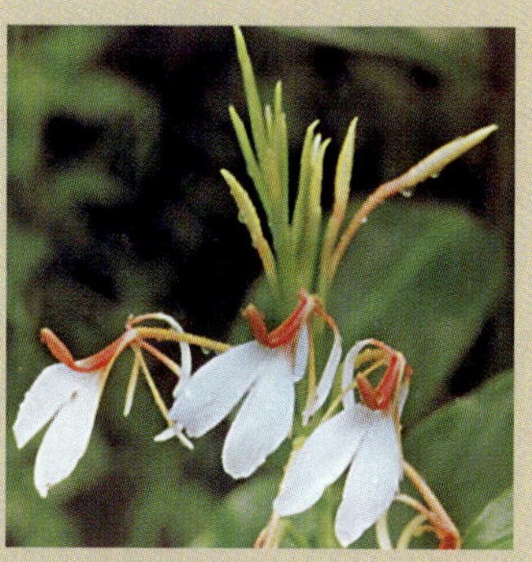

HEDYCHIUM SPICATUM
'White Wings'

A wonderful very different looking Hedychium. Flowers look like small white-winged moths poised to take off at any time. Stamens offer a nice orange contrast. Plant grows 3' to 4' in partial shade. Flowers fragrant. Zone 7 and higher. Supplies limited.

35770 Rhizome............................$10.95
35771 Growing Plant (6" pot)....$15.95

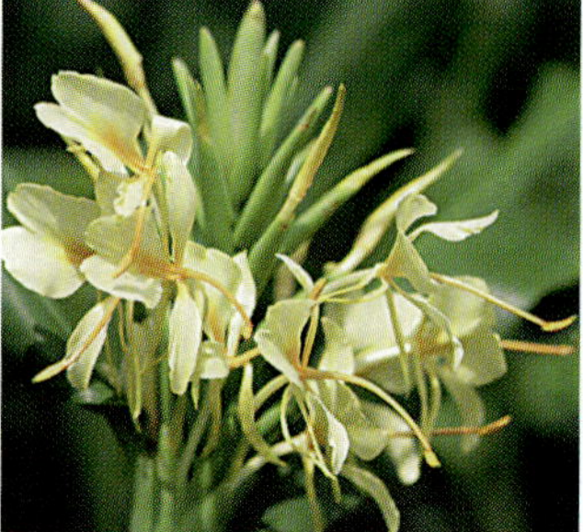

HEDYCHIUM GARDNERIANUM HYBRID 'Yellow'

Often called 'Yellow Kahili' ginger. Has sturdy stems with large wavy leaves. Inflorescence is outstanding with many very fragrant solid-yellow flowers. Prefers medium sun. Grows 6' (1.8m) to 7' (2.1m). Zone 8 and higher.

35150 Rhizome $11.95
35151 Growing Plant (6" pot) $16.95

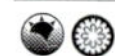

HEDYCHIUM MAXIMUM
'Giant Butterfly'

A splendid large butterfly ginger that can grow to 8'-9' tall in ground. Plant has giant yellow-flowered inflorescence. Flowers have exquisite pink stamens. Many flowers have striking lips that are split into 2 or 3 lobes. Distinctive fragrance. Hardy in zone 8 and higher. Prefers medium shade. Very limited supply. Once you see this plant in bloom, you'll have to have it.

35690 Rhizome $18.95
35691 Growing Plant (6" pot) $23.95

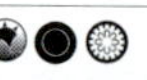

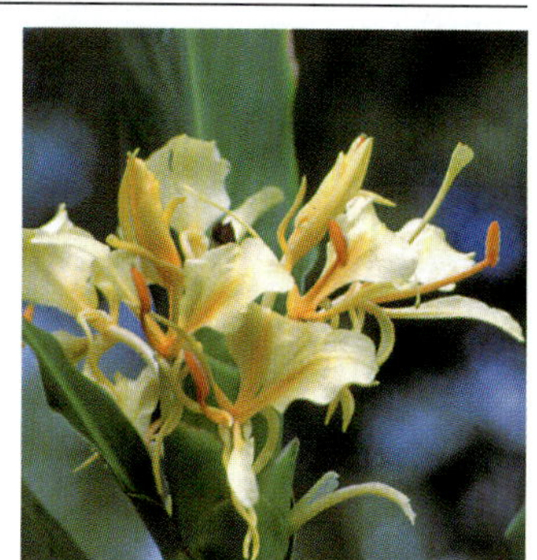

HEDYCHIUM MULUENSE 'Dwarf Borneo Ginger'

Interesting epiphytic species with small flowers. Grows 2' (60cm) in medium sun. Native to Borneo. Zone 10 and higher.

35675 Rhizome $13.95
35676 Growing Plant (6" pot) $18.95

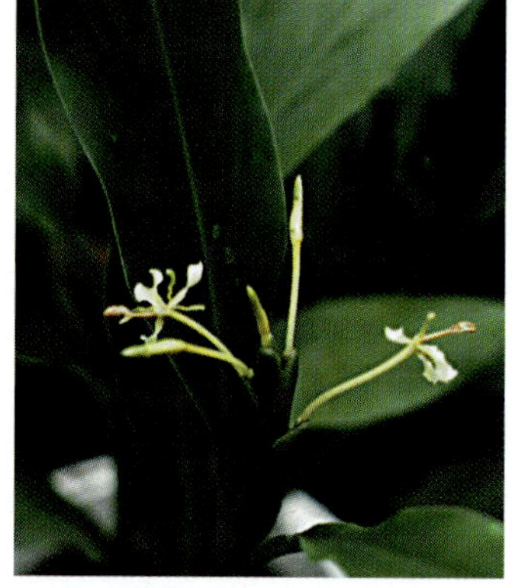

Ginger Collections

Save $5 (Rhizomes only) off listed prices by purchasing entire collection. See pages 66-68.

HEDYCHIUM THRYSIFORME
'Pincushion Ginger'

Also called 'Frilly White' or 'White Pincushion'. Foliage is attractive dark green with wavy texture. Produces large bunches of small white flowers with long white stamens in the fall of the year. Flowers are slightly fragrant; grows 6' (1.8m) to 7' (2.1m). Medium to full sun. Zone 8 and higher.

35710 Rhizome $9.95
35711 Growing Plant (6" pot) $14.95

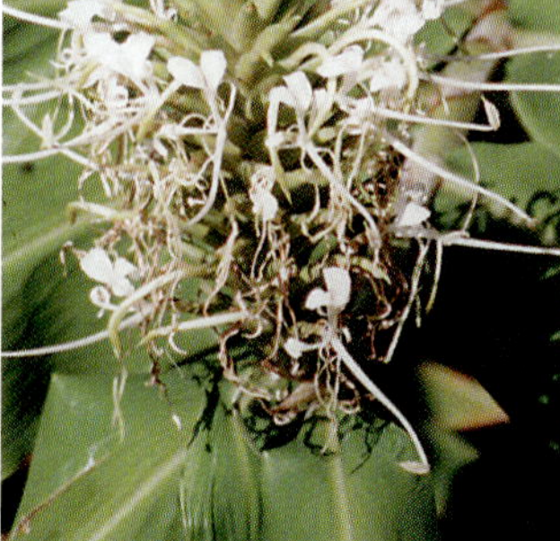

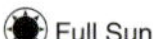 Full Sun   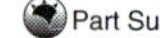 Part Sun    Shade   Extra Water    Fragrant   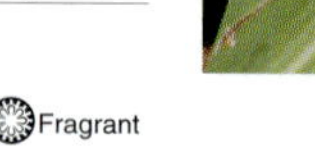 Cut Flower   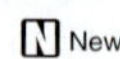 New

TO ORDER CALL **1-800-624-9706**/24 HRS. OR VISIT OUR WEB SITE: www. stokestropicals.com

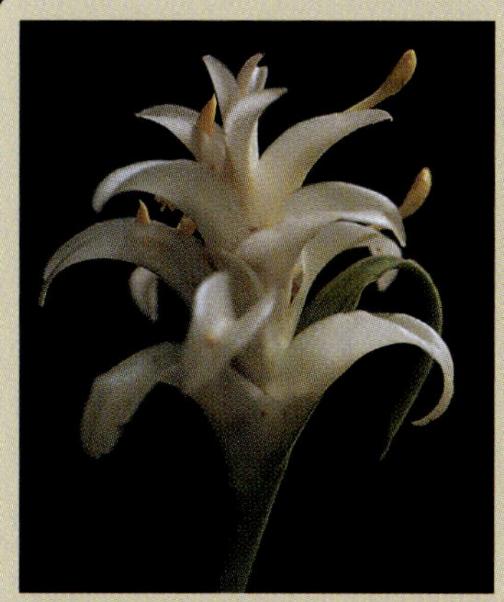

HEDYCHIUM PRADHANII

Another beautiful butterfly ginger species. Tall 4' (1.2m) to 6' (1.8m) and a vigorous grower. Creamy, white flowers with coral pink stamens and delicate fragrance. Medium to full sun. Summer bloomer. Zone 8 and higher.

35700 Rhizome *$11.95*
35701 Growing Plant (6" pot) *$16.95*

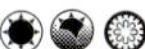

HEDYCHIUM VILLOSUM
TENUIFLORUM 'Sweet Reed'

Fantastic new fragrant butterfly ginger from China. A thin, narrow leafed, epiphyte that has red bracts and white flowers with a very sweet fragrance. The stem has bands of dark red and will bloom in the greenhouse at any time of year. Grow it like an orchid in a mostly bark mix. Its hardiness has not been tested. Probably Zone 9 and higher.

35720 Rhizome *$12.95*
35721 Growing Plant (6" pot) *$19.95*

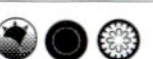

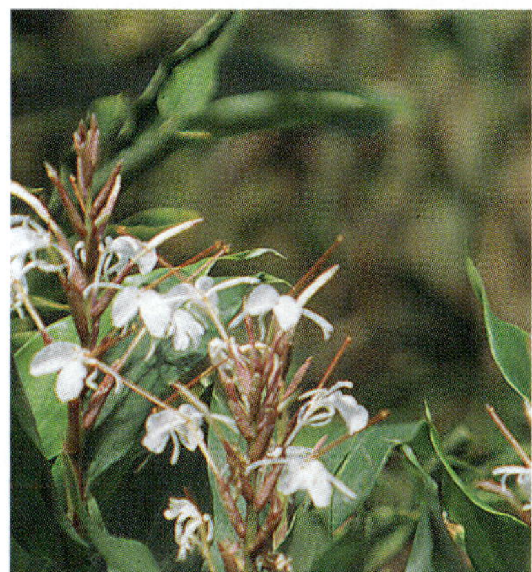

HITCHHENIA SP.
'Siam Platinum'

Hitchhenia is a newly described genus in the ginger family. A majical looking ginger from Thailand with tiers of platinum white bracts from which lovely yellow flowers emerge on long pedicels. Medium to full sun. Plant grows 2'- 3' tall. Floral inflorescence is held above slender leaves. Good cut flower. Probably zone 9 and higher.

35740 Rhizome *$13.95*
35741 Growing Plant (6" pot) ...*$19.95*

KAEMPFERIA SP. 'Alva'

A magnificent looking Kaempferia that has large 8'-10' leaves with a startling brushstroke pattern of brownish maroon edged in white against a lush green leaf. Wonderful violet colored flowers appear almost daily throughout the summer into fall. Grows 10"- 12" tall in full shade. Makes an excellent groundcover. Probably zone 8 and higher.

35790 Rhizome *$6.95*
35791 Growing Plant (6" pot) *$10.95*
35792 Growing Plant (4" pot) *$4.95*

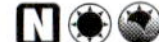

KAEMPFERIA ANGUSTIFOLIA

An elegant little Kaempferia with long, narrow leaves. Produces orchid-like flowers in late spring to early summer. Grows to 7"-8" in shade. Makes good ground cover or pot plant. Zone 8 and higher.

35760 Rhizome *$7.95*
35761 Growing Plant (6" pot) *$11.95*

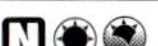

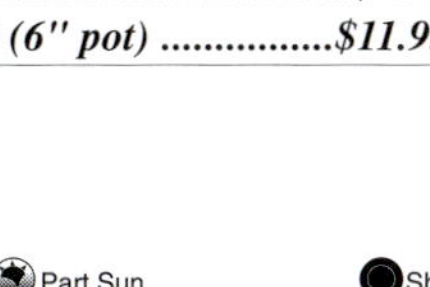

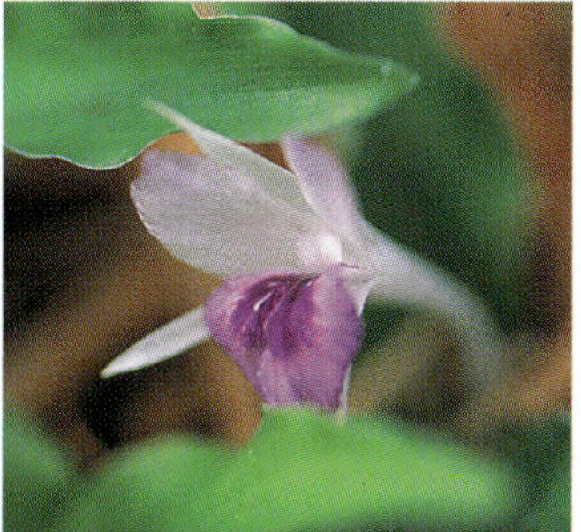

PHONE ORDERS:
1-800-624-9706
24 hours/7days

FAX ORDERS:
1-337-365-6991
24 hours / 7days

FOR CUSTOMER SERVICE:
337-365-6998 - Mon.-Fri.,
8:30 am-4:00 pm C.T.

FOR INTERNET SERVICE:
http://www.stokestropicals.com
24 hours / 7 days

E-MAIL ORDERS / INQUIRIES:
info@stokestropicals.com
24 hours / 7 days

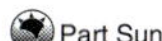 Full Sun   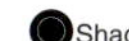 Part Sun   Shade   Extra Water   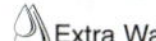 Fragrant   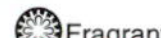 Cut Flower   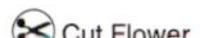 New

Gingers

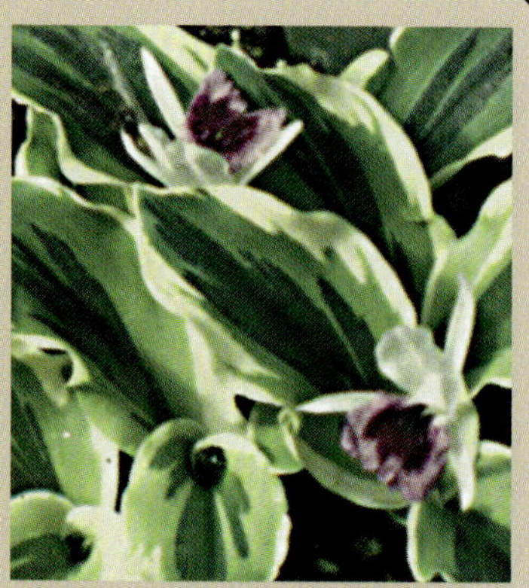

KAEMPFERIA GILBERTII '3-D'

This variety is a sport of *Kaempferia gilbertii*. The leaves are white, dark green, and light green. Small, shade-loving plant with long narrow striped leaves. Blooms late spring into summer; has small white and purple flowers that resemble orchids. Variegated foliage is main attraction. Plant grows to 5". Zone 8 and higher.Goes dormant during winter.
35900 Rhizome..............................$7.95
6($34.95) Save 16%
35901 Growing Plant (6" pot)....$11.95

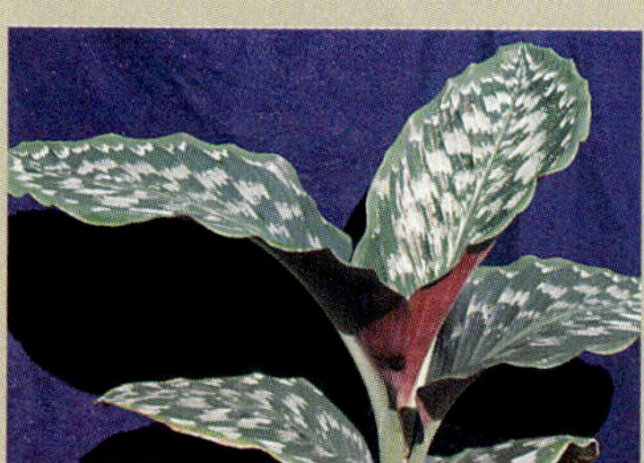

KAEMPFERIA SP. 'Grande'

A majestic Kaempferia that has a wonderful pattern on upper side of leaf with a maroon upper side that is frequently displayed because of its upright growing habit. Grows to 2'-3'. Makes great accent or pot plant. Full to medium shade. Probably zone 8 and higher. Has largest flowers in genus. Flowers are rosy pink.
35870 Rhizome..............................$6.95
35871 Growing Plant (6" pot)....$10.95
35872 Growing Plant (4" pot)......$4.95

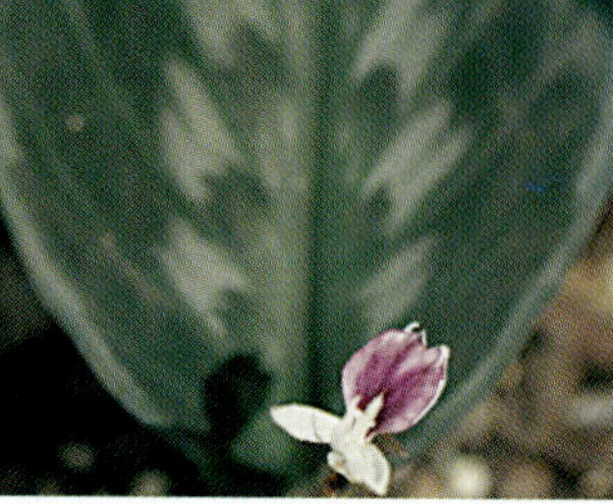

KAEMPFERIA GALANGA

The leaves of this plant are plain green and lay flat on the ground. Grows to 8" (2.5cm) in the shade. The blooms are with two purple spots on the lip. The leaves are large and round on this Asian spice plant grown for its rhizomes. Zone 8 and higher. Goes dormant in winter.
35800 Rhizome $7.95
35801 Growing Plant (6" pot) $11.95
EDIBLE

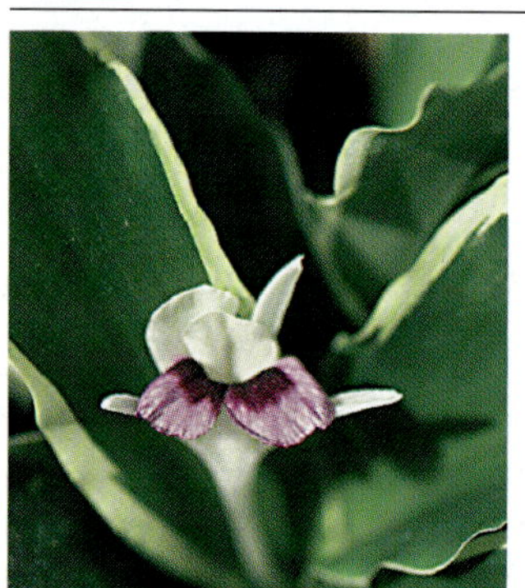

KAEMPFERIA MARGINATA

A great-looking Kaempferia with a large 10"-12"-diameter leaf that is tough and leathery and lies flat on ground. Species gets its name from thin red line along margin of leaves. Produces beautiful violet and white flowers almost daily. Needs lots of shade. Probably Zone 8 and higher.
36020 Rhizomes $7.95
36021 Growing Plant (6" pot) $11.95

KAEMPFERIA ATROVIRENS 'Silver Peacock'

Attractive foliage plant with strikingly patterned leaves; often no green shows through the silver, brown, and black. Flowers white with purple lip. Blooms spring through summer. Grows to 4" (10cm) in shade. Zone 8 and higher. Good groundcover.
35750 Rhizome $7.95
35751 Growing Plant (6" pot) $11.95

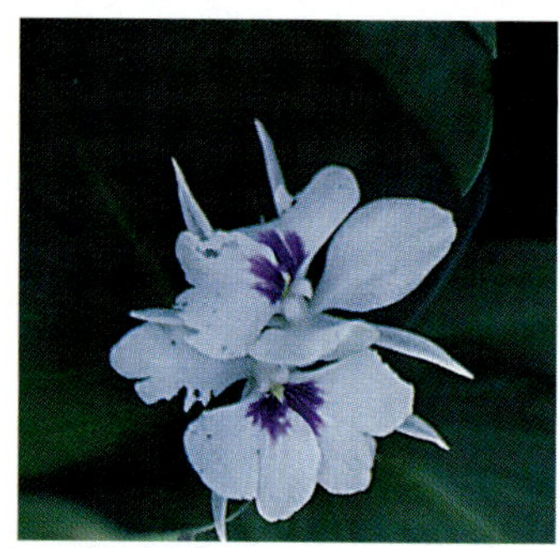

KAEMPFERIA GILBERTII 'Variegated Kaempferia'

Small, shade-loving plant with long narrow striped leaves. Blooms in late spring into summer; has small white and purple flowers that resemble orchids. Variegated foliage is main attraction. Plant grows to 7" (17.5cm). Zone 8 and higher. Goes dormant during winter.
35850 Rhizome $6.95
6($34.95) Save 16%
35851 Growing Plant (6" pot) $10.95

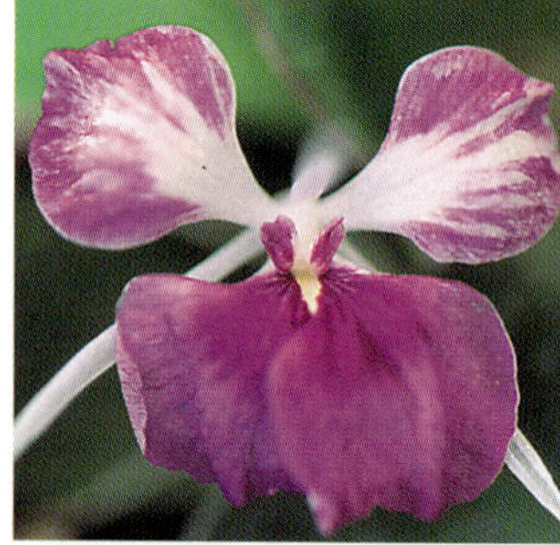

Rhizomes are available only from about December 15th to May 1st . As they must be planted when temperatures are warm; they cannot be kept in dormancy as a rhizome. After May 1st rhizomes will be growing plants. Growing plants of long-day plants (Curcumas, Globbas, Kaempferias, Zingibers, Siphonochilus) are available from May/June through October. Growing plants of bananas, heliconias, certain gingers (Hedychiums, Alpinias, Costus, Monocostus), hibiscus, Siamese lucky plants, bougainvilleas and others are available all year.

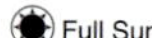 Full Sun 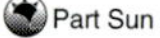 Part Sun 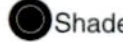 Shade 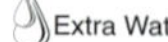 Extra Water 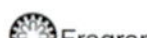 Fragrant 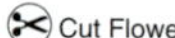 Cut Flower 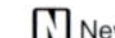 New

KAEMPFERIA PULCHRA 'Bronze Peacock'

Small flat-growing plant, with lavender flowers from spring to fall. Grows 4" (10cm) to 5" (12.5cm) in shade. Has a nice pattern design in the leaves. Background of leaves is bronze color. Good groundcover. Zone 8 and higher. Good substitute for *Hosta* in southern gardens. Goes dormant during winter.

35950 Rhizome *$5.95*
6($34.95) Save 16%

35951 Growing Plant (6" pot) *$9.95*

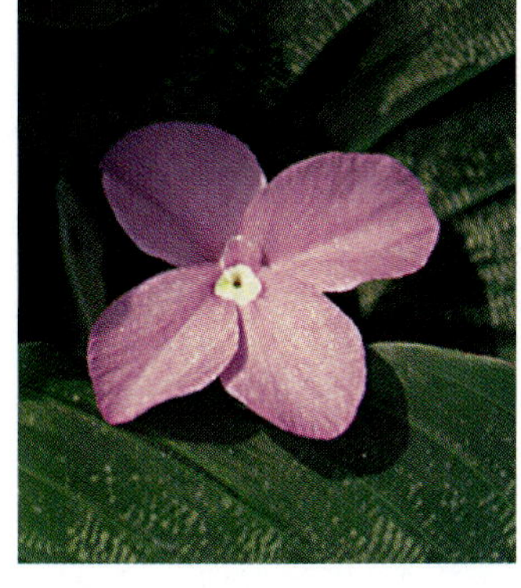

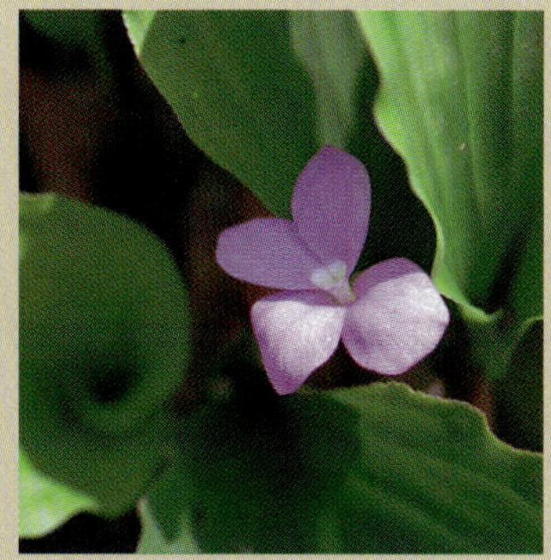

KAEMPFERIA PULCHRA MANSONII

Small plant with ribbed leaves. Grows well in shade to 8" (20cm). Flowers are lavender; blooming occurs daily from spring to fall. Zone 8 and higher. Excellent groundcover. Good substitute for *Hosta* in southern gardens. Goes dormant during winter.

36050 Rhizome..............................*$5.95*
6($28.95) Save 19%;

36051 Growing Plant (6" pot)......*$9.95*

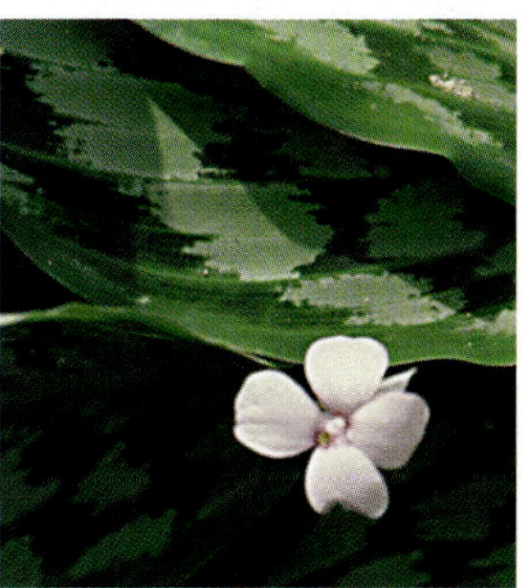

KAEMPFERIA PULCHRA 'Silver Spot'

This unique plant does not go dormant in winter if kept warm. Lavender flowers. The leaves have large silvery patches in a feather pattern. Grows to 5" (12.5cm) in shade. Zone 8 and higher. Good substitute for *Hosta* in southern gardens.

36000 Rhizome *$5.95*
6($28.95) Save 19%;

36001 Growing Plant (6" pot) *$9.95*

KAEMPFERIA SP. AFF. LAOTICA 'Satin Checks'

A low-growing, fascinating plant that makes a great ground cover for deep shade. Plant has bright-green leaves with three rows of dark-purplish checkerboard spots and a very satiny sheen. An exquisite purple flower appears almost daily from midsummer to fall. Zone 8 and higher. Good replacement for Hosta. Goes dormant in winter.

35970 Rhizome *$7.95*
35971 Growing Plant (6" pot) *$11.95*

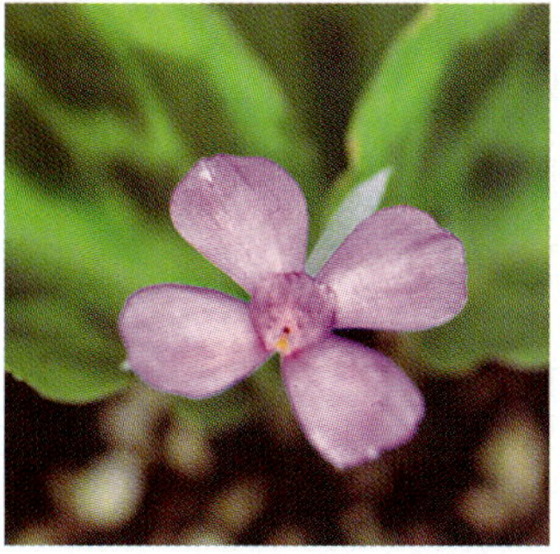

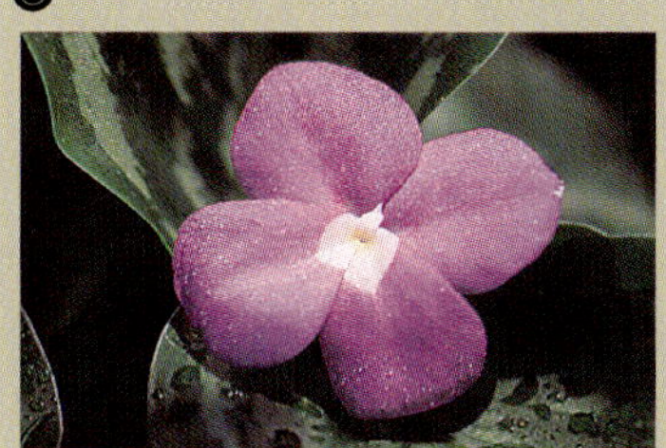

KAEMPFERIA SP. AFF. LAOTICA 'Shazam'

A strikingly beautiful plant with boldly variegated leaves with rows of dark-maroon checks on a silver background and a light-green margin. Stunning 6" leaves are held 4"-5" above ground. Has brilliant purple flowers on reddish stalks. Thrives in deep shade. Another good replacement for Hosta in southern climates. Goes dormant in winter. Zones 8 and higher.

36040 Rhizome...........................*$7.95*
36041 Growing Plant (6" pot)....*$11.95*

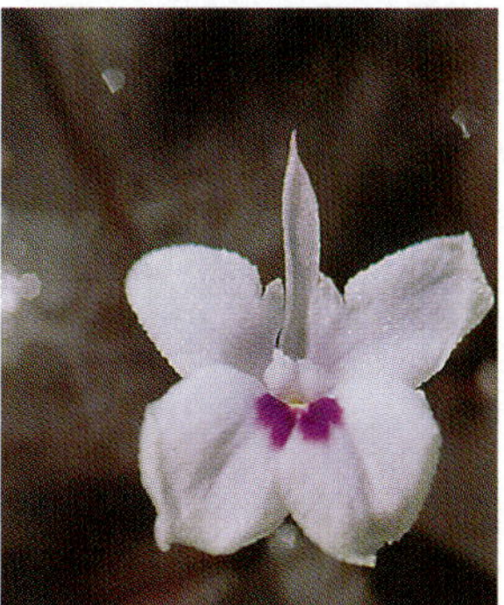

KAEMPFERIA SP. 'Red Leaf'

An amazing Kaempferia species from wilds of Thailand that has a medium-size 6"-7"-round, leathery leaf that lies flat on the ground. Coloration of leaves varies from solid maroon to just a blush of maroon. Produces delicate white flowers with varying degrees of blue markings almost daily. Full shade. Makes a great ground cover. Probably Zone 8 and higher.

36010 Rhizomes *$8.95*
36011 Growing Plant (6" pot)......................*$13.95*

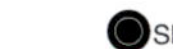
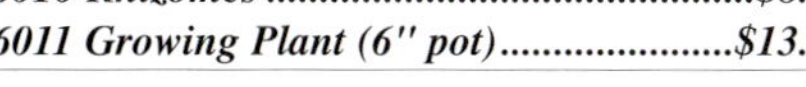
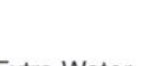
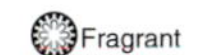
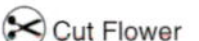
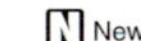

Full Sun · Part Sun · Shade · Extra Water · Fragrant · Cut Flower · New

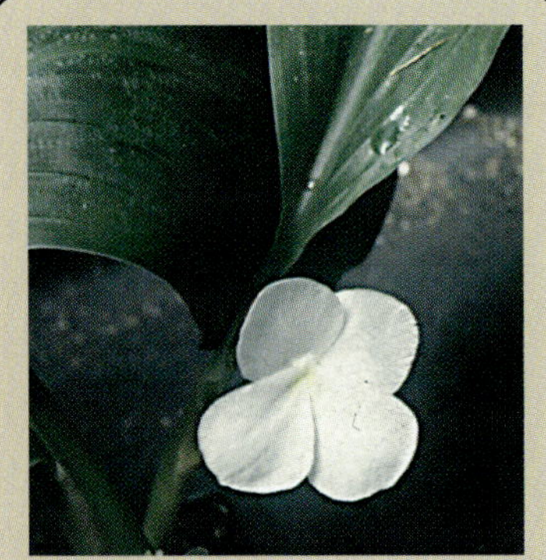

KAEMPFERIA ROSCOEANA

This plant is a relatively new introduction from Thailand. The large-leaves resemble *Kaempferia pulchra* in pattern. Large, white flowers. Grows to 8" (17.5cm). Leaves can be 12" (30cm) to 14" (35cm) across. Full shade. Probably Zone 8 and higher. Goes dormant during winter.

36100 Rhizome............................*$7.95*
36101 Growing Plant (6" pot)..*$12.95*

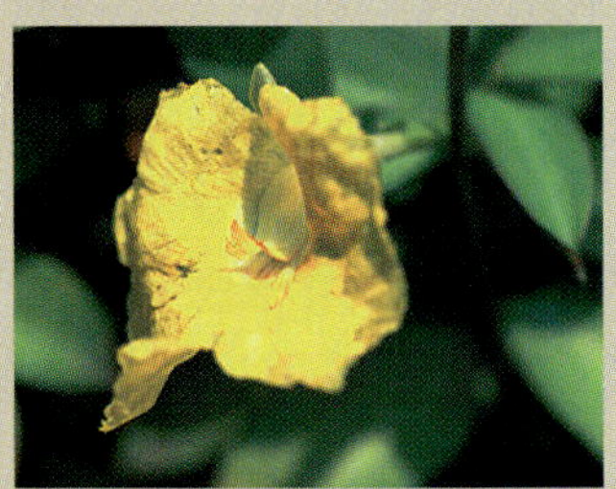

MONOCOSTUS UNIFLORUS

Called 'Yellow Spiral' ginger. Small plant from 18"–24" (45cm to 60cm). Lemon-yellow flowers (2"–3") are borne on slender spiraling canes. Flowers are large for the size of the plant and appear singly in leaves near the top of the stem. Blooms all summer and well into winter. Prefers medium shade. Makes a good pot plant and will do well on a bright windowsill. Zone 9 and higher.

36200 Rhizome............................*$5.95*
6($28.95) Save 19%
36201 Growing Plant (6" pot)......*$9.95*
36202 Growing Plant (4" pot)......*$3.95*

KAEMPFERIA ROTUNDA
'Asian Crocus'

Differs from most Kaempferias in being much taller; grows to almost 2' (60cm) with beautiful long leaves with purple undersides. Flowers are borne at ground level in spring before leaves emerge. Flowers are white, up to 2" (5cm) across with a purple throat, fragrant, and as tall as 3" (7.5cm). Zone 8 and higher. Likes shade and makes a good groundcover. Also excellent pot plant.

36150 Rhizome..*$5.95*   *6($28.95) Save 19%*
36151 Growing Plant (6" pot)..................*$9.95*

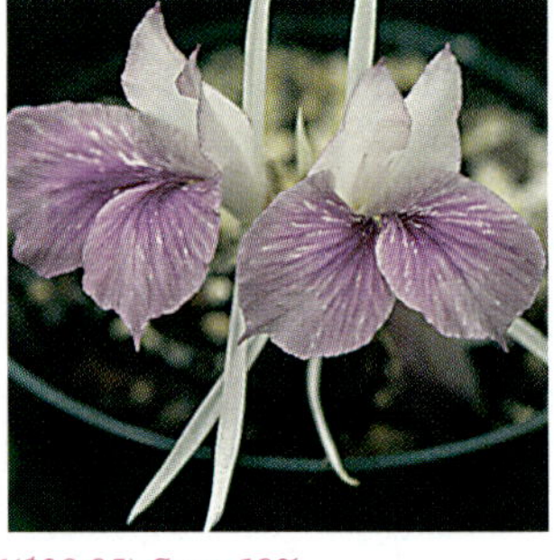

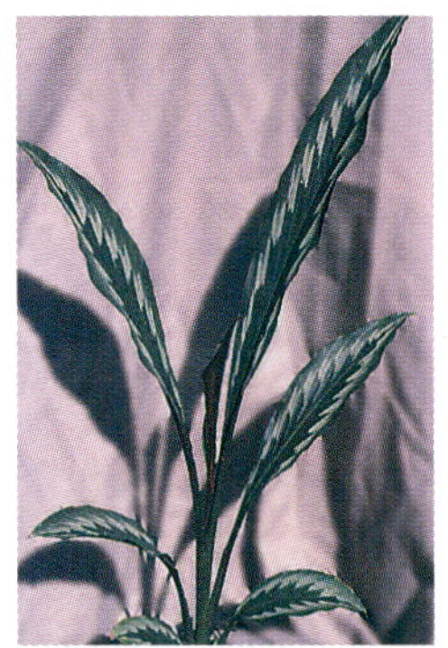

KAEMPFERIA ROTUNDA 'Raven'

One of the best looking Kaempferias. It has tall elegant slim leaves with a striking pattern on the upper surface and a maroon wash on the underside. Plant grows to 18" tall. Full to medium shade. Probably zone 8 and higher. Just like the regular rotunda, fragrant flowers appear first before leaves. From the country of Laos.

36160 Rhizome.......................................*$8.95*
36161 Growing Plant (6" pot)...........................*$14.95*
36162 Growing Plant (4" pot)..............................*$7.95*

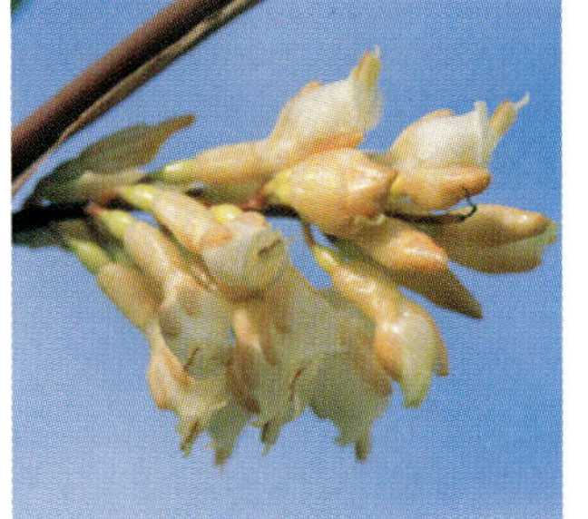

PLEURANTHODIUM HELWIGII
'Golden Bells'

A very striking ginger that originally came from the Solomon Islands. Has a wonderful raceme of creamy, golden shell-like flowers that emerge from a beautiful maroon-colored stem. Flowers are not apical. Medium size plant growing 3'-4' high. Medium sun. Probably zone 8 and higher.

31370 Rhizome.......................................*$17.95*
31371 Growing Plant (6" pot)................*$22.95*

PLEURANTHODIUM SP.
'Pink Pearls'

A marvelous new ginger that grows to 6'-7'. Flowers in spring and summer. Inflorescence consisting of rows of pink pearl flowers held erect. Zone 10 and higher. New.

36170 Rhizome.......................................*$24.95*
36171 Growing Plant (6" pot)................*$31.95*

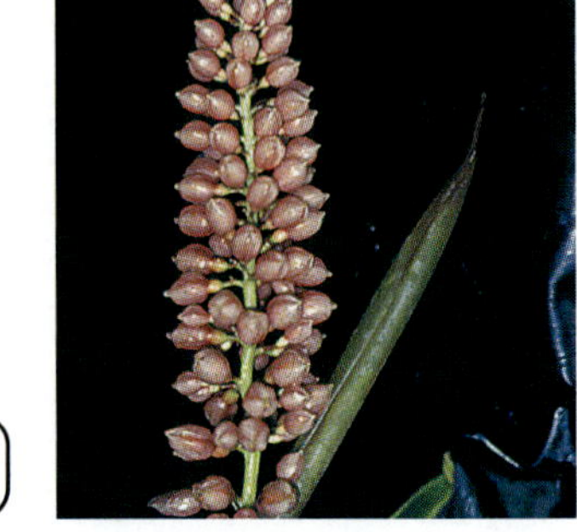

ALL STOKES TROPICALS' PLANTS ARE
EASY-TO-GROW.

RENEALMIA. A large genus of gingers, most of which are native to Central and South America. A few species are known from Africa. Plants superficially resemble Alpinias in growth form and leaf shape and arrangement. Several species of Renealmia have fragrant leaves when crushed like most Alpinia species. Most species have basal inflorescences, however some have terminal inflorescences. All tend to be slow growers and are not cold hardy. All are Zone 10 and higher plants.

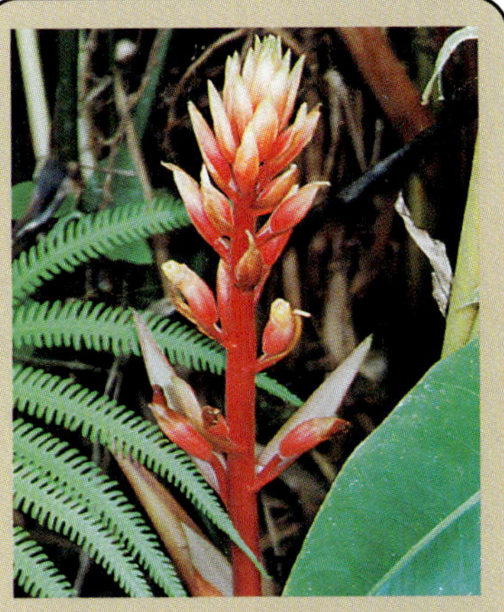

RENEALMIA SP. 'Red Hot'

A magnificent looking species with an Alpinia-looking inflorescence. Grows 4'-5' in medium shade to full sun. Zone 10 and higher. Great plant for collectors. New.

36240 Rhizome............................$14.95
36241 Growing Plant (6" pot)....$19.95

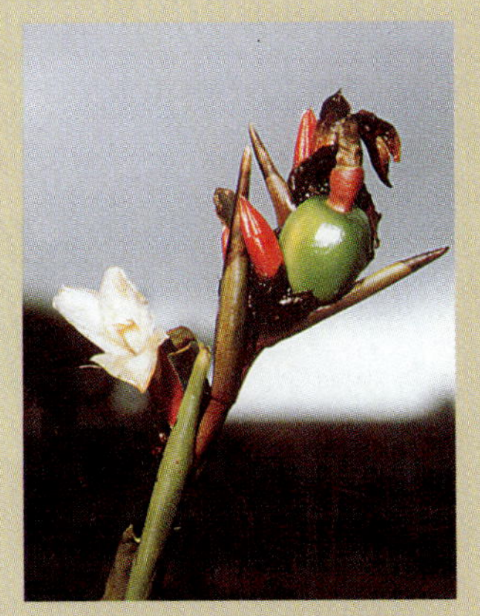

RENEALMIA VENTRICOSA

A native species from Puerto Rico. Great looking plant that has outstanding Alpinia-like foliage. Grows 5'-6' tall. Flowers are also Alpinia-like (white with yellow centers) that mature into attractive red and green seed pods. Zone 10 and higher. Medium shade to full sun. New. Makes very attractive clumps

36260 Rhizome............................$15.95
36261 Growing Plant (6" pot)....$20.95

RENEALMIA ALPINIA

A beautiful species that has a striking inflorescence that superficially resembles an Alpinia, hence the species name. Grows 5'-6' tall. Zone 10 and higher. Shade to full sun. Foliage is outstanding and Alpinia-like. New.

36220 Rhizome $15.95
36221 Growing Plant (6" pot) $20.95

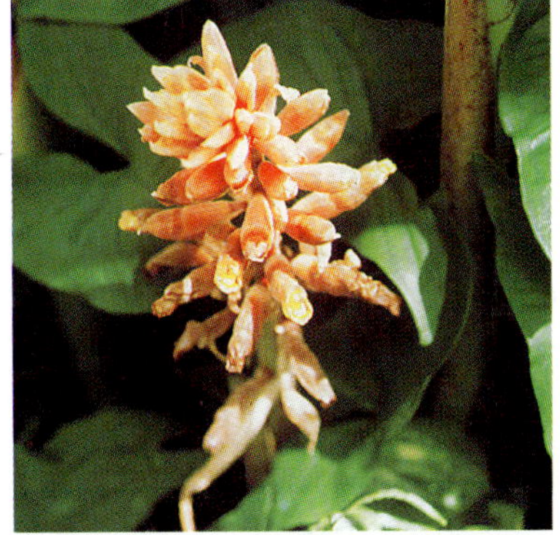

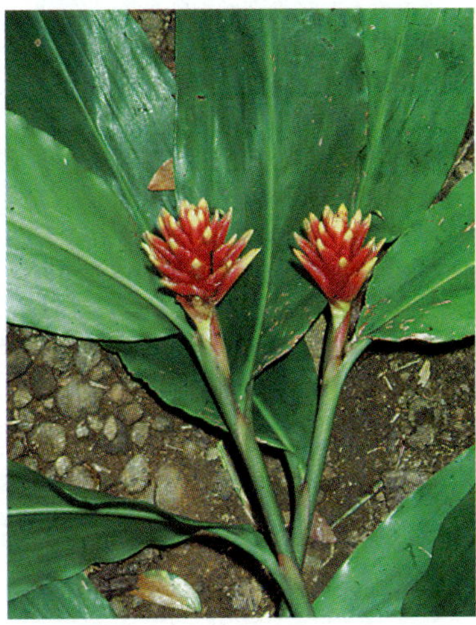

ALL STOKES TROPICALS' PLANTS ARE EASY-TO-GROW.

RENEALMIA CERNUA 'Red Spikes'

A very showy ginger from Ecuador. Grows in tight clumps 5'-7'. Flowers make good cuts. Zone 10 and higher. New.

36230 Rhizome $14.95
36231 Growing Plant (6" pot) $21.95

RENEALMIA CERNUA 'Yellow Spikes'

A great looking plant that grows to 6'-7' in medium sun. Has been grown in Costa Rica for cut flowers. Inflorescence resembles that of certain bromeliads. Bract spikes are very hard and pointed. Gives off distinctive camphory fragrance. Zone 10 and higher. New.

36270 Rhizome $15.95
36271 Growing Plant (6" pot) $20.95

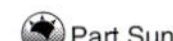 Full Sun 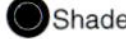 Part Sun 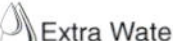 Shade Extra Water 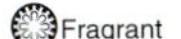 Fragrant 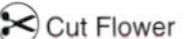 Cut Flower New

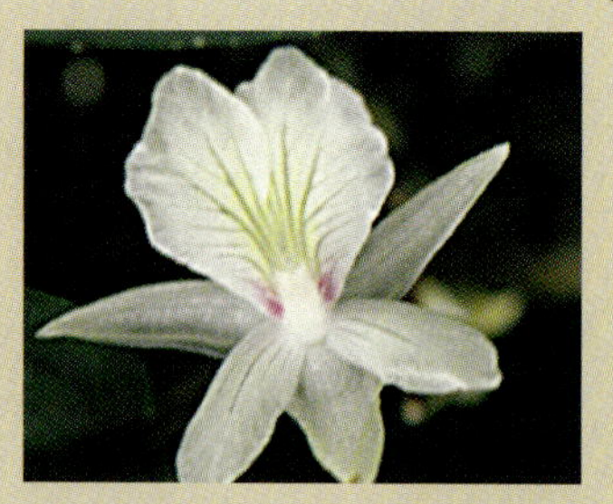

SCAPHOCHLAMYS BILOBA
'Silver Streak Ginger'

Plant has attractive foliage with silver streaked leaves and is the most common of the cultivated species. The leaves have two silver stripes (streaks) that connect at the end; flowers are white. Grows to 5" (12.5cm) in the shade. Zone 10 and higher.

36250 Rhizome............................*$13.95*
36251 Growing Plant (6" pot)....*$18.95*

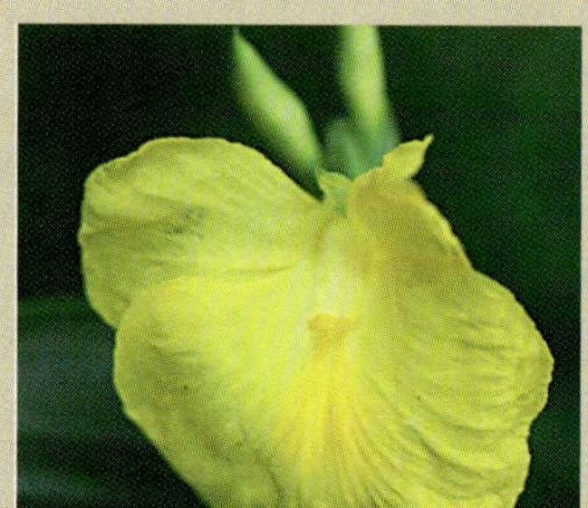

SIPHONOCHILUS DECORA
'Yellow Trumpet'

Called 'Yellow Trumpet' ginger. Short plant (15"–20") (37.5cm to 50cm) with large lanceolate glossy dark leaves with grayish undersides. Separate basal stalk bears a raceme of large canary yellow, funnel-shaped flowers. Prefers 30-50% shade. Blooms between June and July. Zone 8 and higher. An amazing African ginger. Slightly fragrant. Keep dry in winter. Must for the serious collector.

36350 Rhizome............................*$5.95*
6($28.95) Save 19%
36351 Growing Plant (6" pot)....*$10.95*

SCAPHOCHLAMYS KUNSTLERI

Plant resembles a Boesenbergia in form and is a small plant with white flowers. The plant does not have any silver markings and goes dormant in winter. It grows to 7" (17.5cm) in shade. Zone 10 and higher. Good pot plant and house plant.

36300 Rhizome *$12.95*
36301 Growing Plant (6" pot) *$17.95*

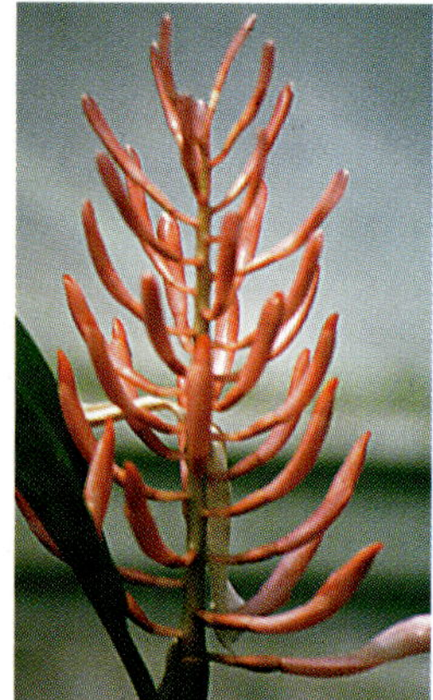

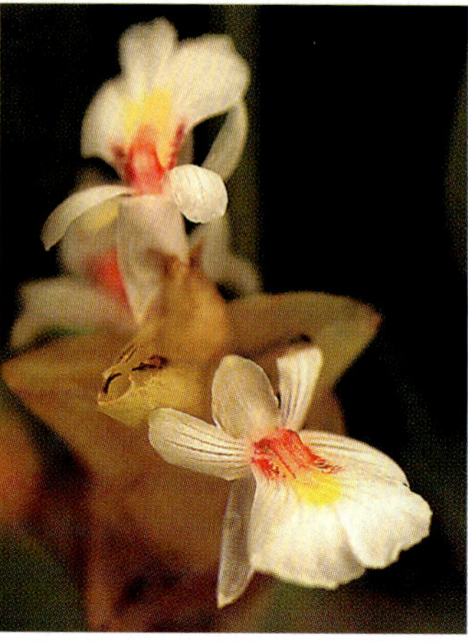

See page 130 for Ginger Fertilizer

RIEDELIA SP.

Very nice species of unknown identity. Native to New Guinea. Beautiful pink flowers and glossy leaves that closely resemble *Alpinia* leaves. Flowers are tubular in shape and are long lasting. Grows to 3' (90cm) in medium sun. Zone 10 and higher.

36210 Rhizome *$15.95*
36211 Growing Plant (6" pot)...........................*$20.95*

SIPHONOCHILUS AETHIOPICUS
'Sunrise Trumpet'

A reedy plant with narrow leaves. that grows in medium sun. In late spring, ground level spikes have giant 5" (12.5cm) mauve flowers that are slightly fragrant. Probably Zone 9 and higher.

36340 Rhizome *$17.95*
36341 Growing Plant (6" pot) *$22.95*

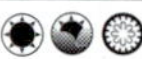

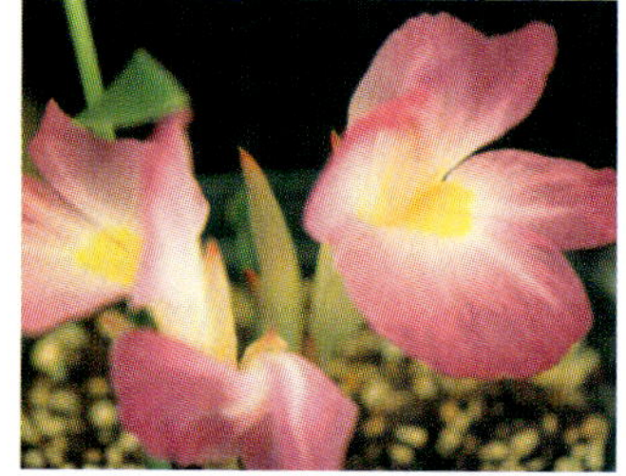

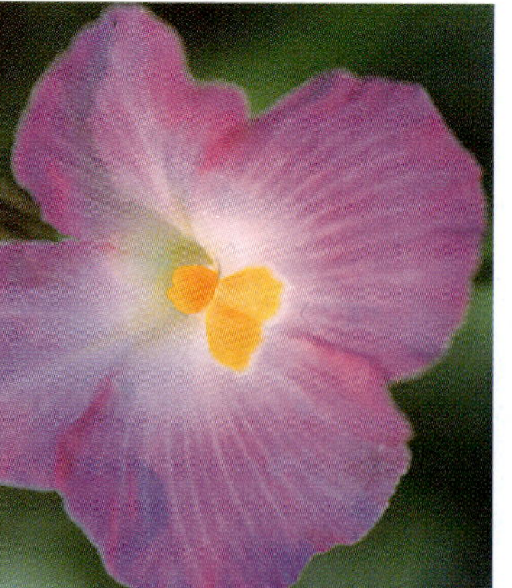

SIPHONOCHILUS KIRKII
'Pink Trumpet'

One of the most beautiful gingers in cultivation, it has a separate bloom spike similar to *S. decora*. The flowers are large and rose-lavender in color. Slightly fragrant. Grows to 18" (45cm) in shade. Zone 9 and higher.

36400 Rhizome........................*$8.95*
6($45.95) Save 15%
36401 Growing Plant (6" pot)$12.95*

 Full Sun 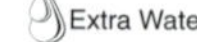 Part Sun 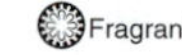 Shade 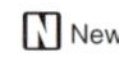 Extra Water Fragrant Cut Flower New

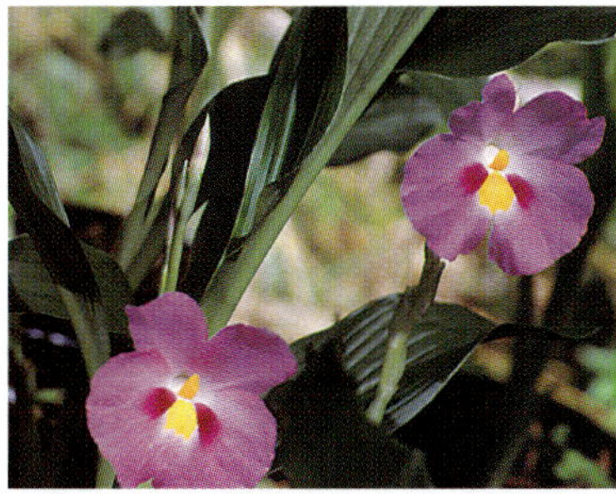

SIPHONOCHILUS KIRKII CARSONII 'Elegant Trumpet'

A compact 2' plant that produces several thin spikes that bear many, large, rose-colored flowers with a yellow central spot flanked by deep maroon spots. It prefers bright shade and well-drained soil. Blooms like clockwork in June. Zone 8 and higher. From Africa. Slightly fragrant.

36360 Rhizome.............................$13.95
36361 Growing Plant (6" pot)......$18.95

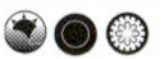

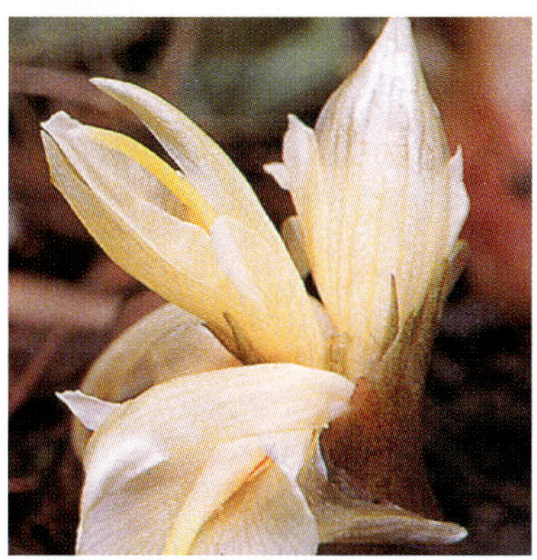

ZINGIBER MIOGA

This edible ginger is grown for its flowers and new shoots. Native to Japan, the light yellow flowers are eaten in tempura and new shoots are used in garnish. Blooms from mid to late summer to late fall on basal inflorescences. This very hardy species is even grown in parts of Canada. Grows to 2' (60cm) in medium sun. Zone 7b and higher.

36600 Rhizome.............................$12.95
36601 Growing Plant (6" pot)......$17.95

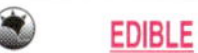
EDIBLE

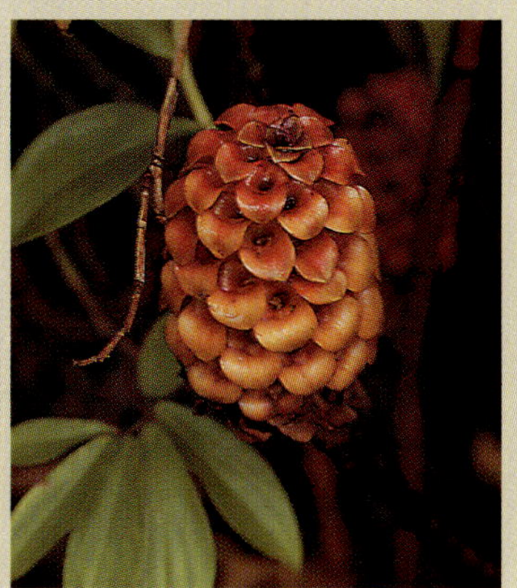

TAPEINOCHILUS ANANASSAE 'Indonesian Wax Ginger'

A fascinating large plant that grows to 12' in medium sun. Plant is grown for its large stiff, waxy inflorescence that makes a good cut flower. Inflorescence appears on tall up to 6', basal spike. Has yellow flowers that emerge from bracts. Zone 10 and higher.

36460 Rhizome.............................$15.95
36461 Growing Plant (6" pot)....$20.95

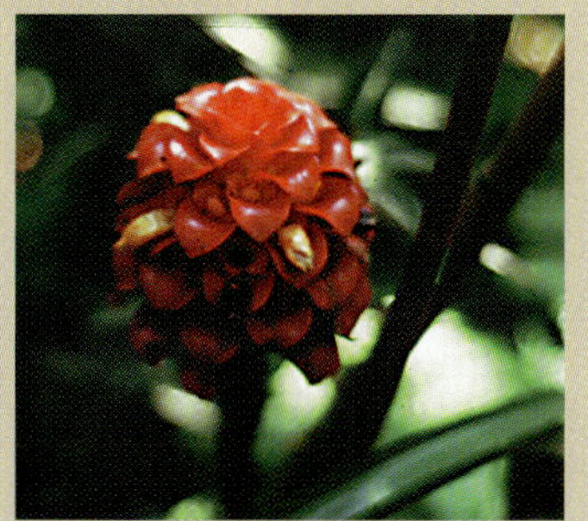

TAPEINOCHILUS QUEENSLANDI

Very closely related to *ananassae* (Indonesian Wax ginger). Native to Northeastern Australia (Queensland). Slight bract differences from *ananassae*. Grows 10' (3m) to 12' (3.6m) in medium sun. Large dark red waxy inflorescence on basal stalk; small yellow flowers appear between bracts. Good cut flower. Zone 10 and higher.

36450 Rhizome.........................$15.95
36451 Bareroot plant (6" pot)....$20.95

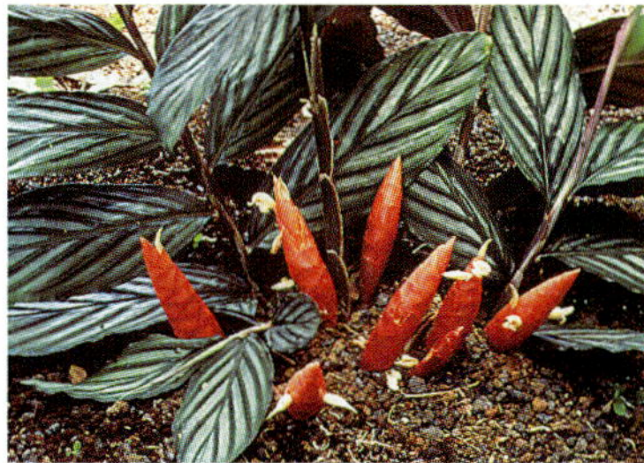

ZINGIBER COLLINSI 'Silver Streaks'

What a showy ginger! Grows 4'-6'. Free flowering in spring and summer with magnificent red basal cones emerging from base of dark green leaves streaked with silver.

36470 Rhizome............................$29.95
36471 Growing Plant (6" pot)....$37.95

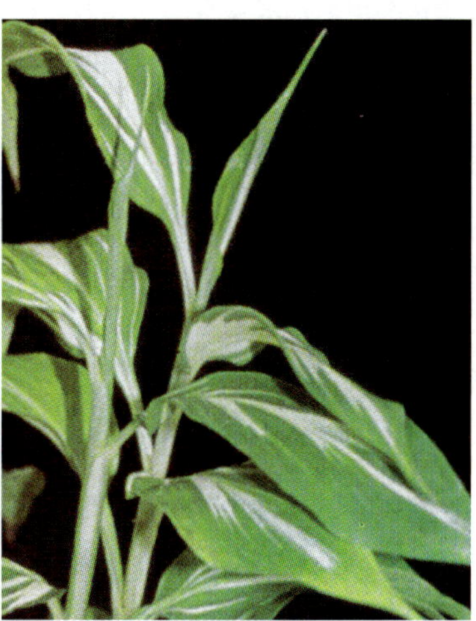

ZINGIBER MIOGA VARIEGATED 'Dancing Crane'

A wonderful new variegated form of one of our most popular zingibers. Has very strong variegation on narrow pointed leaves making it an excellent accent plant. Believed to be as cold-hardy as solid green form. Probably Zone 7b and higher. Grows to 2' in partial shade to medium sun. Flowers are cream colored similar to the regular green mioga.

36760 Rhizome............................$14.95
36761 Growing Plant (6" pot)....$19.95
36762 Growing Plant (4" pot)....$11.95

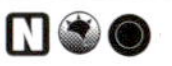
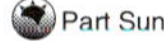
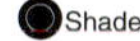
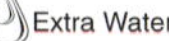

Full Sun   Part Sun   Shade   Extra Water   Fragrant   Cut Flower   New

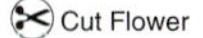

Gingers

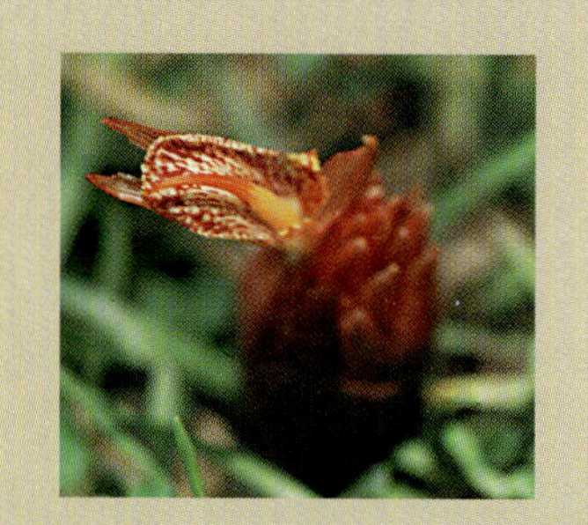

ZINGIBER RUBENS
'Bengal Ginger'

This easy to grow species blooms in mid summer. Blooms appear at ground level as red inflorescences with large red flowers speckled with white and yellow. This medium size species has nice foliage and grows to 4' (1.2m) in medium sun. Zone 7b and higher.

36750 Rhizome..............................$8.95
36751 Growing Plant (6" pot)....$12.95

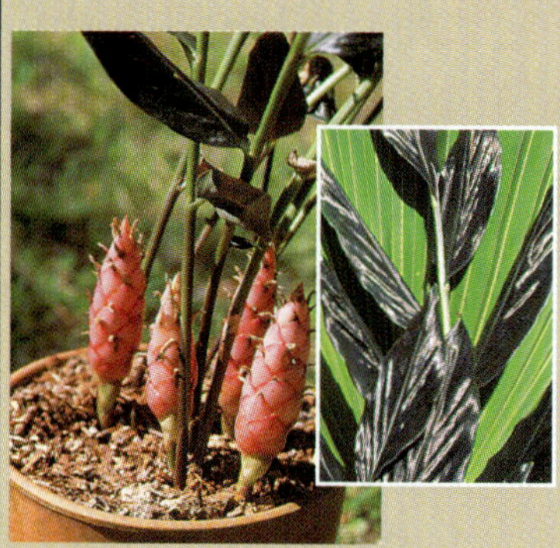

ZINGIBER SP. 'Midnight'

What a great new Zingiber with leaves that appear almost black. Produces basal cones that emerge from the ground sulfur yellow in color and then age as tiny flowers squeeze from tight bracts turning to a delightful pink color. Plants grow to 2'-3'. Dark foliage is main feature. Medium shade. Probably Zone 9 and higher.

36740 Rhizome...........................$14.95
36741 Growing Plant (6" pot)....$18.95
36742 Growing Plant (4" pot)....$13.95

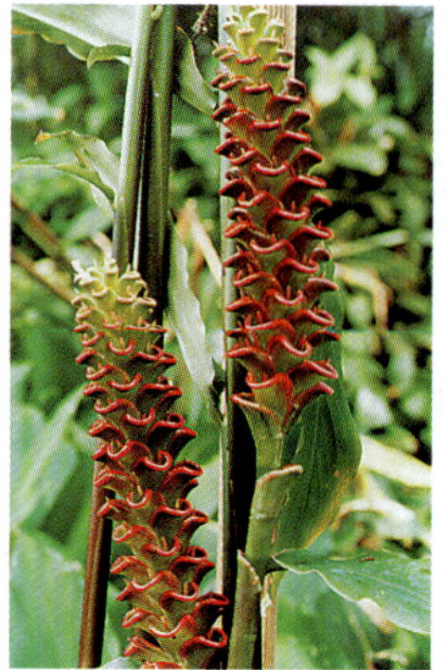

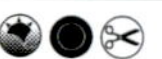

ZINGIBER NEGLECTUM 'Jewel Pagoda'

A miraculous Zingiber with a very tall (up to 12") sculptured inflorescence. From northern Queensland, Australia. Bract tips are ruby red with light-green translucent bases. Emerging from bracts are small purple flowers. Makes a great cut flower. Plant grows 5'-6' in medium shade. Zone 8 and higher. Must to be seen to be believed. Very limited supply only one per customer.

36660 Rhizome $19.95
36661 Growing Plant (6" pot) $24.95
36662 Growing Plant (4" pot) $15.95

ZINGIBER PARISHII 'Ivory Ice'

A new *Zingiber* species from Thailand. The cone inflorescence is a marvelous ivory color and is borne on a basal stem about 2' (60cm) high. Inflorescence makes a nice cut flower. Plant is medium size 3' (90cm) to 4' (1.2m) and grows in medium sun. For the *Zingiber* enthusiast, this is a must. Probably Zone 9 and higher. Very limited quantities.

36780 Rhizome...$20.95
36781 Growing Plant (6" pot) $25.95

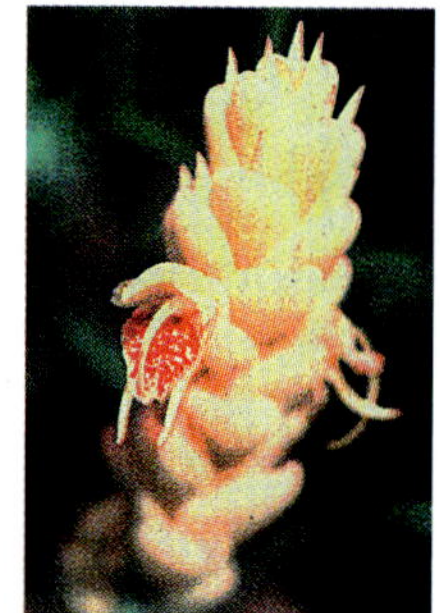

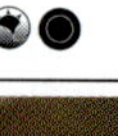

ZINGIBER OTTENSII

An attractive ginger with reddish stems producing a terminal cone that is somewhat similar to shampoo ginger, Zingiber zerumbet. However, cone starts out reddish and has nice orange flowers that emerge from the tight bracts. Grows to 5' in medium sun. Probably Zone 9 and higher.

36710 Rhizome...$15.95
36711 Growing Plant (6" pot)................................$20.95

ZINGIBER OFFICINALE

The common "edible ginger" is grown for its spicy rhizomes used in cooking and medicines. Has thin stems and leaves. Blooms (small green inflorescence with white and maroon flowers) are rare. After blooming green cone does not turn red like most other Zingibers. Blooms basally and terminally. Grows 3' (90cm) to 5' (1.5m) in medium to full sun. Edible rhizome is main attraction. Zone 8 and higher.

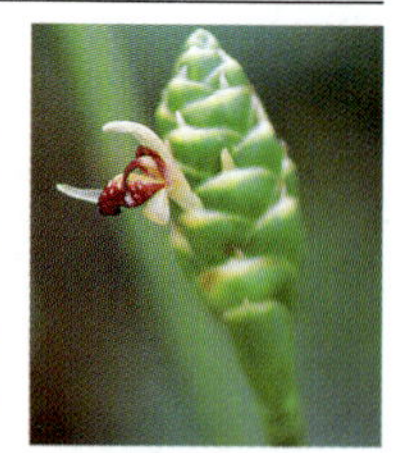

This extremely versatile root is known for its popularity in Oriental and Indian cooking. The Chinese, Japanese and East Indians use ginger root in many forms, including grated and ground. Grown in Jamaica, Brazil, India, Africa, China, Thailand and Hawaii. Ginger root is a gnarled and knobby root that has a tan skin and a pale yellow-green to ivory flesh. Fresh ginger root imparts a pungent, hot and spicy taste to many dishes. Ginger root is also used in baking, confectionery and certain liqueurs.

36700 Rhizome ....$5.95   *6($28.95) Save 19%;*
36701 Growing Plant (6" pot) ....$9.95   *36702 Growing Plant (4" pot)* $3.95

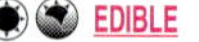

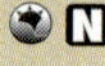 Full Sun   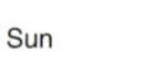 Part Sun   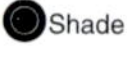Shade   Extra Water   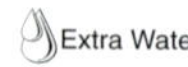Fragrant   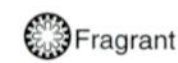Cut Flower   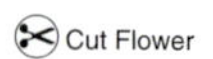 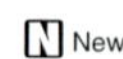New

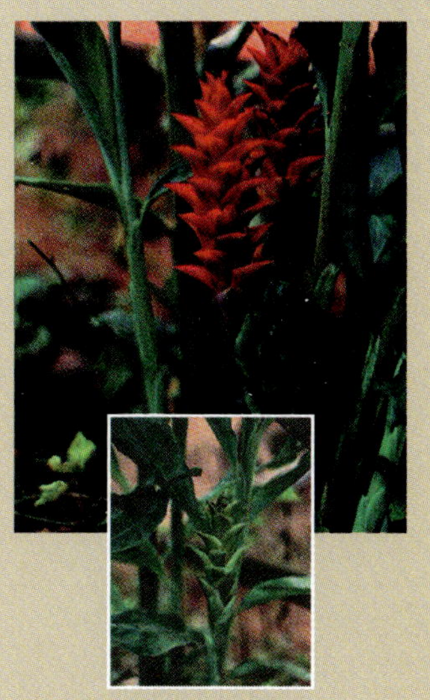

ZINGIBER SP. 'Chiang Mai Princess'

Amazing new *Zingiber* species from Thai-Burma border. We have never seen a *Zingiber* species with sharply pointed bracts on its conical inflorescence. Basal cone with spikes grows 12" (30cm) to 18" (45cm) from ground; new cone is dark emerald green in color. When mature, cone, still with sharp spikes, turns brilliant blood red. Both green and red cones make great cut flowers. Medium to full sun. Grows 3' (90cm) to 4' (1.2m). For the *Zingiber* enthusiast this is a must. Probably Zone 9 and higher.

36770 Rhizome..............................$18.95
36771 Growing Plant (6" pot)....$23.95

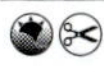

Do you have a shady spot in your garden?
Try growing Kaempferias, Globbas or most any of the gingers.

Do you have a wet area in your yard?
Try growing Variegated Spider Lily, Alpinia aquatica, Hedychium coronarium, Canna 'Cleopatra', or Canna 'Bangkok Yellow'.

ZINGIBER SP. 'Milky Way'

Delightful Zingiber species from Thailand. Compact 2½'-3' plant with light-green foliage that produces late summer through late fall multiple basal inflorescences (tight milky-white cones sometimes suffused with pink). Yellow flowers emerge in a spiral path from bracts for 8-10 weeks. Cones are occasionally produced on stem terminals also. As many as 5-6 cones have emerged from a single 6" pot planting. Medium shade to almost full sun. Probably Zone 8 and higher.

36790 Rhizome $7.95

6($39.95) Save 16%

36791 Growing Plant (6" pot) $12.95
36792 Growing Plant (4" pot) $5.95

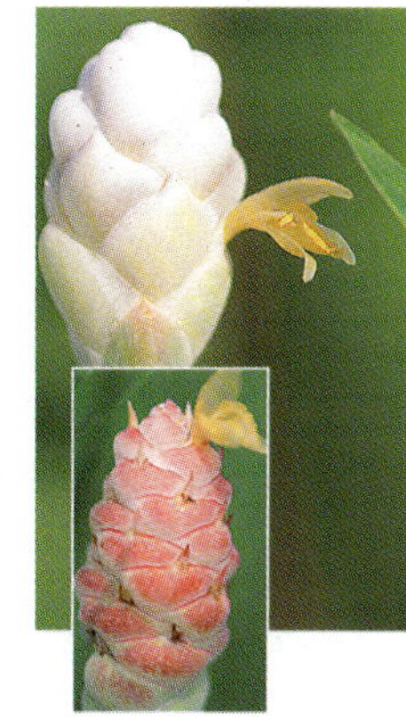

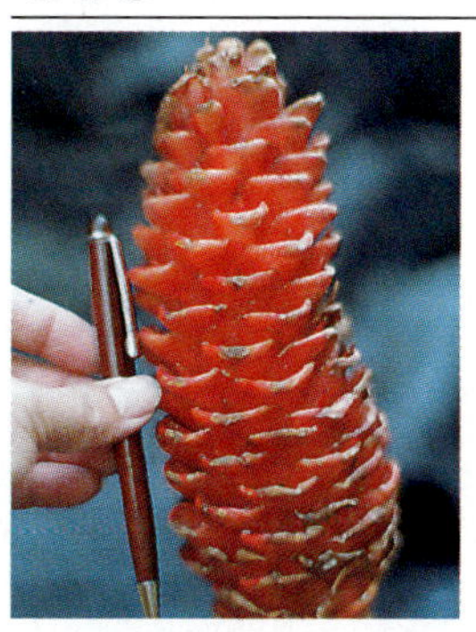

ZINGIBER SP. 'Thai Giant'

A very imposing Zingiber species from Thailand with a 8"-9" x 4"-5" in diameter inflorescence "cone" on a 3 1/2' long stalk. Makes a great cut lasting for weeks. Plant is medium size 4 1/2'-5 1/2'; cone is giant. Medium shade to almost full sun. Probably Zone 9 and higher.

36970 Rhizome.......................................$16.95
36971 Growing Plant (6" pot) $21.95

ZINGIBER SPECTABILE 'Beehive Ginger'

Tall species with large yellow and red inflorescence. This summer blooming plant has tall inflorescence with yellow and black flowers on 3' (90cm) tall stems that are used as a cut flower. Plant grows to 7' (2.4m) in medium sun. Probably Zone 8 and higher.

36900 Rhizome $11.95
36901 Growing Plant (6" pot) $16.95

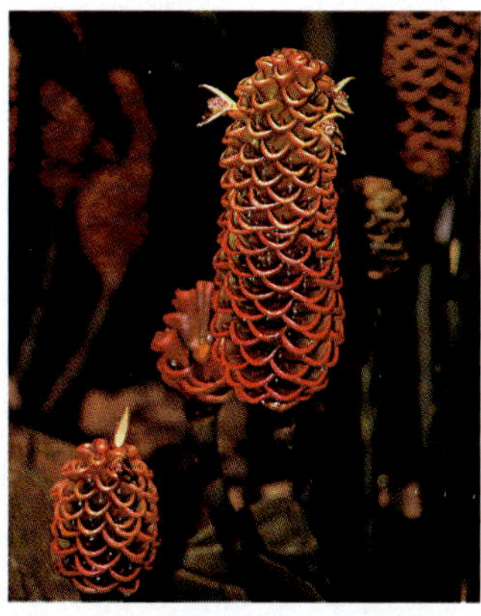

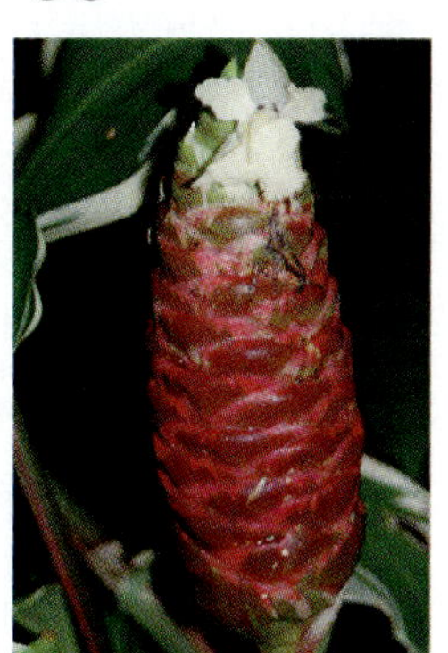

ZINGIBER ZERUMBET 'Darcyi'

Called 'Striped Pine Cone' or 'Variegated Shampoo' ginger. Same as Zingiber zerumbet except with variegated leaves. Outstanding foliage. Grows from 4' to 5' in medium sun. Zone 7 and higher. Produces variegated green cones that turn variegated red. Cones make excellent cut flowers that last for weeks.

37000 Rhizome $5.95
6($34.95) Save 16%
37001 Growing Plant (6" pot) $9.95
37002 Growing Plant (4" pot) $4.95

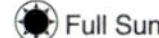 Full Sun 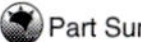 Part Sun 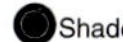 Shade  Extra Water 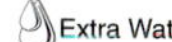 Fragrant 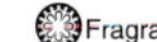 Cut Flower 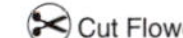 New

Gingers

ZINGIBER ZERUMBET 'Shampoo Ginger'

Also called 'Pine Cone' ginger. Plant grows 6'–8' (8m to 2.4m) in medium sun. Large green cone inflorescences are produced from mid-summer to fall. Small cream yellow flowers appear from under bracts of green cone. After blooming, cone turns brilliant red and lasts for 2–3 weeks. Cones make excellent cut flowers. Zone 7 and higher.

36950 Rhizome ....*$3.95*   *6($18.95) Save 20%*
36951 Growing Plant (6" pot) *$7.95*
36952 Growing Plant (4" pot) *$2.95*

GINGER COLLECTIONS

(Save $5 off listed prices by purchasing entire collection)

Only one collection per customer / Rhizomes only

BEST SELLERS GINGER 5

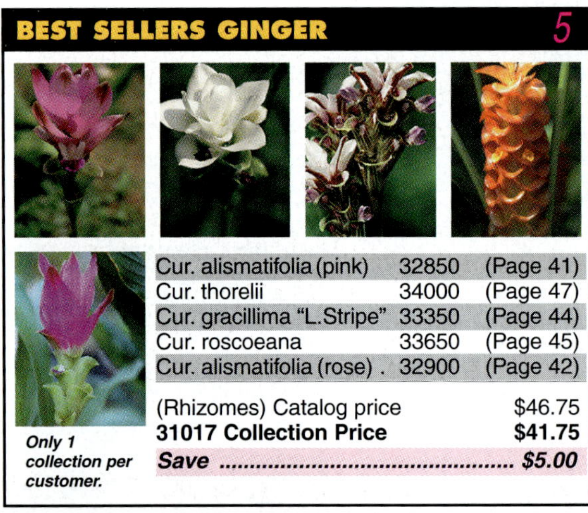

Cur. alismatifolia (pink)	32850	(Page 41)
Cur. thorelii	34000	(Page 47)
Cur. gracillima "L.Stripe"	33350	(Page 44)
Cur. roscoeana	33650	(Page 45)
Cur. alismatifolia (rose)	32900	(Page 42)
(Rhizomes) Catalog price		$46.75
31017 Collection Price		**$41.75**
Save		*$5.00*

Only 1 collection per customer.

COLOR COLLECTION 5

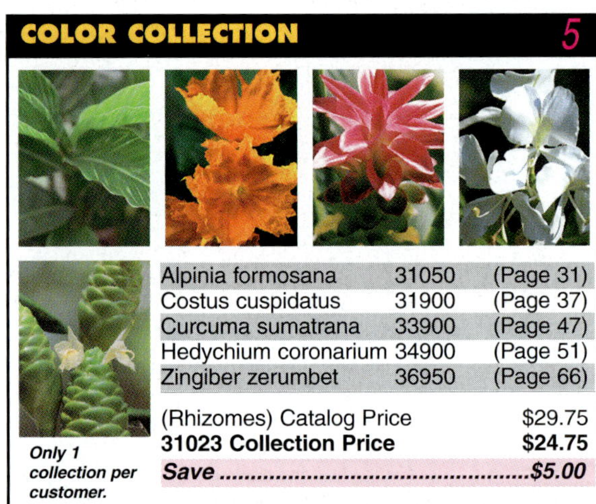

Alpinia formosana	31050	(Page 31)
Costus cuspidatus	31900	(Page 37)
Curcuma sumatrana	33900	(Page 47)
Hedychium coronarium	34900	(Page 51)
Zingiber zerumbet	36950	(Page 66)
(Rhizomes) Catalog Price		$29.75
31023 Collection Price		**$24.75**
Save		*$5.00*

Only 1 collection per customer.

BEGINNER'S COLLECTION 5

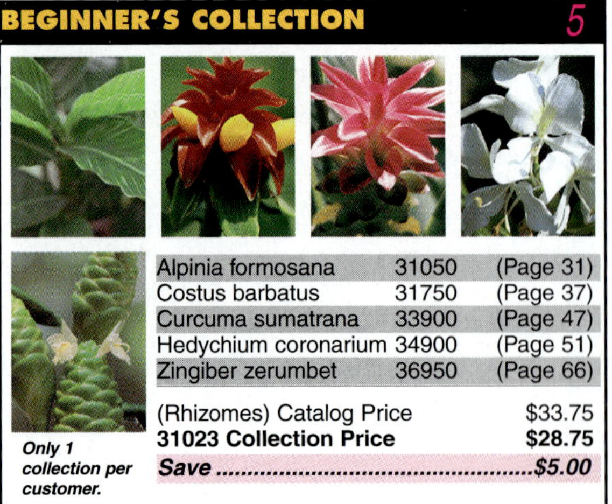

Alpinia formosana	31050	(Page 31)
Costus barbatus	31750	(Page 37)
Curcuma sumatrana	33900	(Page 47)
Hedychium coronarium	34900	(Page 51)
Zingiber zerumbet	36950	(Page 66)
(Rhizomes) Catalog Price		$33.75
31023 Collection Price		**$28.75**
Save		*$5.00*

Only 1 collection per customer.

ALPINIA COLLECTION 5

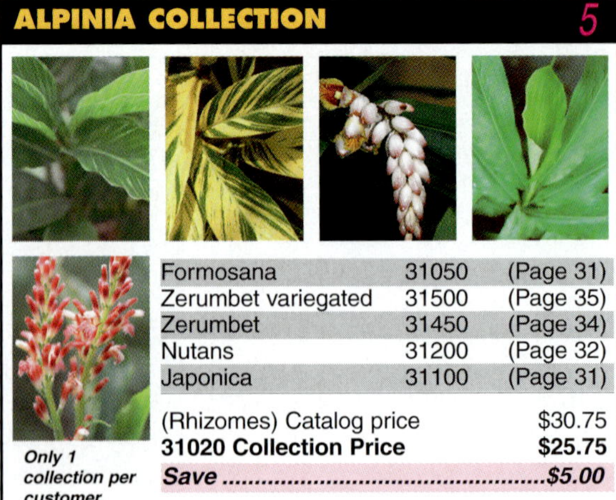

Formosana	31050	(Page 31)
Zerumbet variegated	31500	(Page 35)
Zerumbet	31450	(Page 34)
Nutans	31200	(Page 32)
Japonica	31100	(Page 31)
(Rhizomes) Catalog price		$30.75
31020 Collection Price		**$25.75**
Save		*$5.00*

Only 1 collection per customer.

TO ORDER CALL **1-800-624-9706**/24 HRS. OR VISIT OUR WEB SITE: www. stokestropicals.com

Gingers

CURCUMA COLLECTION 5

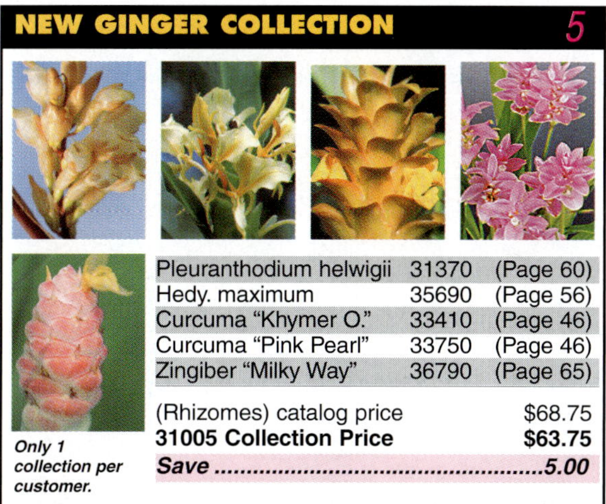

Sumatrana	33900	(Page 47)
Candy Cane	33300	(Page 43)
Cordata	33050	(Page 43)
Inodora	33400	(Page 44)
Aurantiaca	32760	(Page 42)
(Rhizomes) catalog price		$39.75
31021 Collection Price		$34.75
Save $5.00		

Only 1 collection per customer.

SUN COLLECTION 5

Australasica	33000	(Page 42)
Elata	33150	(Page 43)
Ornata	33450	(Page 44)
Barbatus	31750	(Page 37)
Siam Tulip (Pink)	32850	(Page 41)
(Rhizomes) catalog price		$47.75
31003 Collection Price		**$42.75**
Save $5.00		

Only 1 collection per customer.

NEW GINGER COLLECTION 5

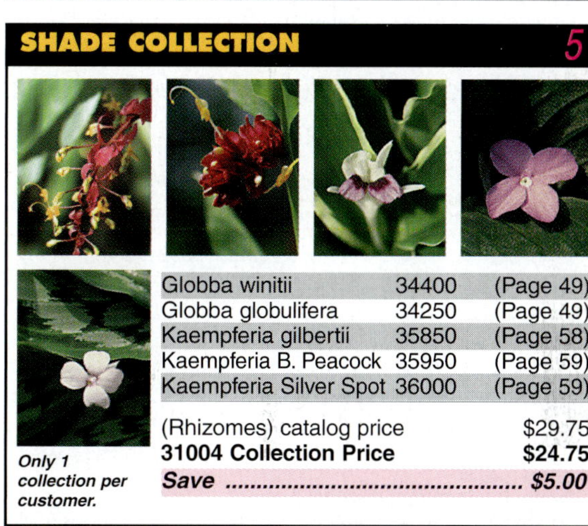

Pleuranthodium helwigii	31370	(Page 60)
Hedy. maximum	35690	(Page 56)
Curcuma "Khymer O."	33410	(Page 46)
Curcuma "Pink Pearl"	33750	(Page 46)
Zingiber "Milky Way"	36790	(Page 65)
(Rhizomes) catalog price		$68.75
31005 Collection Price		**$63.75**
Save 5.00		

Only 1 collection per customer.

SHADE COLLECTION 5

Globba winitii	34400	(Page 49)
Globba globulifera	34250	(Page 49)
Kaempferia gilbertii	35850	(Page 58)
Kaempferia B. Peacock	35950	(Page 59)
Kaempferia Silver Spot	36000	(Page 59)
(Rhizomes) catalog price		$29.75
31004 Collection Price		**$24.75**
Save $5.00		

Only 1 collection per customer.

RARE GINGER COLLECTION 5

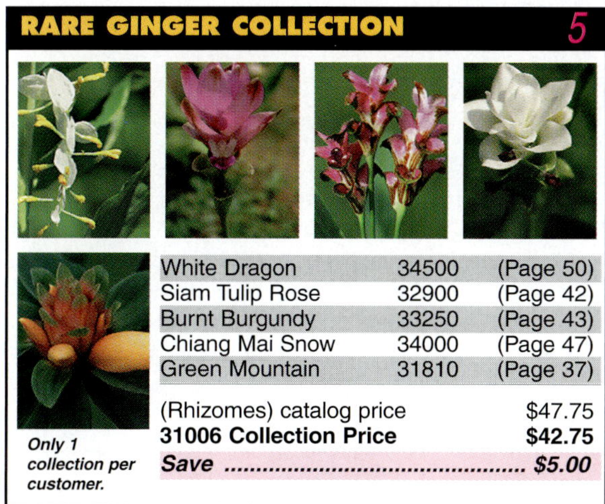

White Dragon	34500	(Page 50)
Siam Tulip Rose	32900	(Page 42)
Burnt Burgundy	33250	(Page 43)
Chiang Mai Snow	34000	(Page 47)
Green Mountain	31810	(Page 37)
(Rhizomes) catalog price		$47.75
31006 Collection Price		**$42.75**
Save $5.00		

Only 1 collection per customer.

FRAGRANT COLLECTION 6

Coronarium	34900	(Page 51)
Kahili	35100	(Page 52)
Filagree	35670	(Page 53)
Kinkaku	35500	(Page 54)
Kewense	35450	(Page 54)
Ayo	34650	(Page 52)
(Rhizomes) catalog price		$59.70
31002 Collection Price		**$54.70**
Save $5.00		

Only 1 collection per customer.

Gingers

SPIRAL GINGER COLLECTION 5

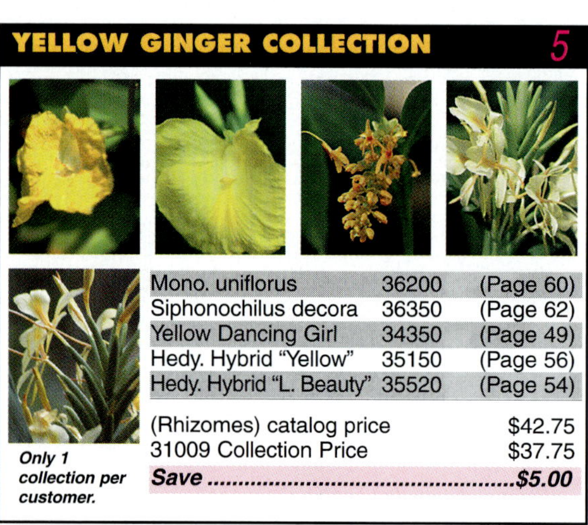

Spicatus	32550	(Page 39)
Barbatus	31750	(Page 37)
Pictus	32050	(Page 38)
Cuspidatus	31900	(Page 37)
Speciosus	32450	(Page 38)
(Rhizomes) catalog price		$38.75
31008 Collection Price		**$33.75**
Save *$5.00*		

Only 1 collection per customer.

VARIEGATED GINGER COLLECTION 5

Curcuma petiolata var.	33600	(Page 45)
Alp. zerumbet var.	31500	(Page 35)
Zingiber zerumbet var.	37000	(Page 65)
Costus speciosus var.	32500	(Page 39)
Costus amazonicus	31700	(Page 36)
(Rhizomes) catalog price		$47.75
31007 Collection Price		**$42.75**
Save *$5.00*		

Only 1 collection per customer.

YELLOW GINGER COLLECTION 5

Mono. uniflorus	36200	(Page 60)
Siphonochilus decora	36350	(Page 62)
Yellow Dancing Girl	34350	(Page 49)
Hedy. Hybrid "Yellow"	35150	(Page 56)
Hedy. Hybrid "L. Beauty"	35520	(Page 54)
(Rhizomes) catalog price		$42.75
31009 Collection Price		$37.75
Save *$5.00*		

Only 1 collection per customer.

MULTI-COLOR GINGER 5

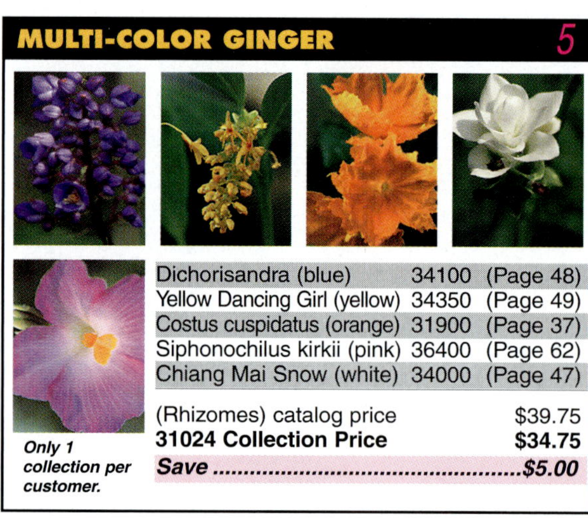

Dichorisandra (blue)	34100	(Page 48)
Yellow Dancing Girl (yellow)	34350	(Page 49)
Costus cuspidatus (orange)	31900	(Page 37)
Siphonochilus kirkii (pink)	36400	(Page 62)
Chiang Mai Snow (white)	34000	(Page 47)
(Rhizomes) catalog price		$39.75
31024 Collection Price		**$34.75**
Save *$5.00*		

Only 1 collection per customer.

EDIBLE GINGER COLLECTION 5

Kaempferia galanga	35800	(Page 58)
Curcuma domestica	33100	(Page 43)
Curcuma zedoaria	34050	(Page 47)
Zingiber mioga	36600	(Page 63)
Zingiber officinale	36700	(Page 64)
(Rhizomes) catalog price		$50.75
31013 Collection Price		$45.75
Save *$5.00*		

Only 1 collection per customer.

Put yourself or a friend on our mailing list. A phone call is all it takes to bring the beautiful STOKES TROPICALS' Plant Guide/Catalog into your home —or a friend's home. Free! For just $7.95 charged to your credit card or a personal check you get the catalog with a guarantee of $7.95 free merchandise with your first purchase. So in effect the catalog is free. Our catalogs are becoming a collector's item because of their scientific value as a pictorial and descriptive reference of rare tropical plants. Foreign catalogs will be $7.95 & actual cost of postage.

HELICONIAS

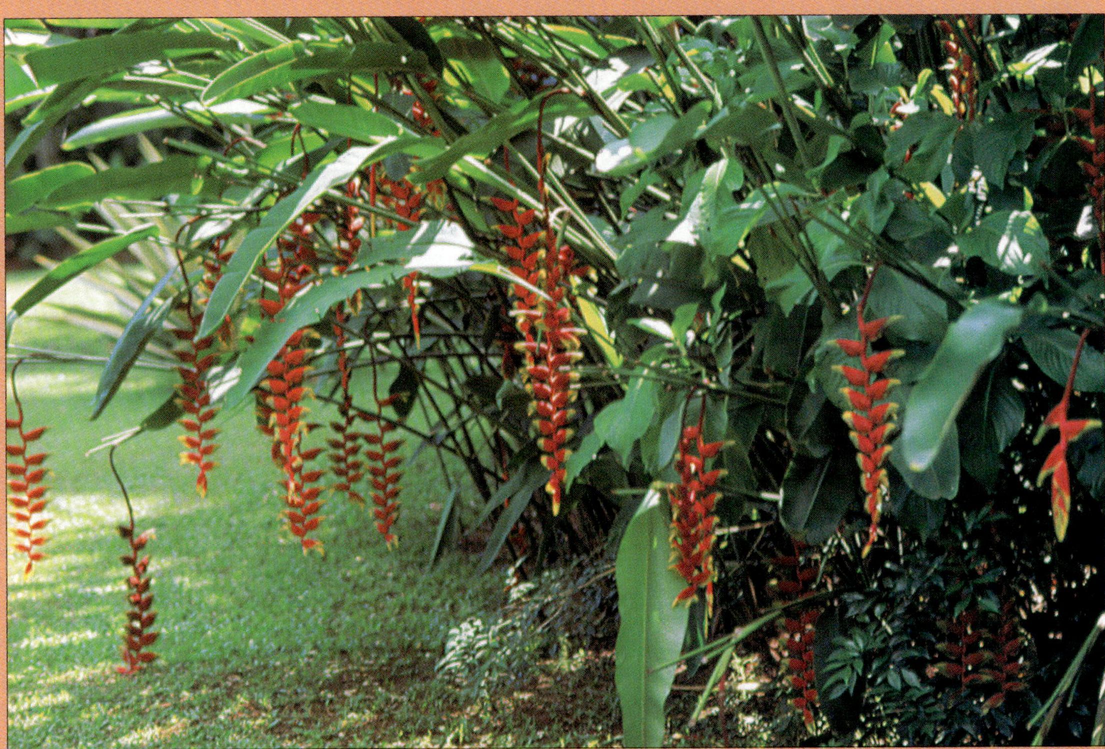

HELICONIAS are remarkable tropical plants of princely dimension with great stems and leaves and beautiful ornamental flowers. Heliconias are native to Central America, the Caribbean islands, South America, and some of the islands of the South Pacific. However their easy growth and brilliant and exotic show have made them favorite garden subjects throughout the tropics and subtropics.

They are becoming increasingly popular as landscaping plants and also as potted plants and cut flowers in regions where they cannot be garden grown. There are over 450 species, varieties, hybrids and cultivars of heliconia. Depending on variety, heliconias will range in height from two to twenty feet, often with extensive rhizomatous growth. The flower or inflorescence of heliconias is nearly always terminal and may last from several days to several months. The inflorescence bracts are usually red, yellow or both, but they are sometimes green or even pink. Heliconias like water, rich soil, and sunlight. They can be grown in any area where temperatures do not fall below 40 degrees F. (4.4 Celsius) for any length of time. The smaller heliconia varieties can be grown as indoor potted plants or in any atrium environment where ideally, temperatures are maintained in the 60° F (18.5 Celsius) to 70° F (28.66 Celsius) range. Heliconias are generally free of diseases.

Heliconias make exceptional cut flowers, cut stems, and cut leaves. Every swimming pool should have a heliconia because of its tropical and exotic form, its grace in movement produced by breezes, and its exceptional reflections. Stokes Tropicals' Heliconia blend (9-3-6) is a good fertilizer source for these fantastic plants.

Heliconias are an excellent choice for a container plant that can be grown indoors for the winter and outdoors during the summer. Heliconias derive their beauty from highly modified leaves or bracts. Thus we cannot call a heliconia bloom a flower; it is actually an inflorescence or cluster of bracts. Dogwood, artichokes, proteas, poinsettias and other plants similarly display colorful bracts. Heliconias as cut flowers are particularly desirable because of their long lasting characteristics. The following heliconia varieties have been selected for their easy-to-bloom quality in an ordinary household pot.

Heliconias

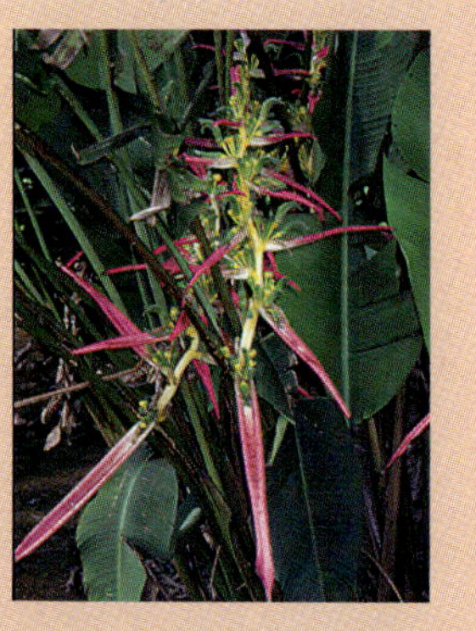

HELICONIA AEMYGDIANA
'Lavender Storm'

A magnificent pendulous heliconia from Peru that grows 4'-6' tall. Blooms year-round. A must for collectors. Zone 10 and higher. New.
41160 Rhizome...........................$24.95
41161 Growing Plant (6" pot)....$31.95

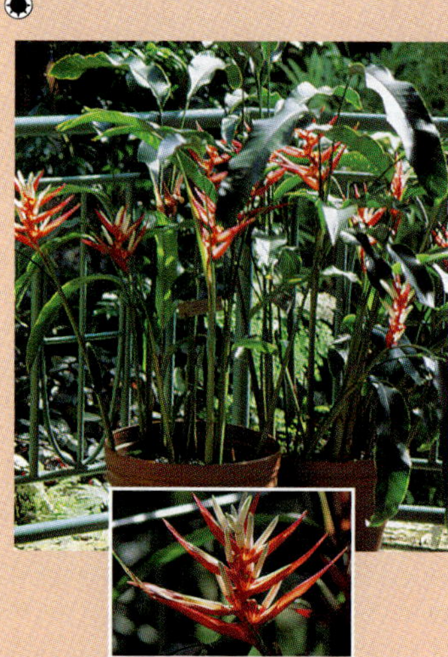

HELICONIA ANGUSTA
'Red Holiday'

A miraculous cultivar of Heliconia angusta from Brazil. Bracts are a deep, blood-red with soft white flowers. Blooms during the holiday (Christmas and New Years) season, hence the name. A short plant (1'-2') that prefers shade. Zone 9 and higher. An absolutely delightful plant for the holiday season.
41330 Rhizome.............................$9.95
41331 Growing Plant (6" pot)...$16.95

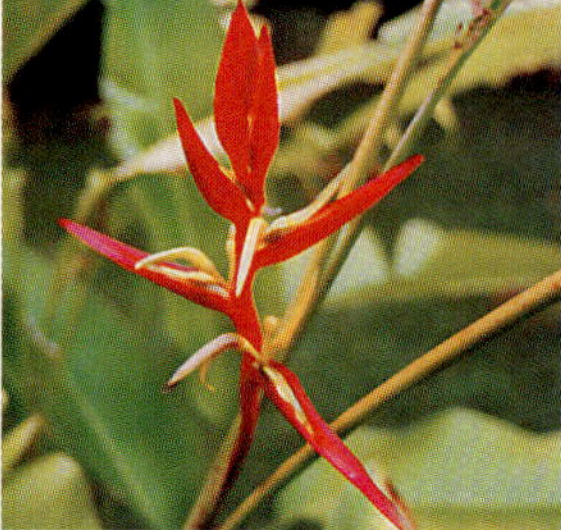

HELICONIA AFF. SCHEIDEANA
'Fire and Ice' ™

An amazing new heliconia that was collected from northern Mexico at high elevation. Has survived fires, snow and ice. A real horticultural breakthrough. Now for first time, a heliconia will survive in the ground outside in Zone 9 and possibly Zone 8. Plant is even more attractive because it is short (4' to 5'), compact, and erect in growth. Blooms in early spring. Full sun to 20% shade. Very limited supply.
41170 Rhizome...............................$49.95   *41171 Growing Plant (6" pot)* $59.95

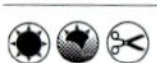

HELICONIA ANGUSTA
'Orange Christmas'

A magnificent cultivar of *Heliconia angusta* from Brazil. Blooms during "Christmas" period, thus its name. Has wonderful rich orange bracts from which emerge soft white flowers. A short plant growing 1'-2'. Brightens your Christmas season. Zone 9 and higher. Prefers shade. Very limited supply.
41340 Rhizome $12.95
41341 Bareroot Plant $19.95

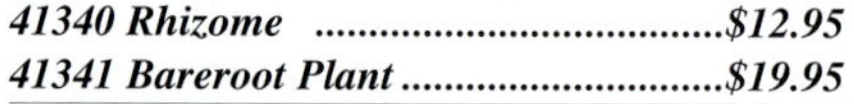

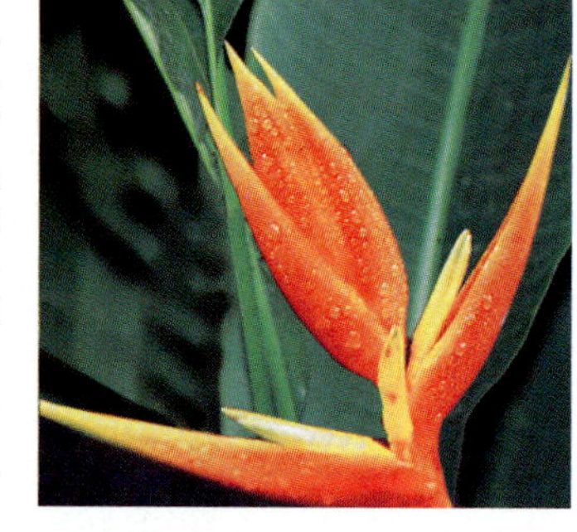

HELICONIA ANGUSTA
'Yellow Christmas'

Another of the 3 delightful *angusta* cultivars, also from Brazil, that has yellow bracts with soft white flowers. Blooms during the Christmas season. Prefers shade. A short (1'-2') plant with small dark green leaves. Zone 9 and higher. Very limited supply.
41320 Rhizome $19.95
41321 Growing Plant (6" pot) $26.95

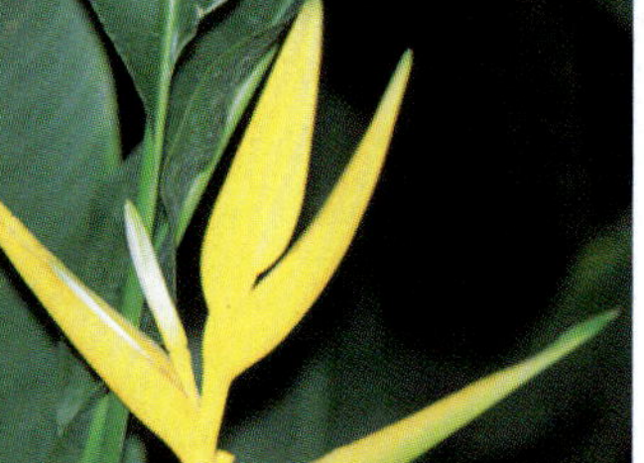

HELICONIA CARIBEA X BIHAI
'Bubble Gum'

A marvelous new heliconia with wonderful bubblegum-colored bracts. Grows 8'-10'. Flowers year round. Zone 10 and higher. New.
41370 Rhizome $44.95
41371 Growing Plant (6" pot) $51.95

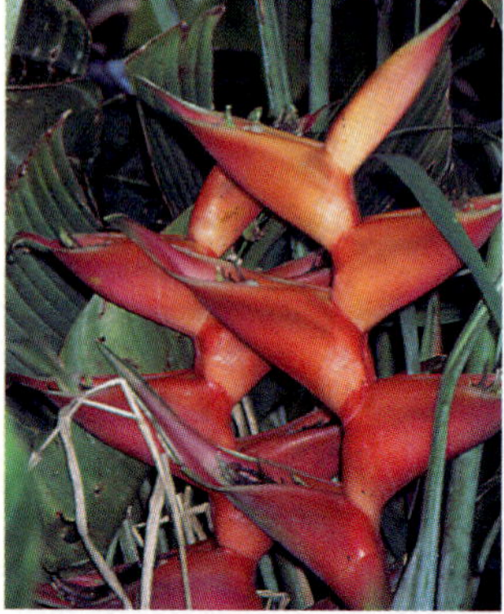

ALL STOKES TROPICALS' PLANTS ARE EASY-TO-GROW.

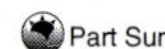 Full Sun   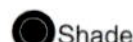 Part Sun   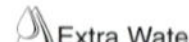 Shade   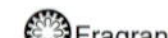 Extra Water   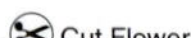 Fragrant   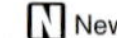 Cut Flower   New

TO ORDER CALL **1-800-624-9706**/24 HRS. OR VISIT OUR WEB SITE: www. stokestropicals.com

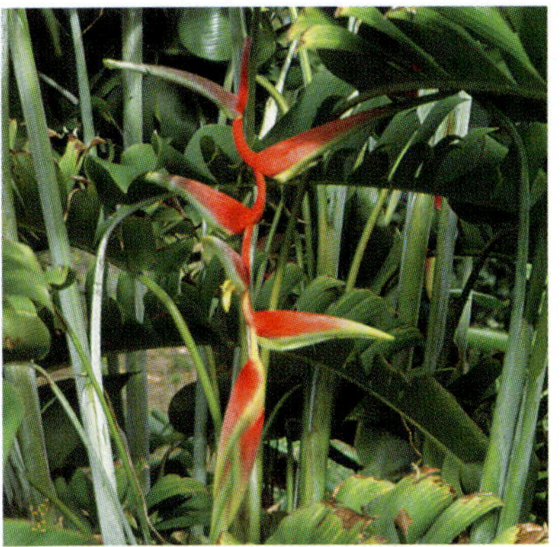

HELICONIA CHARTACEA X PLATYSTACHYS 'Temptress'

A miraculous pendulous heliconia that grows 10'-12'. Flowers year round. A very vigorous plant. Zone 10 and higher. New.

41380 Rhizome *$29.95*
41381 Growing Plant (6" pot) ..*$37.95*

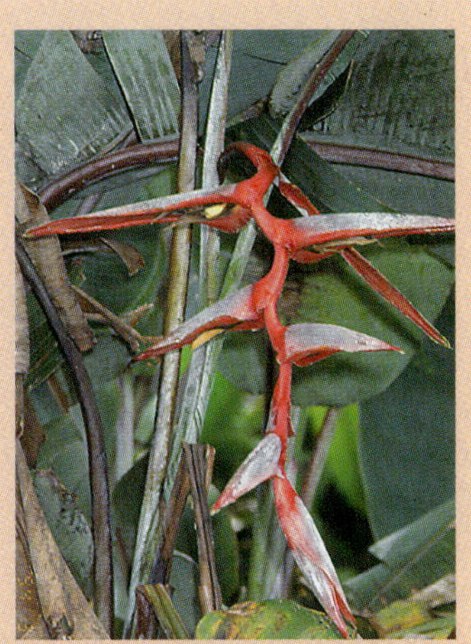

HELICONIA EPISCOPALIS

A different looking heliconia in that its inflorescence consists of tightly overlapping bracts with flowers squeezing out between them; it is flat and pointed like an arrowhead. Native of Amazonia in S.A. Blooms all year in warm areas. Medium size $2^{1}/_{2}$-7' (75cm) to (2.1m). Grows in full sun to 70% shade. Bracts are suffused with yellow, orange-yellow and red that are delicately blended together.

41300 Rhizome *$10.95*
41301 Growing Plant (6" pot) *$17.95*

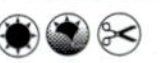

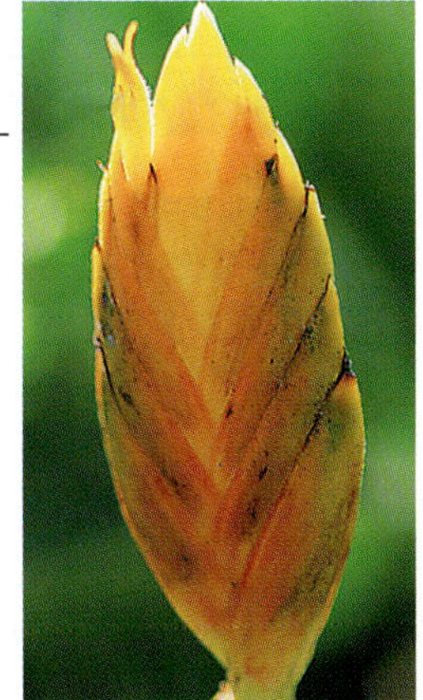

HELICONIA GRIGGSIANA 'Angry Moon'

A spectacular large heliconia with pendulous inflorescence. Grows 8'-10'. Makes a great cut flower. Zone 10 and higher. New.

41140 Rhizome *$39.95*
41141 Growing Plant (6" pot) *$47.95*

HELICONIA FARINOSA 'Rio'

What a spectacular new heliconia. Erect inflorescence with dark red bracts containing creamy yellow florets. Grows 6'-7'. Flowers year round. Zone 10 and higher. New.

41130 Rhizome *$15.95*
41131 Growing Plant (6" pot) *$22.95*

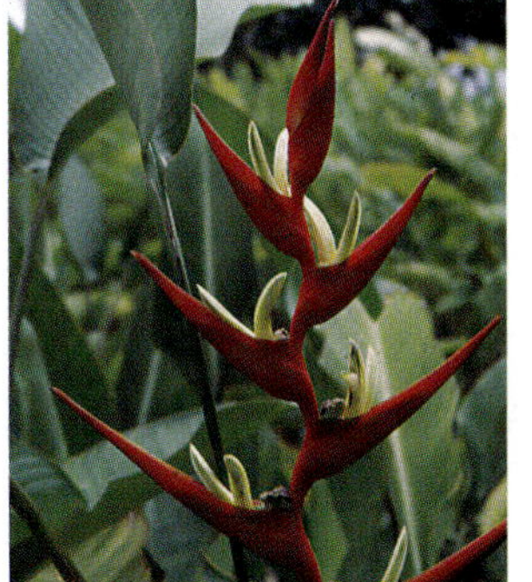

HELICONIA GLORIOSA 'Satin Glory'

A very special heliconia from Peru. Grows 6'-8'. Flowers the year round. One of the rarest heliconia in the world. Inflorescence is different from all other heliconias. Zone 10 and higher. Dark green satin foliage with purple undersides. New.

41020 Rhizome *$249.95*
41021 Growing Plant (6" pot) *$275.95*

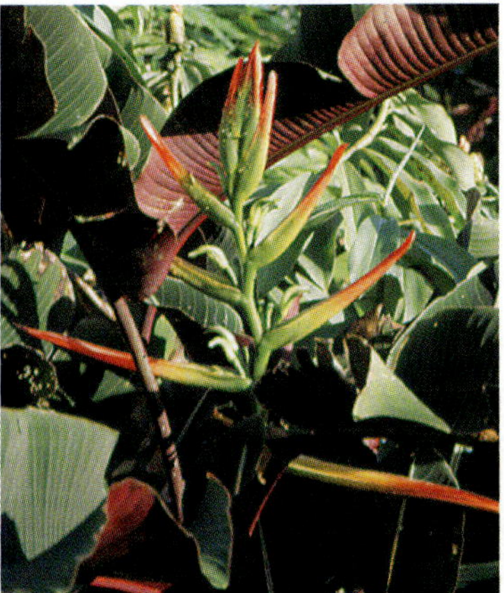
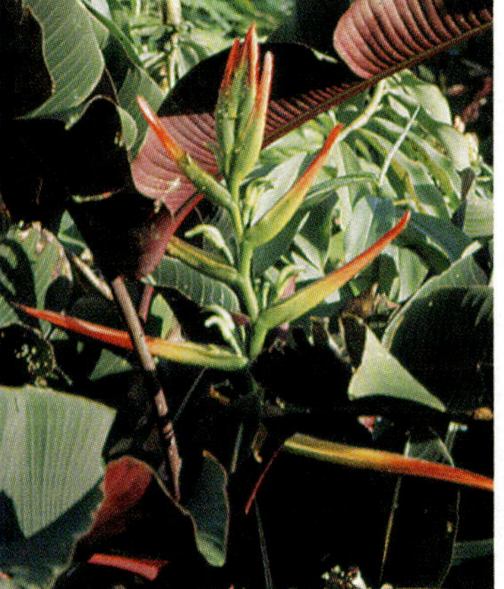
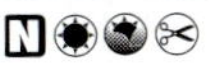

HELICONIA: AN IDENTIFICATION GUIDE

By Fred Berry and W. John Kress
1991 334 pp.

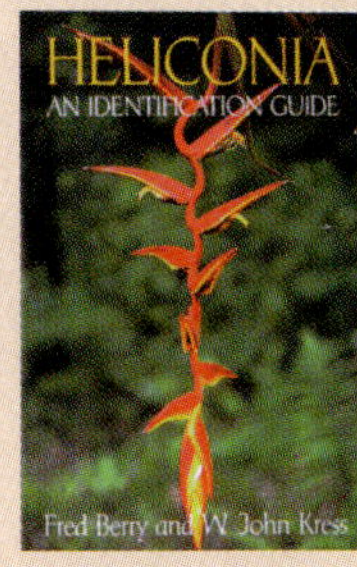

The bible on heliconia by two of the world's authorities on heliconia. Two hundred different varieties of heliconia are covered in this handy handbook-size publication. An absolute must for the heliconia grower and enthusiast.

75000 ....*$21.00*

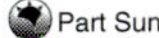 Full Sun   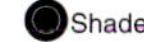 Part Sun   Shade   Extra Water   Fragrant   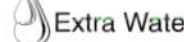 Cut Flower   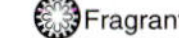 New

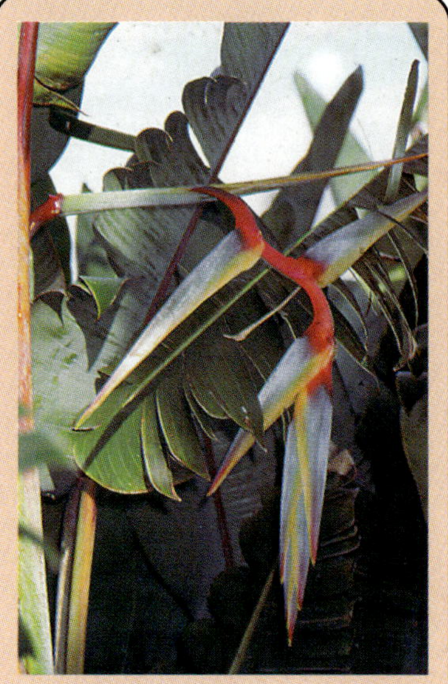

HELICONIA GRIGGSIANA
'Full Moon'

A spectacular large heliconia with pendulous inflorescence. Grows 8'-10'. Makes a great cut flower. Zone 10 and higher. New.

41180 Rhizome $39.95
41181 Growing Plant (6" pot)....$47.95

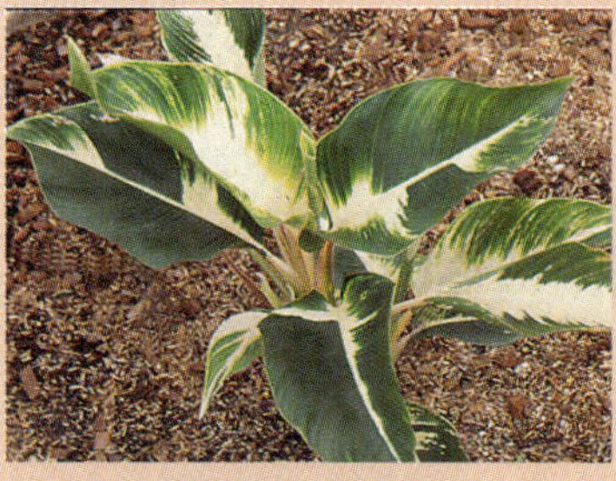

HELICONIA INDICA
'Bangkok'

A spectacular variegated form of indica that only grows 4'-6' high. Strikingly colored leaves are main features. Seldom flowers. Zone 10 and higher. New.

41390 Rhizome $29.95
41391 Growing Plant (6" pot)....$37.95

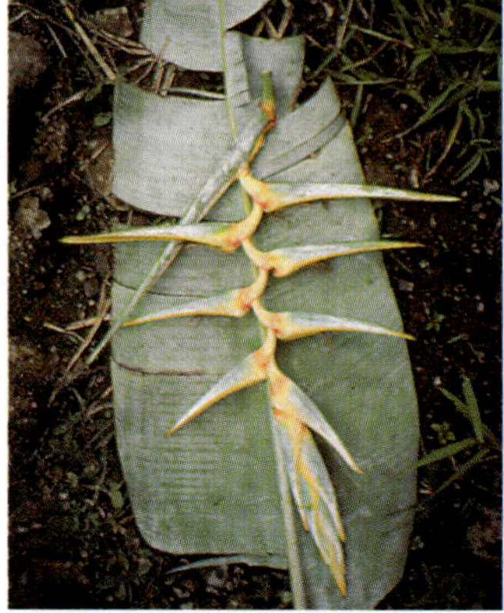

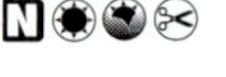

HELICONIA GRIGGSIANA
'Harvest Moon'

A spectacular large heliconia with pendulous inflorescence. Grows 8'-10'. Makes a great cut flower. Zone 10 and higher. New.

41190 Rhizome $39.95
41191 Growing Plant (6" pot) $47.95

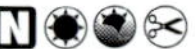

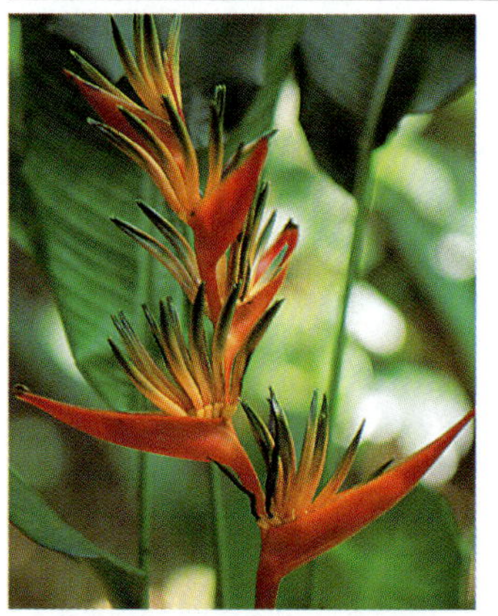

HELICONIA NICKERIENSIS
(H. PSITTACORUM X H. MARGINATA)

A very nice medium size heliconia species that grows from 4' (1.2m) to 8' (2.4m) in full sun to 40% shade. Blooms from June to November. Native to Guyana and Suriname. Classic looking inflorescence with 5-9 bracts that are pink-red in color over most of keel and cheek with yellow on lip, tip and, small part of base. Sepals gold in color.

41050 Rhizome $12.95
41051 Growing Plant (6" pot) $19.95

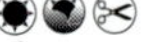

HELICONIA GRIGGSIANA
'Blue Moon'

A spectacular large heliconia with pendulous inflorescence. Grows 8'-10'. Makes a great cut flower. Zone 10 and higher. New.

41210 Rhizome $39.95
41211 Growing Plant (6" pot) $47.95

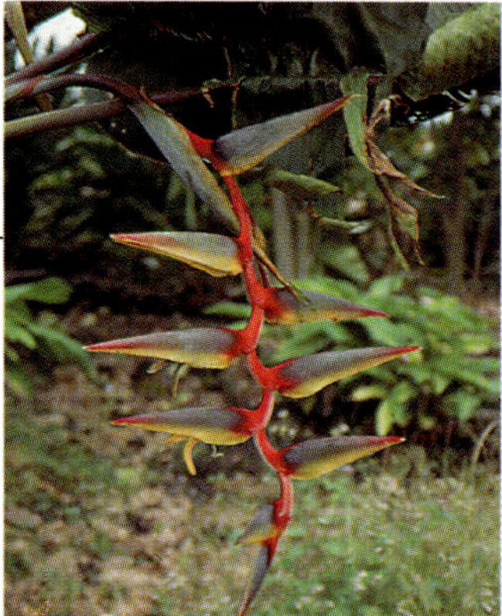

HELICONIA GUYANA

In some people's mind one of the most beautiful heliconias. Bracts are wide and stout with rich red keels with orange edges, literally stuffed with flowers. Sepals light yellow proximally then darkening to butter yellow distally with emerald green bands at tips. Bracts smartly arranged spirally around reddish orange peduncle (stem). Medium size plant reaching 5' (1.5m) to 6' (1.8m). Vigorous grower. Full sun to medium shade.

41030 Rhizome $12.95
41031 Growing Plant (6" pot) $19.95

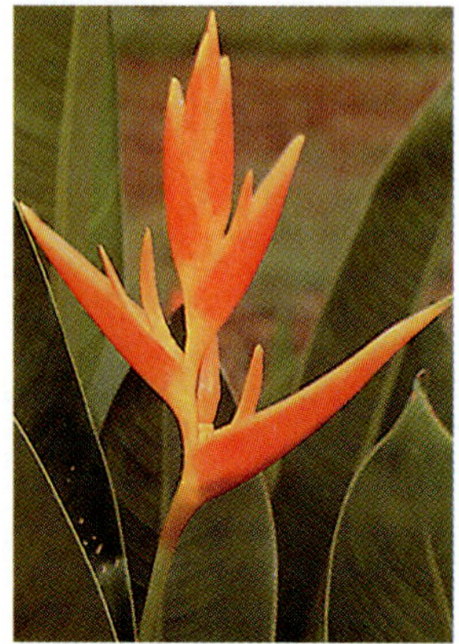

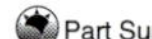 Full Sun   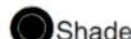 Part Sun   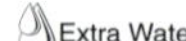 Shade   Extra Water   Fragrant   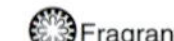 Cut Flower   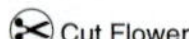 New

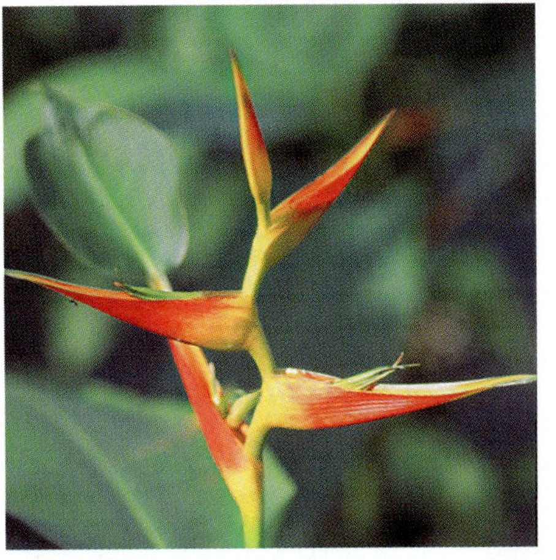

HELICONIA LATISPATHA CV. 'Distans'

A superb-looking heliconia with bracts that are spirally arranged. Blooms all year with an April-to-September peak. Semi-dwarf 1½'-5½' high. Easy to bloom in a pot. Full sun to 40% shade. Bracts are red on distal half and yellow proximally with pale yellow-green sepals. Zone 10 and higher.

41040 Rhizome *$9.95*
41041 Growing Plant
(6" pot)................................*$16.95*

HELICONIA LINGULATA

A beautiful heliconia with bracts displayed in a single plane. Blooms all year with spring and late summer peaks. Medium to full sun. Grows 5'-7' tall. Zone 10 and higher.

41110 Rhizome *$13.95*
41111 Growing Plant (6" pot) *$20.95*

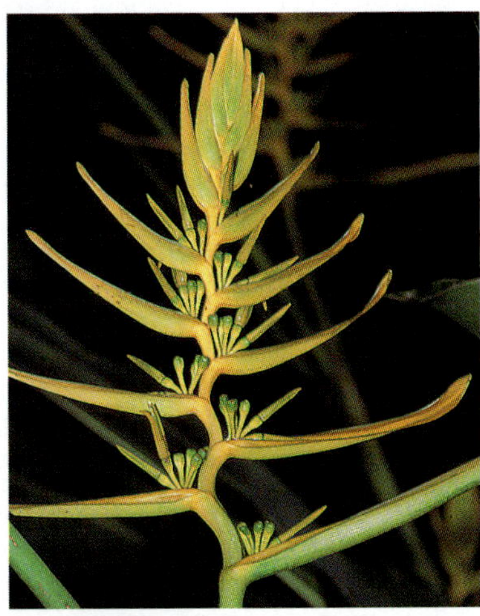

SAVE $10.00

Save off listed prices by buying a collection. See page 79..

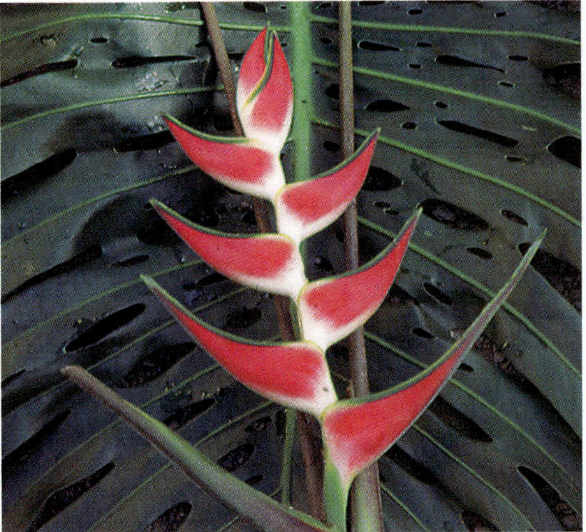

HELICONIA ORTHOTRICA 'Imperial'

A spectacular heliconia that grows to 5'-7' and flowers year round. From Ecuador. A great cut flower. Zone 10 and higher. New.

41120 Rhizome . *$24.95*
41121 Growing Plant
(6" pot) *$31.95*

FLOWERING TROPICALS BLEND (7-9-5)

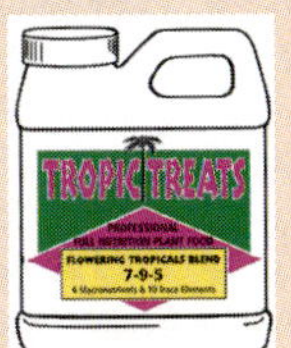

An excellent general purpose nutrient solution with 6 macronutrients and 10 essential trace elements that all our need. This growth formula will give your tropicals healthy leaf and stem growth; also works well for vegetables, fruits and lawns. Use as a rapid cure for nutrient deficiencies! Mixed at dilute concentrations Flowering Tropical Blend is quick acting as a foliar spray. It is ideal for poor soils and container- grown plants. The low soluble salts and slightly higher phosphorus makes this a great all-year tropical plant formula for those who don't want to switch formulas to promote flowering. Works well on African violets, orchids and houseplants in general.

6070 (8 oz) bottle **$5.00**
6071 (Qt.) bottle **$10.75**

MULTI METER

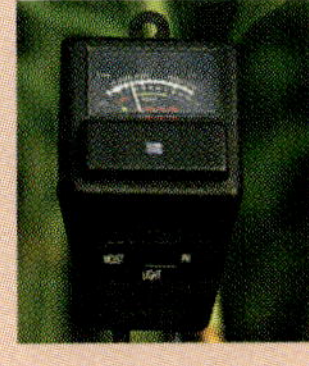

This meter has a 3-setting switch that lets you test light, moisture and pH for indoors and out. No battery required.

80100......................................*$19.95*

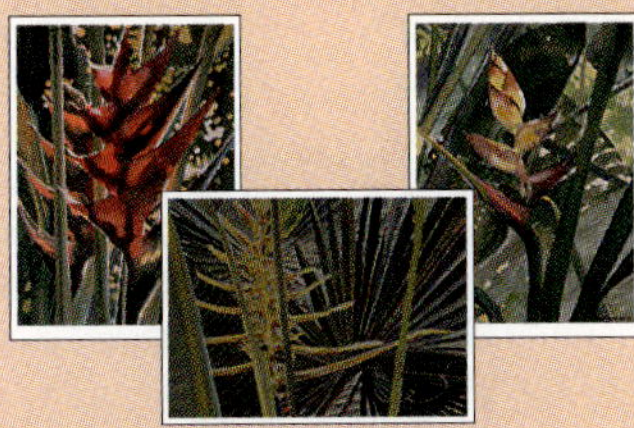

GREETING CARDS (5X7)

Breathtaking watercolor images of 6 species of Heliconia. Packed in sets of 6, with envelopes included.

9000 set of 6...........................*$12.00*

Heliconias

PSITTACORUMS

The psittacorum (or parrot's beak) heliconias are small, dainty and exotically tropical. They bloom abundantly all year. "Flower heads" appear to be handpainted and glow with brilliant colors. The psittacorums rarely exceed 3' (90cm) to 5' (1.5m) in height. The floral bracts arise from the same point on the stem with psittacorums. They resemble birds-of-paradise more than other heliconias. Bright, banded florets curve gracefully with the bracts for added visual appeal. Psittacorums don't seem to mind cool temperatures as much as other heliconias, but do best in warm, humid areas or micro environments. The cut inflorescence lasts 2 to 3 weeks. Cutting the bracts before 8:00 a.m. and immediately submersing the "cut end" in water along with recutting every few days extends their life. The Psittacorum is fast becoming a darling of the floriculture trade. If you only have room for a little bit of the tropics, a psittacorum fits the bill perfectly requiring little space and little care and produces large rewards.

HELICONIAS: LLAMARADAS DE LA SELVA COLOMBIANA

By John Kress, Julio Betaneur, Beatriz Echeverry
1999 200 pp.

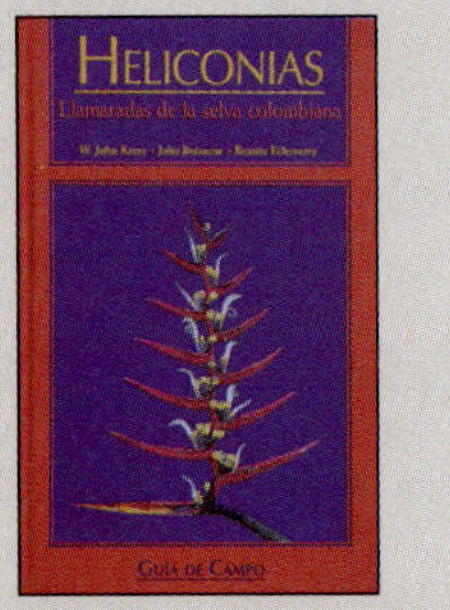

73950 ....$40.00
See page 128 for details.

HELICONIA PSITTACORUM CV. 'Andromeda'

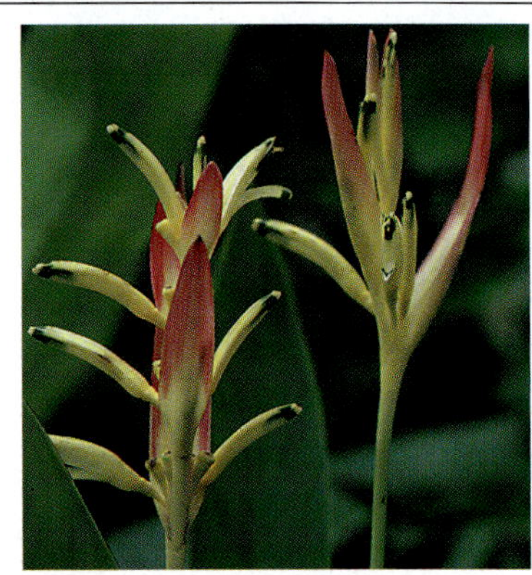

The 'Andromeda' is a very attractive semi-dwarf bursting with orange-red shading to pink bracts and white frosting color at base of green tips. Sepals orange with distal metallic black or green band and orange tips. Flowers are very long lasting. Blooms all year in full sun to 50% shade. Height 4' to 5'. Most cold hardy of psittacorums.
41100 Rhizome $9.95
41101 Growing Plant (6" pot) $17.95

HELICONIA PSITTACORUM CV. 'Blush'

'Blush' has delicately colored bracts, light pink distally with cream pale green proximally. Sepals are gorgeous yellow with dark green band and yellow tip. Blooms all year in full sun to 50% shade. Height 3' (90cm) to 5' (1.5m).
41150 Rhizome $9.95
41151 Growing Plant (6" pot) $17.95

HELICONIA PSITTACORUM CV. 'Choconiana'

'Choconiana' blooms all year. Grows up to 5' (1.5m); in pots 2' (60cm) to 3' (90cm). Has beautiful orange inflorescence with orange bracts and orange sepals with distal black bands and yellow and white tips. Flowers are long lasting. Full sun to 50% shade. Originally from the Guianas.
41200 Rhizome $9.95
41201 Growing Plant (6" pot) $17.95

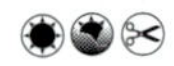

HELICONIA PSITTACORUM CV. 'Double B Red'

A very striking cultivar with an outstanding inflorescence. Obtained from Guyana. Long, stout bracts that are deep red, both inside and outside, with rounded points. Sepals are yellowish green with distal dark green bands and white tips. Full sun to 50% shade.
41250 Rhizome $10.95
41251 Growing Plant (6" pot) $18.95

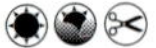

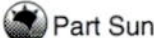 Full Sun   Part Sun   Shade   Extra Water   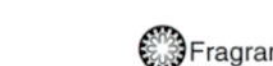 Fragrant   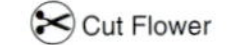 Cut Flower   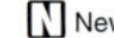 New

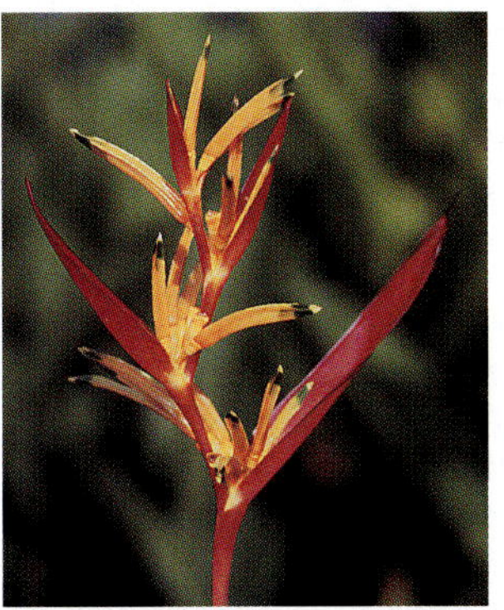

HELICONIA PSITTACORUM CV. 'Kathy'

This is rapidly becoming one of our most popular psittacorums. It's long dark-red bracts filled with orange florets tipped with dark green bands and the outstanding open architecture of the inflorescence all combine to make it a dynamite plant. Grows 2'-4' in height. Blooms April to November in full sun to 40% shade. Zone 10 and higher.

41260 Rhizome *$10.95*
41261 Growing Plant (6" pot) *$18.95*

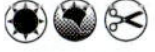

HELICONIA PSITTACORUM CV. 'Keanea Red'

A majestic new psittacorum hybrid from Hawaii. What a dramatic statement: deep red bracts filled with tangerine-colored florets. A great addition to the parrot's beak group of dwarf heliconias. Grows from 4'- 5'. Full sun to 40% shade. Zone 10 and higher.

41220 Rhizome *$10.95*
41221 Growing Plant (6" pot) *$18.95*

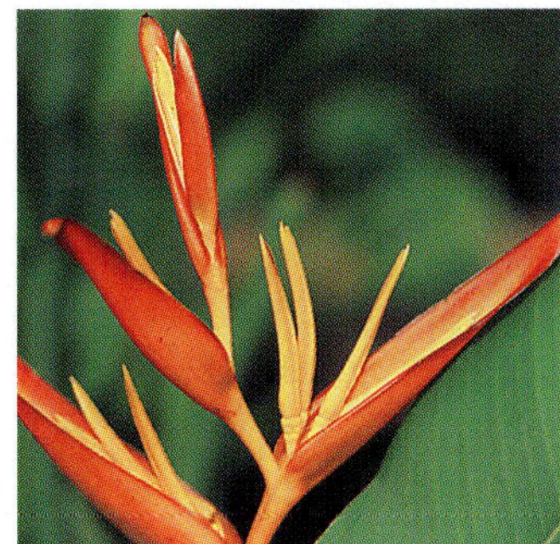

HELICONIA PSITTACORUM CV. 'Lady Di'

'Lady Di' may be the most beautiful of the psittacorums, with dark rose red bracts and cream—yellow sepals with dark green bands and white tips which create a dramatic color display. Grows 2' (60cm) to 5' (1.5m) in height. Long lasting blooms on stalks that are only 8 weeks old. Blooms April to November in full sun to 40% shade.

41350 Rhizome *$9.95*
41351 Growing Plant (6" pot) *$17.95*

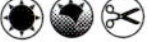

HELICONIA PSITTACORUM CV. 'Petra'

Has one of the largest inflorescences of the psittacorums. Its inflorescence is a larger version of an 'Andromeda'. We obtained this outstanding cultivar from Guyana. Sepals are bright orange with black bands distally and yellow orange tips. One of our best sellers. Full sun to 50% shade.

41500 Rhizome *$9.95*
41501 Growing Plant (6" pot) *$17.95*

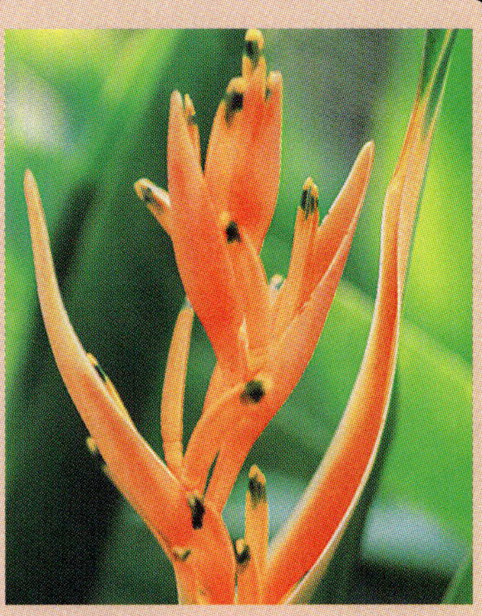

HELICONIA PSITTACORUM CV. 'Sherbet'

Our biggest selling psittacorum with its orange sherbet colors. Free flowering. Obtained from Puerto Rico. Very similar growth characteristics to 'Choconiana' except 1'-2' taller with larger inflorescence. If you like 'Choconiana,' you'll love 'Sherbet.' Zone 10 and higher.

41700 Rhizome *$9.95*
41701 Growing Plant (6" pot) *$17.95*

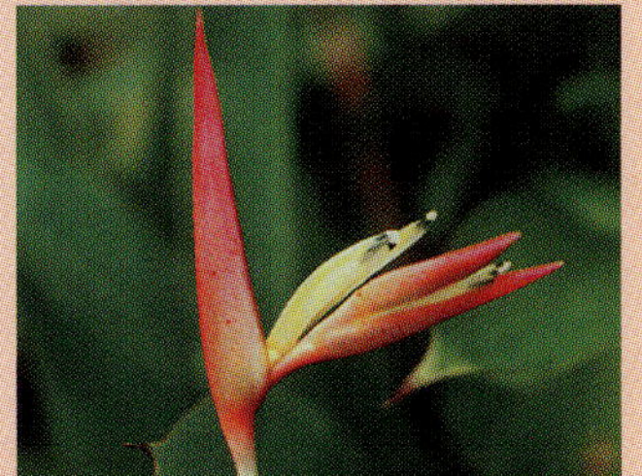

HELICONIA PSITTACORUM CV. 'Pinky'

A very beautiful cultivar with lovely pinkish bracts. Similar growing characteristics as the other psittacorums. Obtained from Hawaii. Bracts are delicate pinkish red with bases of keels pale yellow; sepals yellowish cream color with narrow green bands distally and white tips. Full sun to 50% shade.

41550 Rhizome *$9.95*
41551 Growing Plant (6" pot) *$17.95*

Heliconias

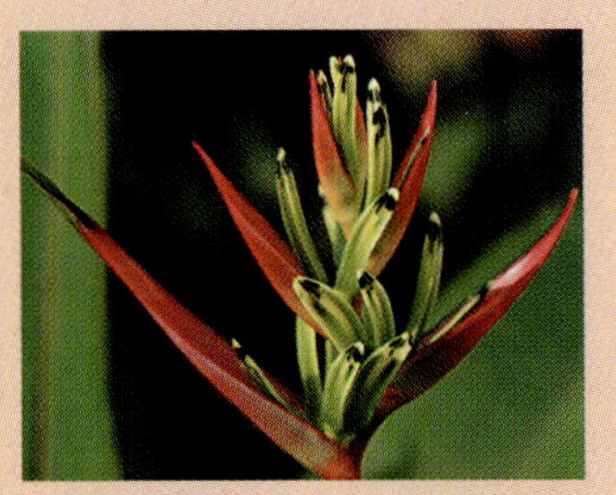

HELICONIA PSITTACORUM CV. 'Rosi'

'Rosi' is a nice cultivar with bracts rosy pink distally and light pink proximally. Sepals are beautiful light green with yellow cream stripes and dark green bands and cream tips. Blooms all year in full sun to 50% shade. Height 3' (90cm) to 6' (1.8m).

41600 Rhizome *$9.95*
41601 Growing Plant (6" pot)..$17.95

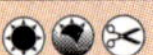

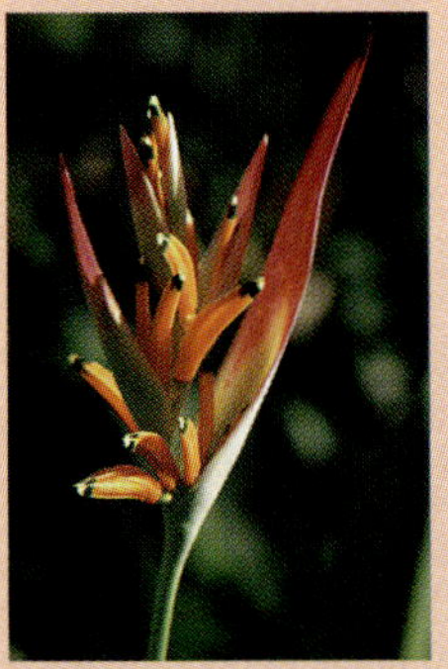

HELICONIA PSITTACORUM CV. 'Sassy'

Sassy is a wonderful variety with delicate coloring. Bracts are pale green or cream at base and reddish pink distally. Sepals are orange with distal green-black bands and white tips. Blooms from April to November. Grows 3' (90cm) to 5' (1.5m) in full sun to 40% shade.

41650 Rhizome............................*$9.95*
41651 Growing Plant (6" pot)..$17.95

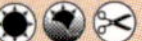

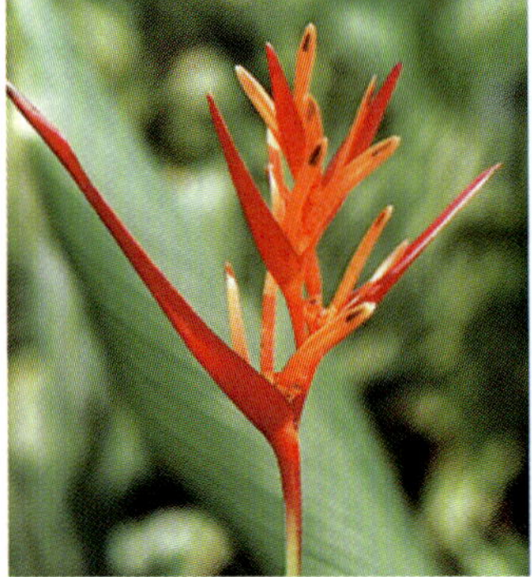

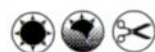

HELICONIA PSITTACORUM CV. 'Strawberries & Cream'

A very beautiful parrot's beak heliconia with a delicate distinctive inflorescence. Similar to other psittacorums in growth characteristics: blooms all year, 3'(90cm) to 5'(1.5m), full sun to 40% shade, and vigorous grower. Bracts strawberry colored distally and cream proximally. Sepals pale yellow with distal dark green bands and white tips. Obtained from Hawaii.

41800 Rhizome *$9.95*
41801 Growing Plant (6" pot) *$17.95*

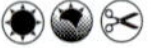

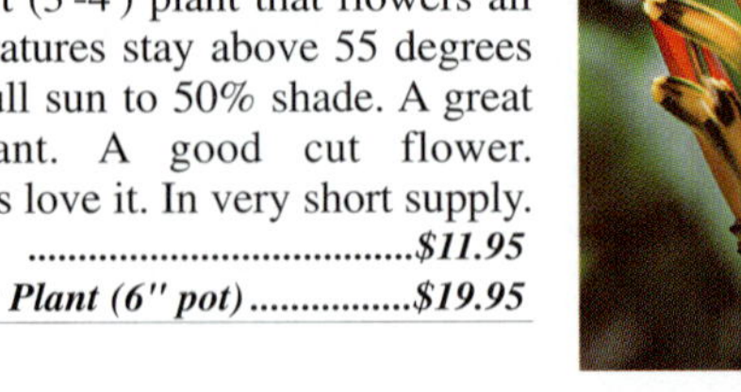

HELICONIA PSITTACORUM CV. 'Tangerine'

A marvelous dwarf psittacorum Heliconia. Small banana-like flowers are tinged in delicious tangerine and lime green. Bracts are beautifully shaded gold and orange. A very nice short (3'-4') plant that flowers all year if temperatures stay above 55 degrees F. Will take full sun to 50% shade. A great container plant. A good cut flower. Hummingbirds love it. In very short supply.

41830 Rhizome *$11.95*
41831 Growing Plant (6" pot) *$19.95*

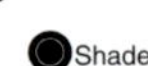

HELICONIA PSITTACORUM CV. 'St. Vincent Red'

'St. Vincent Red' is a very attractive variety similar to Andromeda but without the bract frosting and deep red color. The beautiful red color of the bracts blends into the stems. Flowers year-round on bright orange-red bracts. Grows 2 1/2' (75cm) to 6' (1.8m) in height. Full sun to 40% shade. Originally from island of St. Vincent.

41750 Rhizome *$11.95*
41751 Growing Plant (6" pot) *$19.95*

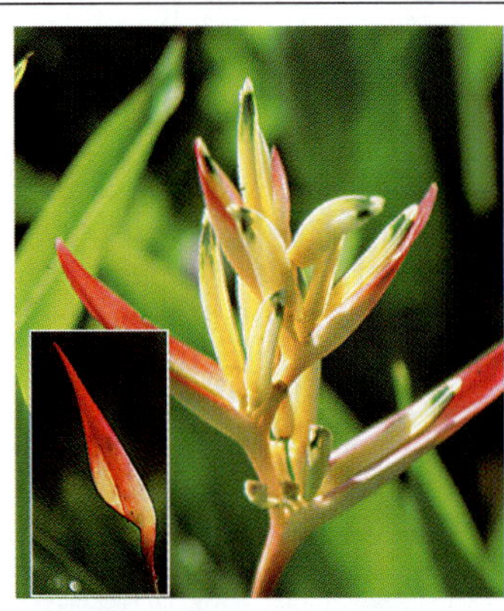

HELICONIA PSITTACORUM X SPATHO-CIRCINATA CV. 'Golden Torch'

'Golden Torch' has extremely large golden boat-shaped bracts with butter yellow flowers. Inflorescence like rigid golden sun rays with excellent color longevity and durable texture. Somewhat larger than most other psittacorums. 2½' (75cm) to 7' (2.1m) in height in full sun to 40% shade. Originally from Guyana.

41850 Rhizome *$9.95*
41851 Growing Plant (6" pot) *$17.95*

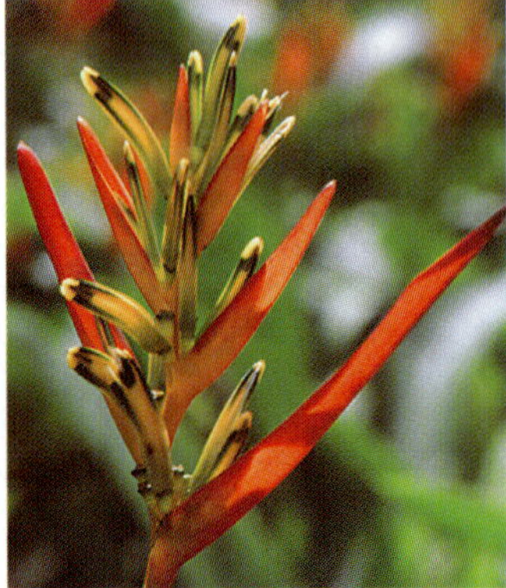

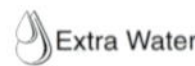
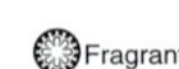

Full Sun   Part Sun   Shade   Extra Water   Fragrant   Cut Flower   N New

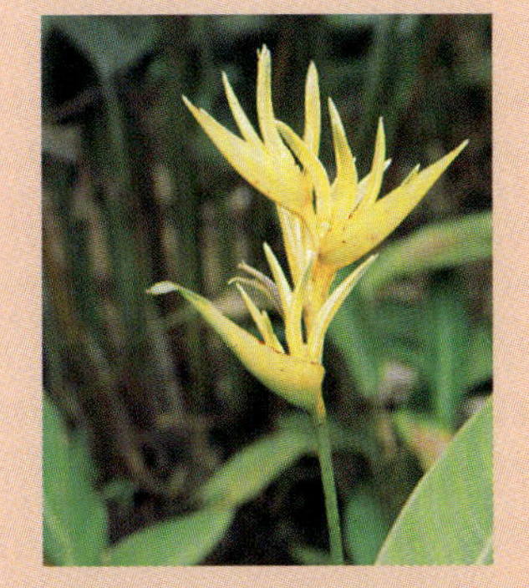

HELICONIA PSITTACORUM X SPATHO-CIRCINATA CV. 'Tortuga'

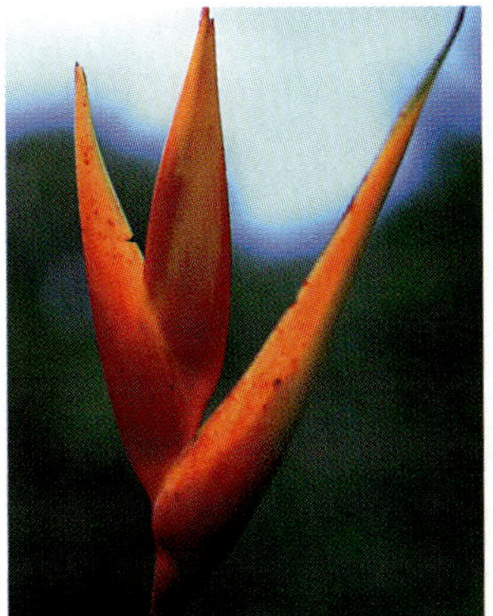

'Tortuga' is our introduction that is strikingly beautiful. Bracts fiery orange red at base with yellow-gold ends with splashes of red. Sepals golden yellow with faint green distally. Blooms all year in full sun to 20% shade. Grows to 3$1/2$' (1.05m) to 5' (1.5m) in height. Stems with dark red spots. Flowers are proudly held up above foliage.

41950 Rhizome *$11.95*
41951 Growing Plant (6" pot)........................*$19.95*

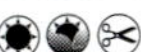

HELICONIA PSITTACORUM X SPATHOCIR-CINATA CV. 'Tropica'

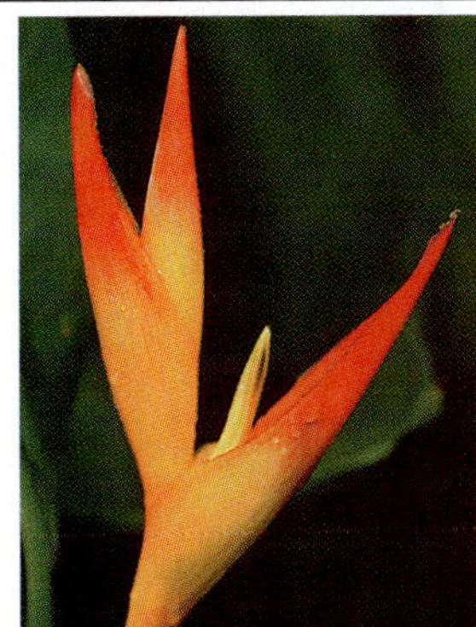

A visually appealing cultivar from Puerto Rico. Very similar to 'Golden Torch Adrian'. Blooms January to October. Grows to 5' (1.5m) in full sun to 20% in shade. Bracts pointed with outer bases golden yellow fading to reddish orange midway up bract. Sepals creamy yellow with wide dark distal bands that are barely showing through and with yellow tips.

42000 Rhizome *$11.95*
42001 Growing Plant (6" pot)........................*$19.95*

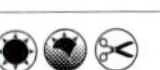

HELICONIA X SPATHOCIRCINATA CV. 'Richardiana'

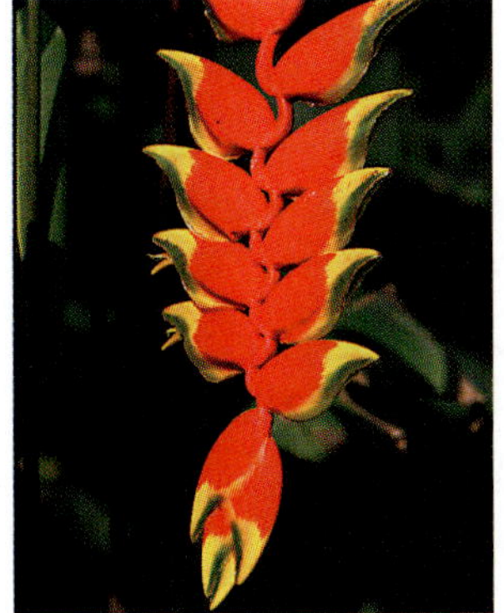

A very beautiful medium size heliconia species. Blooms from June to November. Reaches 3' to 6'. Grows in full sun to 40% shade. Distributed from Venezuela, through Guianas to eastern Brazil. Has 4-7 bracts that are yellow-green over most of bract with small red or pink-red area at base. Rachis is red or orange. Sepals light green with yellow flush bent abruptly backwards near base. Ovaries red.

42040 Rhizome *$11.95*
42041 Growing Plant (6" pot) *$19.95*

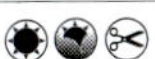

HELICONIA ROSTRATA

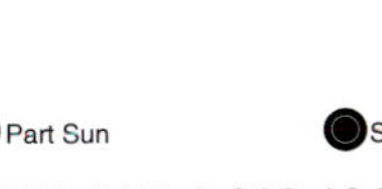

This traditional and most recognized heliconia is called 'Pendula Lobster Claw'. Blooms are pendulous or hanging up to 3' (90cm) in length with striking red and yellow bracts. Blooms all year. 3' to 10' in height. In pots will flower at 5' (1.5m) to 6' (1.8m). Full sun to 50% shade. Originally from the Amazon.

42050 Rhizome *$11.95*
42051 Growing Plant (6" pot) *$19.95*

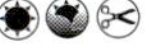

HELICONIA PSITTACORUM X SPATHOCIRCINATA 'Yellow Parrot'

A magnificent new form of 'Golden Torch'. Flowers year-round. Grows 3'-5'. Zone 10 and higher. New.

41870 Rhizome *$9.95*
41871 Growing Plant (6" pot)....*$16.95*

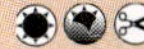

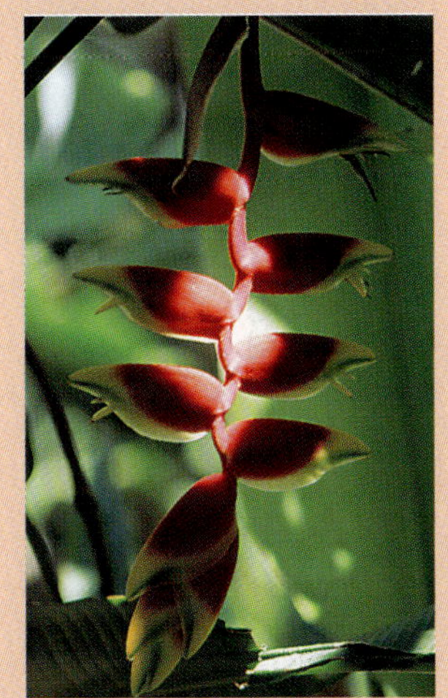

HELICONIA ROSTRATA 'Dwarf'

This is dwarf form of the standard *H. rostrata* that we recently obtained from Puerto Rico. It flowers easily at 5' to 6' and will flower in a pot. Has same appearance and growing characteristics as standard rostrata except its flower size is smaller. We are very excited about this new cultivar. Full sun to 50% shade.

42100 Rhizome..............................*$12.95*
42101 Growing Plant (6" pot)....*$20.95*

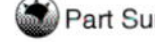 Full Sun   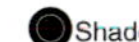 Part Sun   ● Shade   Extra Water   Fragrant   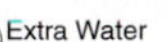 Cut Flower   N New

Heliconias

STRICTAS

The strictas have an exotic inflorescence that mimics shish kebobs of lobster claws. The crimson claws are rigid and retain their shape and color for weeks. Just as lobsters from different seas come in an array of shapes, sizes, colors, so do their floral counterparts. The lobster claws are one of the most diverse groups of the heliconias. Colors of inflorescence range from red, gold, orange, maroon, and green singularly or in combination. Smaller lobster claws are slimmer, shorter stemmed and more refined in shape than the larger lobster claws. There are several smaller lobster varieties whose bracts tend to be flat-sided rather than rounded. These exotic tropicals are ideal for small arrangements as their inflorescences range from 5" (12.5cm) to 12" (30cm) long and are not too heavy.

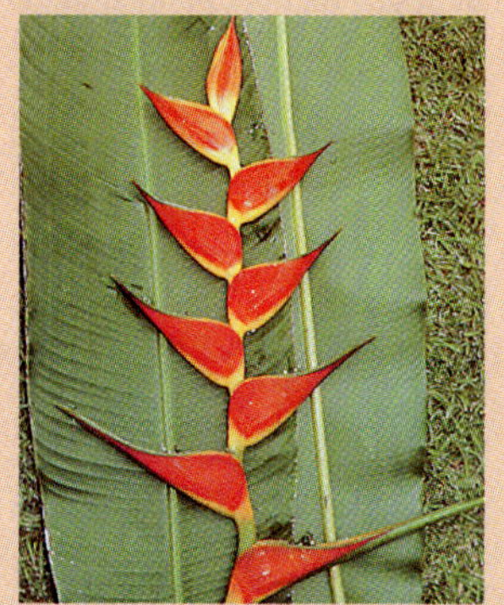

Photo with permission from Berry & Kress' *Heliconia: An Identification Guide.*

HELICONIA STRICTA 'Tagami'

A very sharp looking medium size heliconia with an inflorescence that is eyestopping. Plant grows to 4'-5' in containers. Inflorescence is erect with deep orange-red bracts that have basel keels painted yellow. Small florets peak from inside bracts. Good cut flower. medium to full sun. Zone 10 and higher.

42300 Rhizome............................$17.95
42301 Growing Plant (6" pot)....$24.95

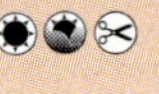

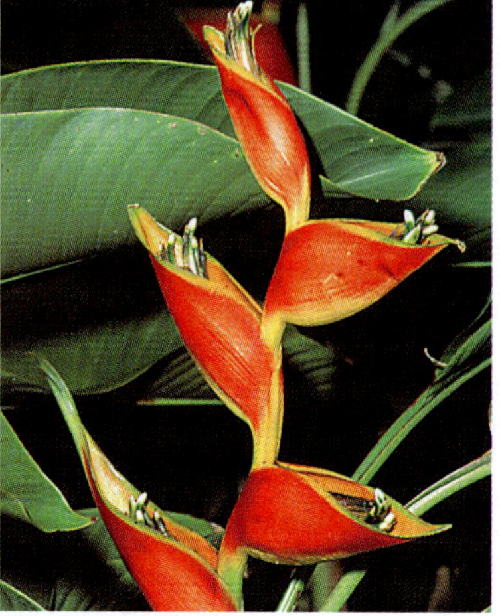

HELICONIA STRICTA CV. 'Dwarf Jamaican'

'Dwarf Jamaican' is a real beauty that is small 1½' (45cm) to 3' (90cm) high and does well in pots. Very beautiful 5" (12.5cm) dainty inflorescence that are deep rose-colored and evenly grade from pale to deep hues. Each bract is ridged with green on its upper edge, matching the tiny green and white striped sepals. Blooms year-round with a winter peak. Adapts beautifully to variable temperatures. Grows in full sun to 60% shade.

42150 Rhizome $9.95
42151 Growing Plant (6" pot) $17.95

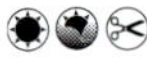

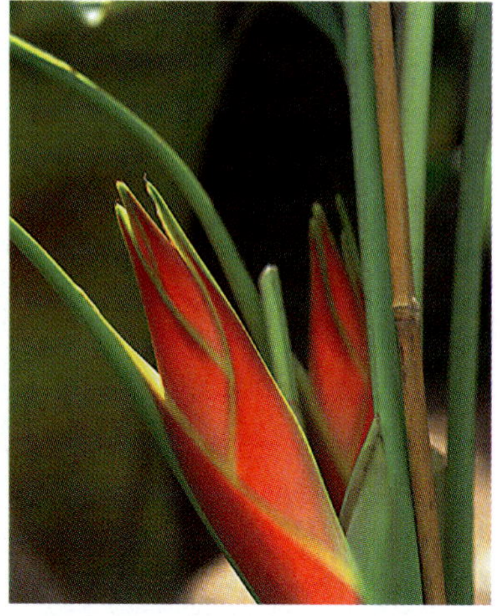

HELICONIA STRICTA CV. 'Sharonii'

'Sharonii' is a real prize. It's broad foliage is borne proudly on stiff red stalks. Blooms late July to February. A shade loving heliconia. Enjoys low light up to 80% shade. Height 3' (90cm) to 6' (1.8m). Sensational red, yellow, and green inflorescence that stands erect. Foliage is spectacular with red wine coloring on undersides of broad dark green leaves. Will burn in full sun.

42200 Rhizome $11.95
42201 Growing Plant (6" pot) $20.95

GIFT CERTIFICATES

Purchase a Stokes Tropicals' Gift Certificate as the ultimate gift for a birthday, special occasion, Christmas, Wedding Anniversary, Valentine's Day, Mother's Day, Father's Day, Graduation, or other special reason. You choose the amount. Then the recipient selects the plant or product and we will ship directly to them.

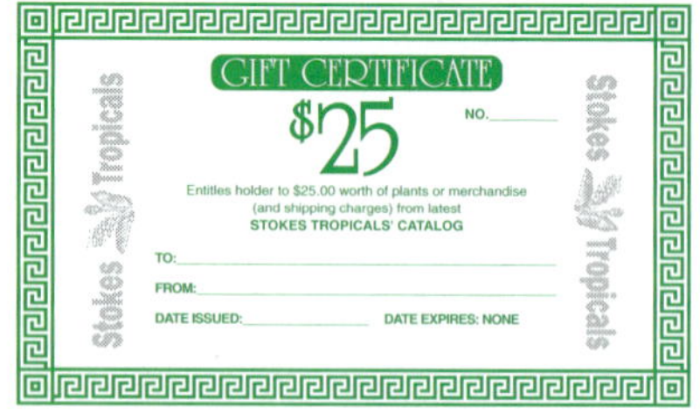

We have gift certificates in the denomination of $25.00. Of course multiple gift certificates can be purchased. Certificate totals include shipping. For example, if the plant cost $19.00 and shipping is $5.95, then a $25.00 gift certificate would be adequate. If the cost of plant selected and shipping is less, then the difference will be refunded. Or if amount is more, then the difference will be billed to the gift certificate holder. See page 134 for details.

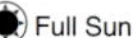 Full Sun   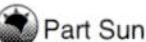 Part Sun   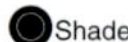 Shade   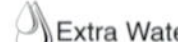 Extra Water   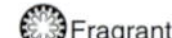 Fragrant   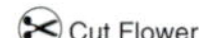 Cut Flower   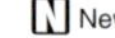 New

Heliconias

HELICONIA COLLECTIONS

(Save $10 off listed prices by purchasing entire collection)
Only one collection per customer / Rhizomes only

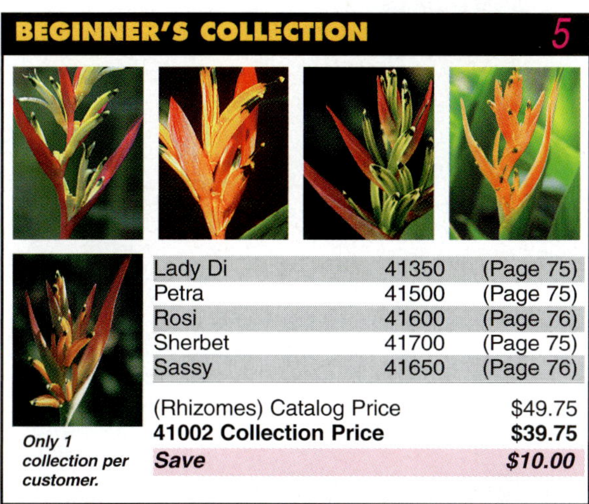

BEGINNER'S COLLECTION 5

Lady Di	41350	(Page 75)
Petra	41500	(Page 75)
Rosi	41600	(Page 76)
Sherbet	41700	(Page 75)
Sassy	41650	(Page 76)
(Rhizomes) Catalog Price		$49.75
41002 Collection Price		**$39.75**
Save		*$10.00*

Only 1 collection per customer.

PSITTACORUM COLLECTION 5

Andromeda	41100	(Page 74)
Lady Di	41350	(Page 75)
Strawberries & Cream	41800	(Page 76)
Petra	41500	(Page 75)
Choconiana	41200	(Page 74)
(Rhizomes) catalog price		$49.75
41000 Collection Price		**$39.75**
Save		*$10.00*

Only 1 collection per customer.

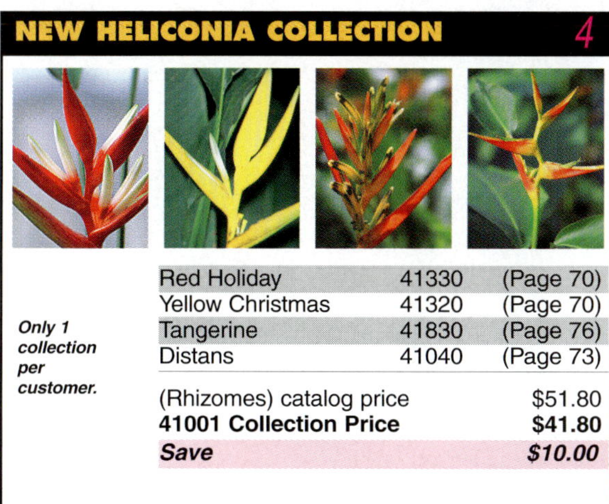

NEW HELICONIA COLLECTION 4

Red Holiday	41330	(Page 70)
Yellow Christmas	41320	(Page 70)
Tangerine	41830	(Page 76)
Distans	41040	(Page 73)
(Rhizomes) catalog price		$51.80
41001 Collection Price		**$41.80**
Save		*$10.00*

Only 1 collection per customer.

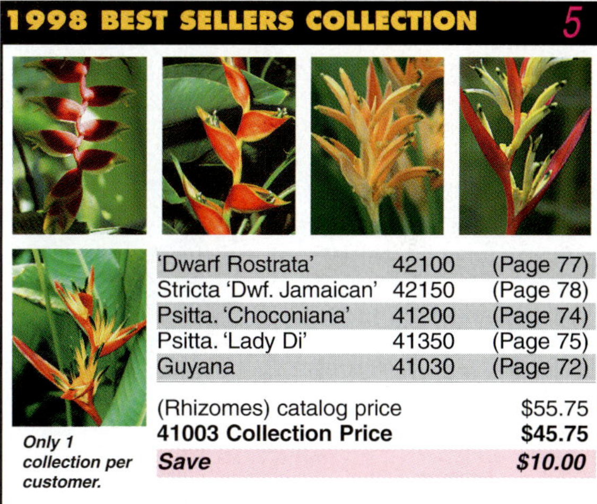

1998 BEST SELLERS COLLECTION 5

'Dwarf Rostrata'	42100	(Page 77)
Stricta 'Dwf. Jamaican'	42150	(Page 78)
Psitta. 'Choconiana'	41200	(Page 74)
Psitta. 'Lady Di'	41350	(Page 75)
Guyana	41030	(Page 72)
(Rhizomes) catalog price		$55.75
41003 Collection Price		**$45.75**
Save		*$10.00*

Only 1 collection per customer.

NEED A LECTURER ON TROPICAL PLANTS?

If you have a special function and are in need of an expert lecturer on tropical plants with great slides (of the same quality you find in our Guide/Catalog), please inquire. Advance notice is required. Or maybe you need an expert to advise you on growing or using tropical plants.

Telephone (337) 365-6998
or write to:
Stokes Tropicals, P.O. Box 9868, New Iberia, LA 70562-9868

FAX ORDERS:
1-337-365-6991
24 hours / 7days

FOR CUSTOMER SERVICE:
337-365-6998 - Mon.-Fri.,
8:30 am-4:00 pm C.T.

E-MAIL ORDERS / INQUIRIES:
info@stokestropicals.com
24 hours / 7 days

TO ORDER CALL **1-800-624-9706**/24 HRS. OR VISIT OUR WEB SITE: www. stokestropicals.com

WOODEN FLOWERS FROM MORO

'If you can't grow it, you can show it'
(Lengths may vary by 4")

We exclusively offer the handpainted wooden flowers by famed Haitian artist Moro. We offer 8 different 'flowers' that we commissioned by Moro. You won't find them anywhere else. Moro's other hand painted wooden flower and banana creations are found in gift shops throughout the Caribbean Islands and Southern Florida, including Key West. And if you have taken a Caribbean cruise in the last 5 years, you have seen, admired and may have bought his wonderful wooden art creations. So if you can't 'grow it', you can 'show it'. And wooden flowers don't need water, fertilizer, soil and warm temperatures. They are so realistic in appearance that they can be mixed with real flowers.

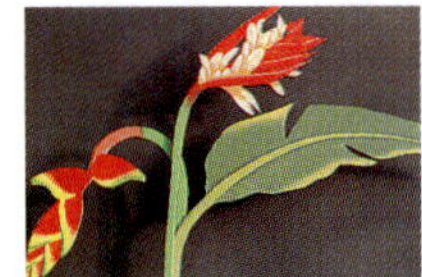

**(Left to right)
Heliconia rostrata, Heliconia psittacorum 'Lady Di' and Heliconia leaf**
*9145 ....$9.95
9135 ....$9.95
9190 ....$9.95*

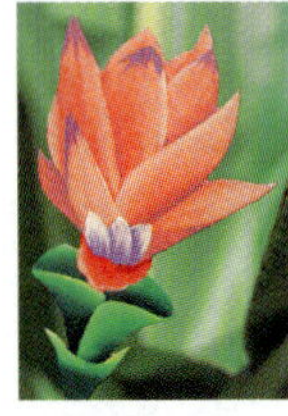

**Siam Tulip ginger—
'Curcuma alismatifolia'
(40")**
9160 ....$9.95

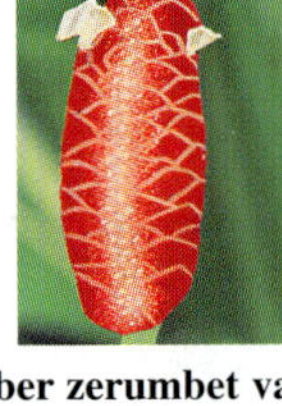

Zingiber zerumbet variegated 'Darcyi' (ripe variegated pine cone ginger) (36")
9180 ....$9.95

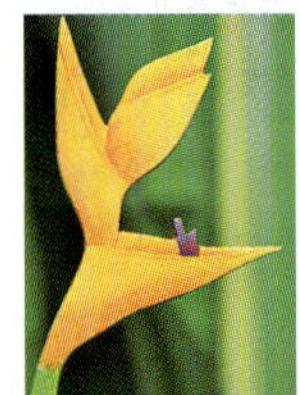

Heliconia 'Yellow Caribaea' erect (35")
9120 ....$9.95

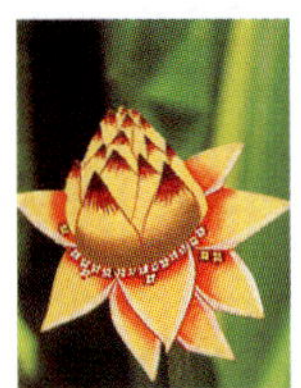

**Musella lasiocarpa—
'Chinese Yellow banana' (37")**
9150 ....$9.95

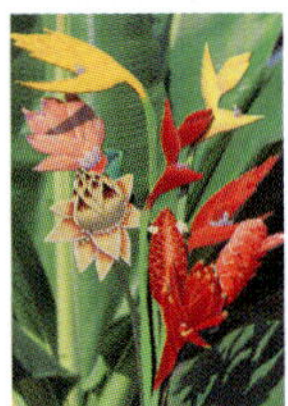

Flower Arrangement of all 8
*9170 ....$69.60**
*(save $10.00)

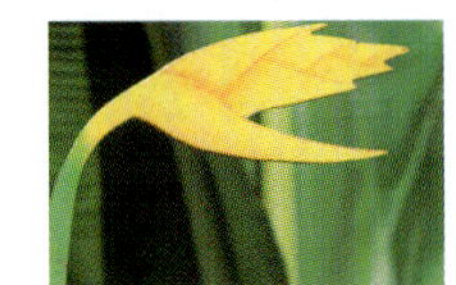

Heliconia 'Yellow Caribaea' sideways (41")
9130 ....$9.95

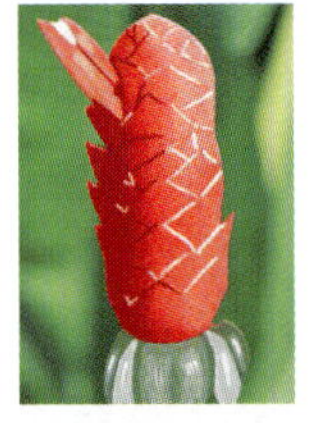

**Costus spicatus ginger—
'Indianhead ginger' (45")**
9100 ....$9.95

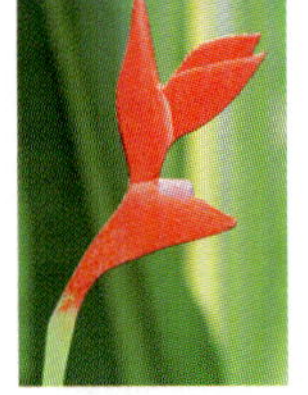

Heliconia 'Red Caribaea' (38")
9110 ....$9.95

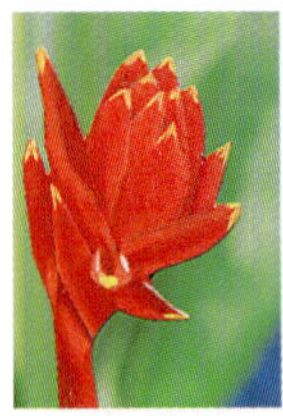

**Musa uranoscopus—
'Red flowering Thai banana' (41")**
9140 ....$9.95

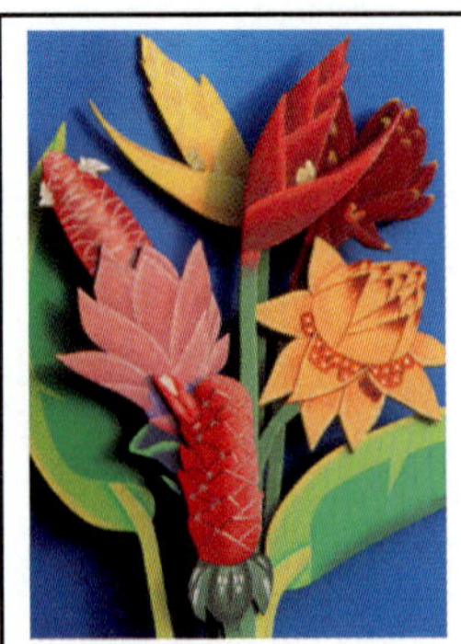

Buy the Tropical Arrangement of All 8 And SAVE $10

HIBISCUS

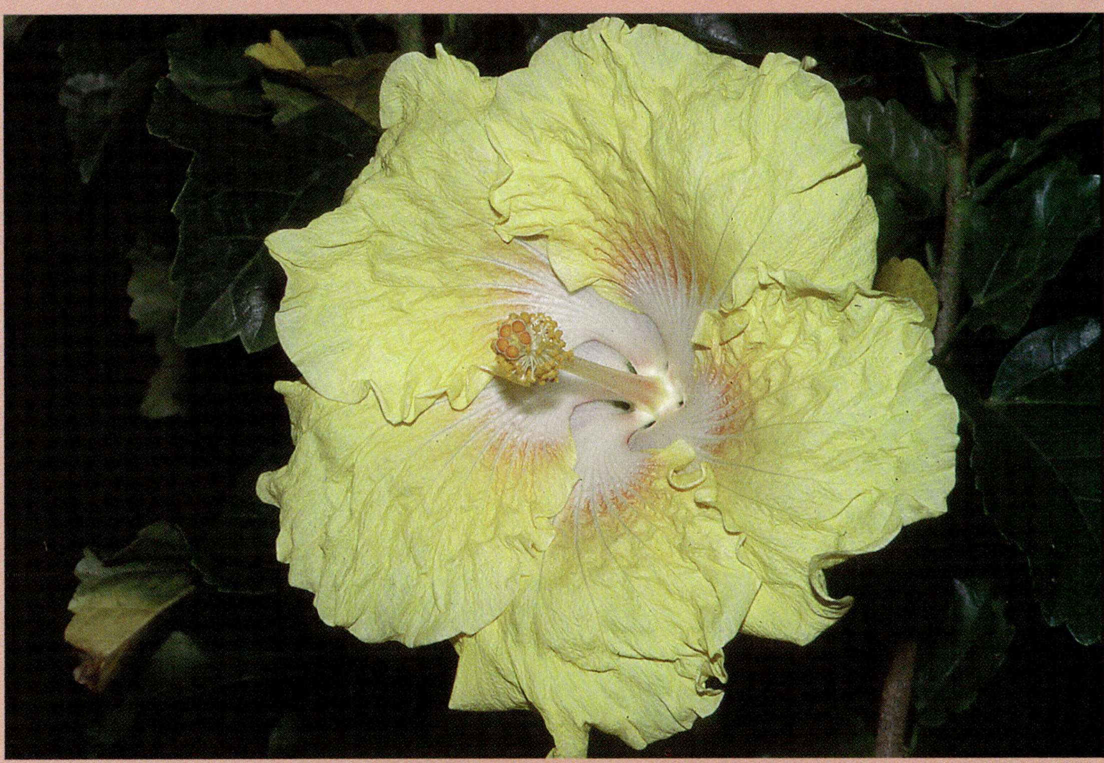

Hibiscus are great plants for tropical blooms and foliage.They can be grown year-round in the northern U.S. and Canada -noting greenhouses. Although you can't expect the same lush growth and bloom numbers while your plants are over-wintering inside under less-than-tropical conditions, they will be ready to reward you once placed outside when warm weather arrives. Cultural directions for normal growing and over-wintering are included with each order.

All our hibiscus are grafted to superior root stock and supplied as 8"-12" plants with leaves in 4" pots.

All our hibiscus are American Hibiscus Society sponsored show winners and all are proven garden performers.

Hibiscus

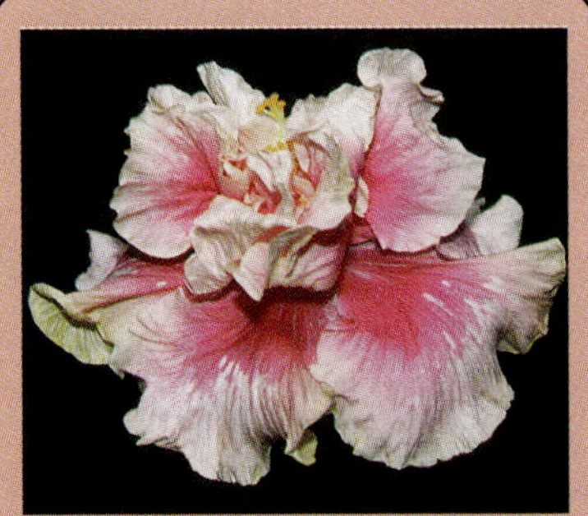

AMBER SUZANNE

Striking 8" double, pink flower with white edges and lots of white spots on the petals. Tall upright plant that is good a bloomer.
82005 Grafted Plant....................$14.95
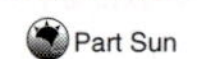 ☀

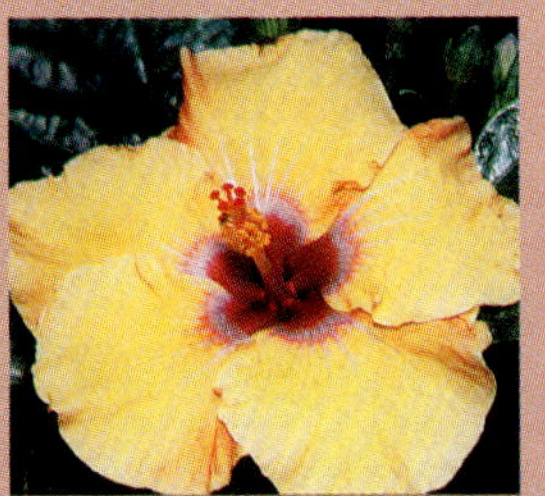

ED FLORY

6" single gold color with a center of dark red, dark grey and bright pink. Great grower and bloomer.
82030 Grafted Plant....................$13.95
☀

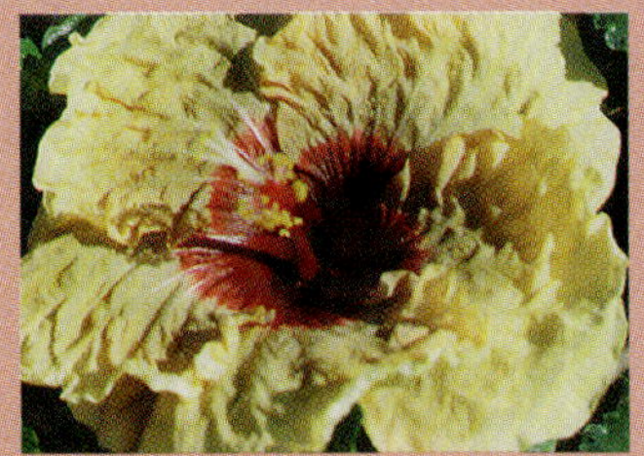

HERM GELLER

Single flower with dark wine eye and lighter oranges and yellows toward edges. Best brown ever. Tall grower. 8"-10" flower. Good bloomer. Spectacular bush!
82000 Grafted Plant....................$12.95
☀

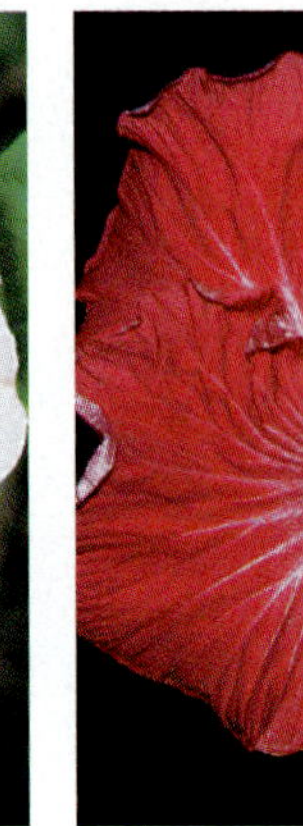

DOLORES DEL RIO

A remarkable 4" double lavender color with light pink edges, and a deeper pink center. Good upright grower and good bloomer.
82010 Grafted Plant $13.95
☀

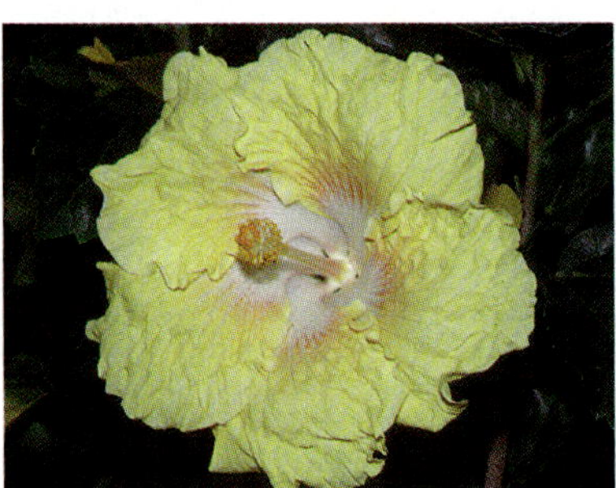

5TH DIMENSION

A brilliant 7" single, gun-metal grey flower with tangerine edges. White rays extend from the dark red center. Color fades throughout the day. A great blooming medium sized plant.

82025 Grafted Plant....
$14.95
🅝 ☀

DRAGON'S BREATH

Spectacular 8" single, ruffled, dark-blood red flower with white streaks radiating from the dark red center. Medium height and a great bloomer.
82015 Grafted Plant $14.95
🅝 ☀

EYE OPENER

Amazing 7" single, crepey and ruffled, bright-yellow flower with a white center and pink rays coming from the center. Medium size plant that is a very good bloomer.
82020 Grafted Plant $14.95
🅝 ☀

ALL STOKES TROPICALS' PLANTS ARE EASY-TO-GROW.

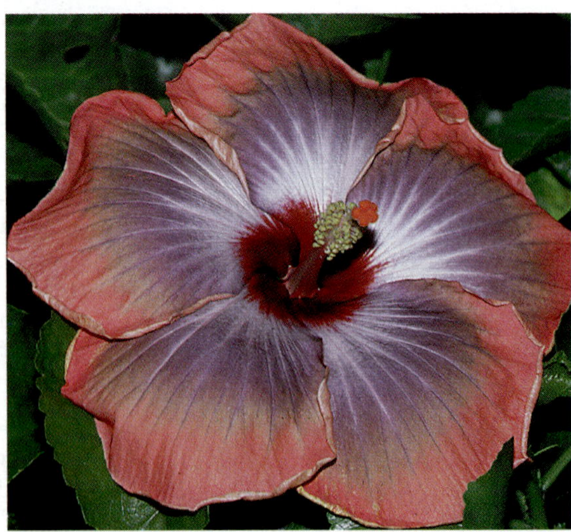

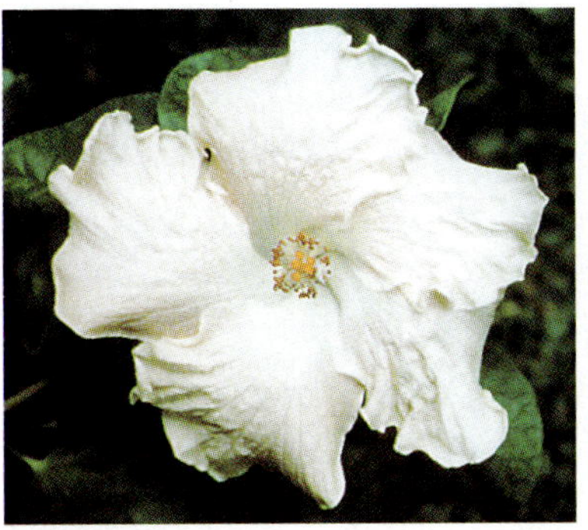

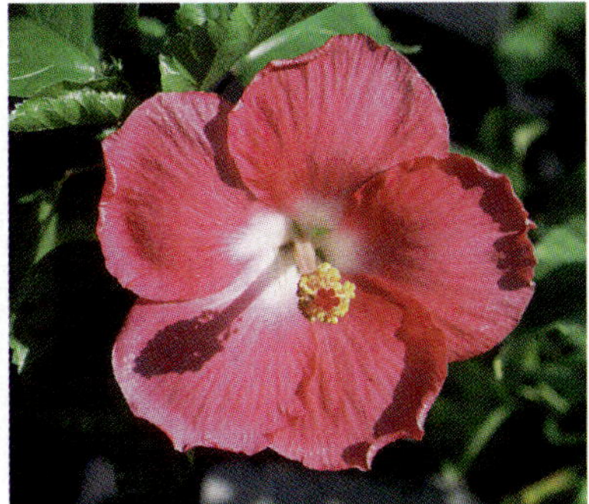

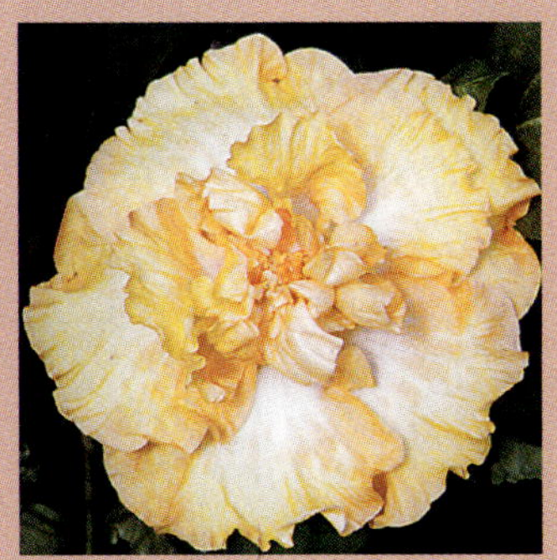

IVORY COAST

One of the most striking flowers that we have ever seen. A very distinctive 7" single cream color with light veins of pink. Very strong grower and good bloomer.

82050 Grafted Plant $13.95

LINDA BORINCANA

Wonderful 7" single, bright pink flower with a nice white center. Excellent hybrid from Puerto Rico. Tall, great blooming plant.

82040 Grafted Plant $14.95

ORANGE PINEAPPLE

A truly amazing 7" double yellow color with orange edges and a white center. Good grower and bloomer.

82120 Grafted Plant....................$13.95

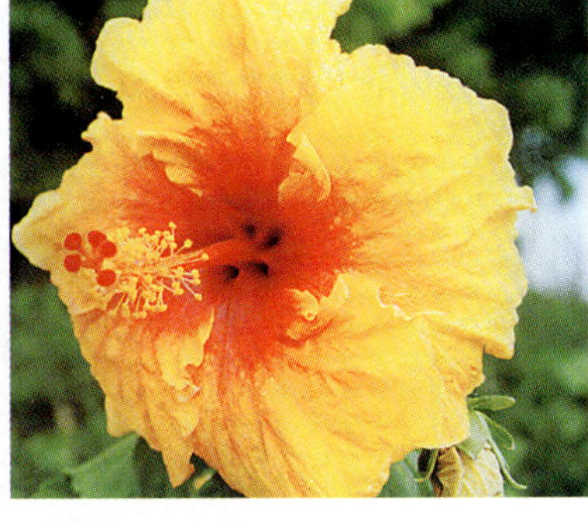

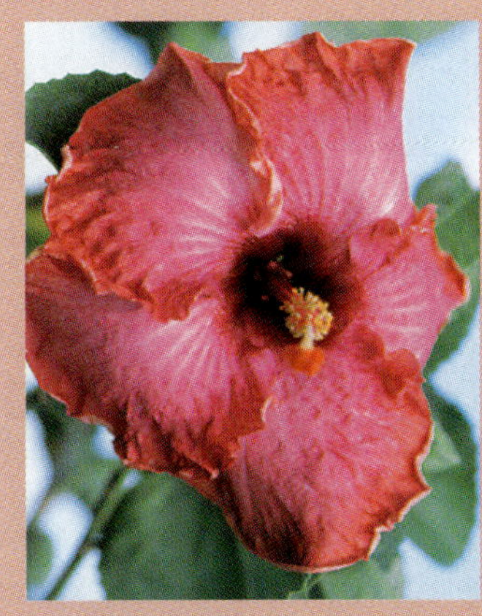

ME TARZAN

Smashing 7-8" single, orange flower fading to a yellow edge with a dark red center. Medium size, good blooming plant.

82045 Grafted Plant $14.95

ORANGE SPICE™

Single yellow-orange with diffuse reddish center. 7" flower. Great grower and bloomer. Very popular.

82100 Grafted Plant $14.95

ROJANNA™

Single with dark black eye on ruffled petals that are pink with an orange overlay. 8" flower. Great bloomer. A smashing plant.

82200 Grafted Plant....................$14.95

ROYAL BONNET

A startling 8" single orange/red color with tan edge with darker red center. Good grower and bloomer.

82140 Grafted Plant $13.95

For information on The American Hibiscus Society see page 135.

SAVE $10.00 Get 5 of our fantastic new Hibiscus at an unbeatable savings by buying a collection. **See page 84.**

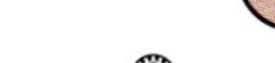

Full Sun Part Sun Shade Extra Water Fragrant Cut Flower New

TO ORDER CALL **1-800-624-9706**/24 HRS. OR VISIT OUR WEB SITE: www. stokestropicals.com

Hibiscus

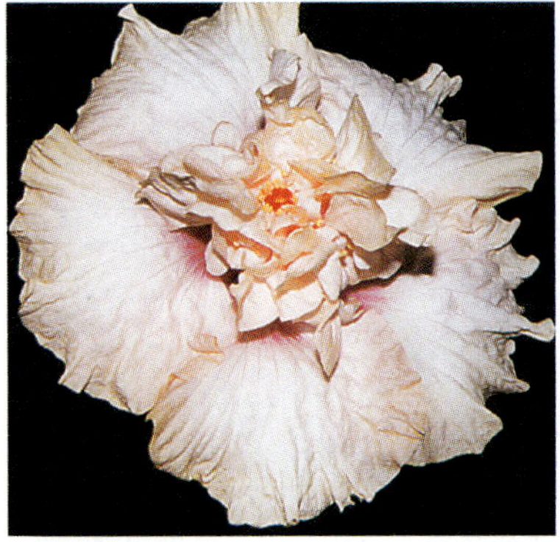

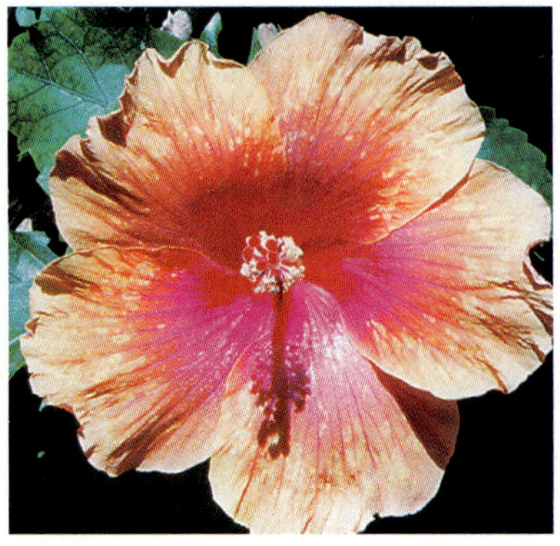

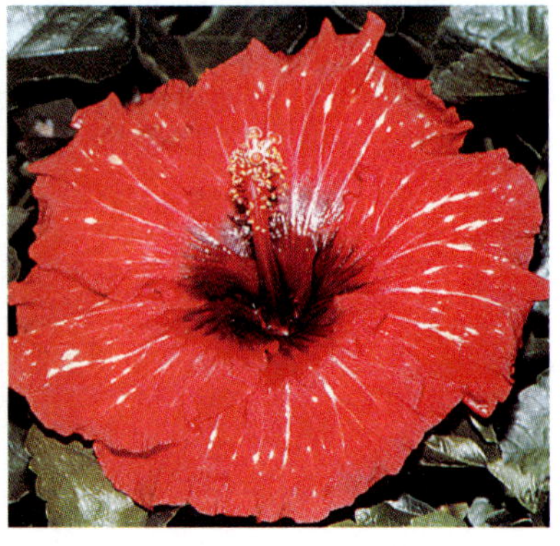

SILVER CHARM

A great 7" double cream color with a light pink center. Great grower and bloomer.

82230 Grafted Plant *$13.95*

TEQUILLA SUNRISE

Has to be seen to be believed. 5" single, pink color with orange edge and yellow splashes on the petals. Great grower and bloomer.

82250 Grafted Plant *$13.95*

VOLCANO

One of our favorites. 6" single red color with streaks of gold radiating from the dark red center. Good grower and bloomer. You have to see to believe.

82280 Grafted Plant *$13.95*

HIBISCUS COLLECTIONS

(Save $10 off listed prices by purchasing entire collection)

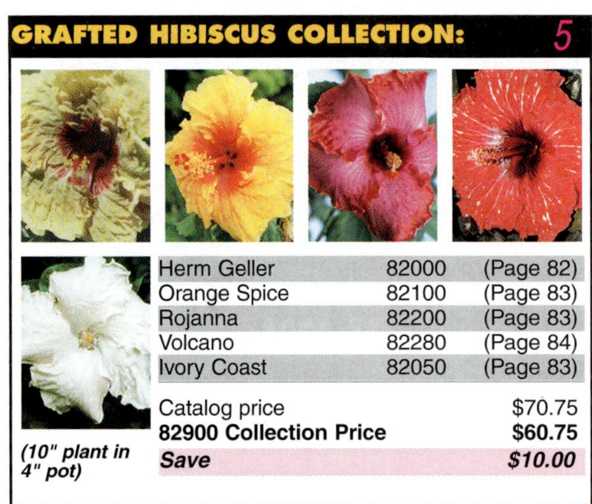

GRAFTED HIBISCUS COLLECTION: 5

Herm Geller	82000	(Page 82)
Orange Spice	82100	(Page 83)
Rojanna	82200	(Page 83)
Volcano	82280	(Page 84)
Ivory Coast	82050	(Page 83)
Catalog price		$70.75
82900 Collection Price		**$60.75**
Save		*$10.00*

(10" plant in 4" pot)

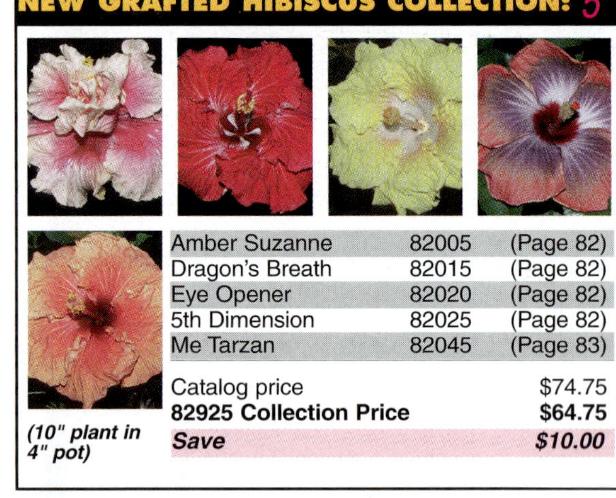

NEW GRAFTED HIBISCUS COLLECTION: 5

Amber Suzanne	82005	(Page 82)
Dragon's Breath	82015	(Page 82)
Eye Opener	82020	(Page 82)
5th Dimension	82025	(Page 82)
Me Tarzan	82045	(Page 83)
Catalog price		$74.75
82925 Collection Price		**$64.75**
Save		*$10.00*

(10" plant in 4" pot)

STOKES TROPICALS' HIBISCUS BLEND

Controlled Release Fertilizer
(3-Month Formula)
ANALYSIS 10-4-12 w/minors plus iron.

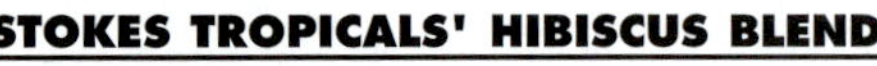

6010 (1 lb. Bucket) $6.00
6011 (4 lb. Bucket) $17.00

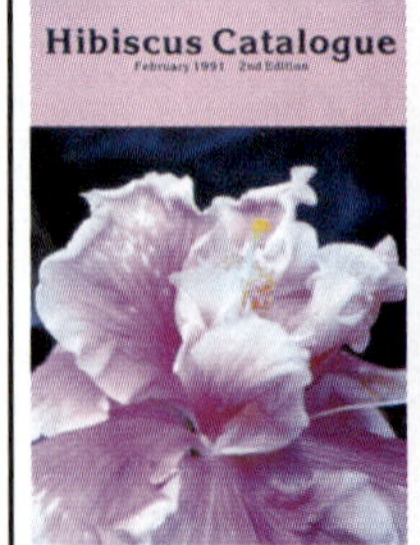

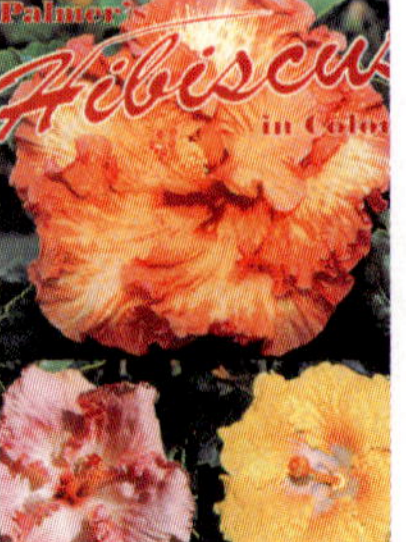

See pages 126,127 for these books and others on Hibiscus.

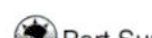 Full Sun   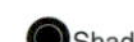 Part Sun   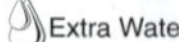 Shade   Extra Water   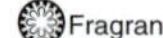 Fragrant   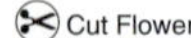 Cut Flower   N New

PLUMERIAS

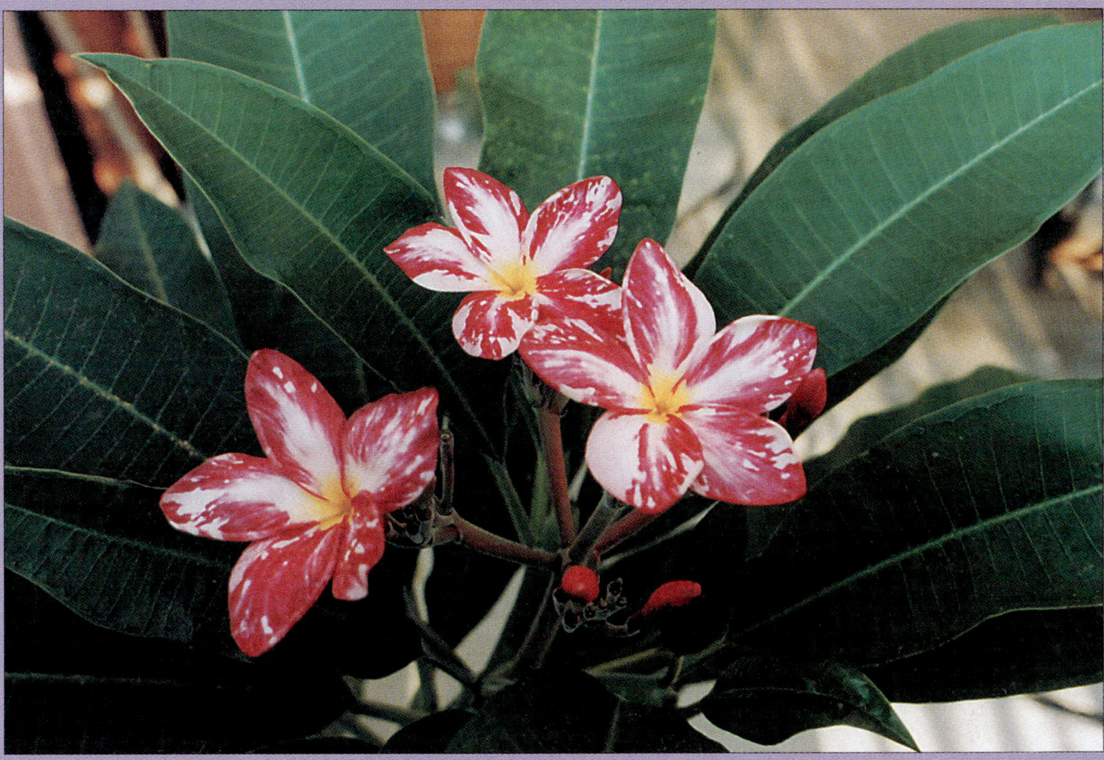

Princess Victoria™, new seedling variety (available 2001)

PLUMERIAS (also called frangipanis) are at once the most beautiful and fragrant trees in the plant world. They are all natives of the New World tropics. The word plumeria connotes perfume. There are 7 species and over 200 named varieties. From their native habitat in the American tropics they have been introduced to all tropical areas of the world with great success. Plumeria flowers are what leis are made of in Hawaii.

Their growth habits, shape and leaf and floral beauty are unrivaled among trees. With proper care and attention plumeria can be successfully grown throughout the U.S. They make wonderful pot plants. Foolproof cultural methods are available.

Plumerias have very few insect or disease problems. Just feed and water and protect from freezing temperatures and they do great. The fragrances of plumeria flowers are legend ranging from coconut to jasmine and including citrus, rose, honeysuckle, raspberry, spice, apricot and peach. Flower color varies from pure white to deep red with yellows, golds, oranges, roses, pinks and all combinations in between.

The plumeria is unique among trees, it can be lifted from the soil in the colder months and stored in a basement, garage, greenhouse or other enclosure for the winter, replanted after the last frost, and then brought into bloom. The plumeria plant goes dormant in the winter losing its leaves and requires no care. They grow and bloom well in the ground or in containers. In containers they are wonderful for creating tropical floral highlights in gardens, or on patios or decks, and along walkways. But plumerias need protection when temperatures drop below 38 degrees. Stokes Tropicals' Plumeria Blend (8-14-10) fertilizer is the very best fertilizer source for these miraculous plants.

When you order a plumeria cutting from Stokes Tropicals you will receive a "rooting cutting". This is a cutting that we have specially prepared for you. It takes 4-10 weeks depending on the time of year and variety to fully root a cutting. When you order we remove the rooting cutting from its growing medium, gently pack to prevent roots from drying, and ship to you. We ship rooting cutting from March 1st to November 1st.

Stokes Tropicals brings together the best of the Hawaiian and the best of the Floridian hybrids along with the newest seedling hybrids for one of the premier collections of plumerias in the world.

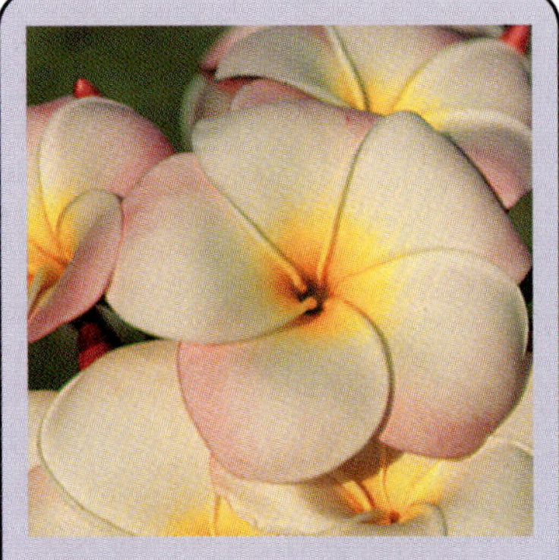

ABIGAIL ™

A great new seedling from Maui Beauty. A white flower suffused with pink and a dark-yellow center. Petals are short and barely pointed. Reverse side of petals is a uniform deep pink. Flowers are 2 1/2" across. A nice sweet fragrance; compact grower. In very short supply.

51021 Rooting Cutting..................$49.95

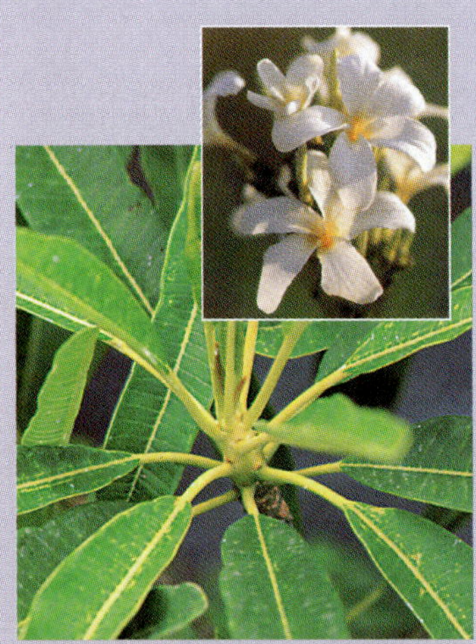

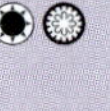

BAHAMAENSIS

Believed to be a species form. Has small white flowers with yellow center about 1¹/₂"-2" across. Has sweet fragrance. Leaves are long with rounded tips and thick texture. Branches are very long and thin; leaf scars close together. In very short supply.

51171 Rooting Cutting..................$49.95

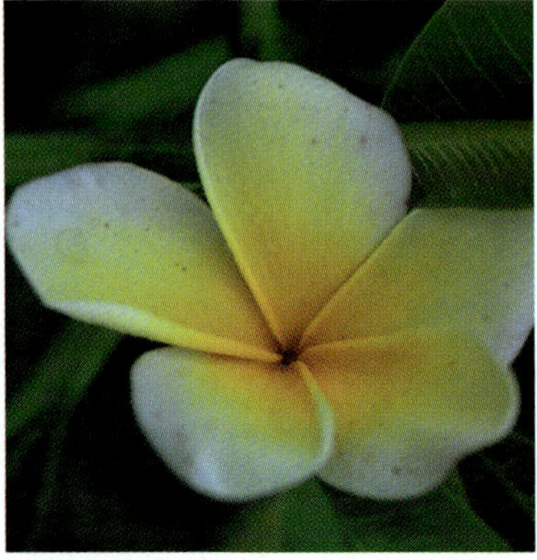

ANGUS #3 SELECTION

A wonderful hot pink flower with dark radiating lines. Petals fold back on themselves. Gold bleeds from the center. Flowers are 1¹/₂" across. A nice, sweet fragrance.

51011 Rooting Cutting..................$38.95

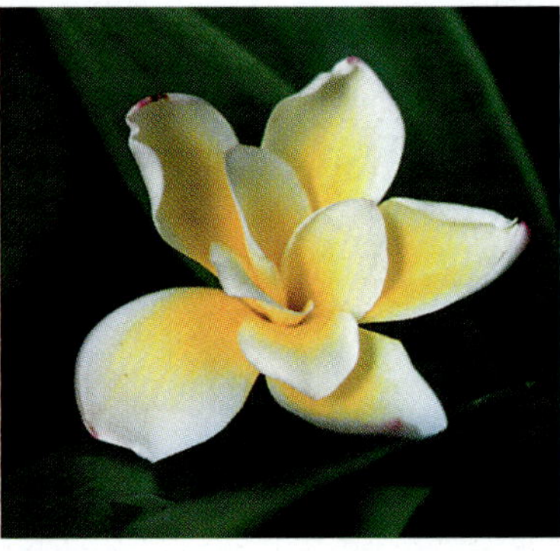

BALI WHIRL

The only double-flowered plumeria with ten petals. Colored similar to a Celadine, rich bright yellow, with the edges of the petals bordered white. The flower is about 3¹/₂" (8.5cm) across. The plant blooms easily and is easy to grow. A must for collectors.

51151 Rooting Cutting..................$49.95

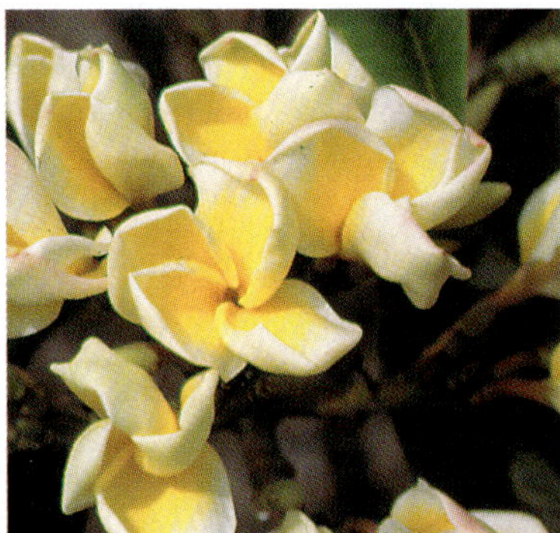

AZTEC GOLD

A marvelous large buttercup-yellow flower 4" (10cm) that shades to white, with faint pink edging showing through from back. A unique fragrance of ripe peaches. Flowers are very large, long-lasting and have a long blooming period.

51101 Rooting Cutting..................$29.95

BALI PALACE

A magnificent plumeria. A heavy golden-yellow on both sides of the flower with a pagoda type tip to its heavy textured petals. It has a sweet medium fragrance and averages around 2" across. Discovered by Jim Little in King Gunadhi's Palace garden in Bali, Indonesia. Flowers occur in large clusters that are pendulous. Looks like a yellow version of Japanese Lantern. Recently found in Singapore.

51041 Rooting Cutting..................$49.95

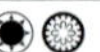

 Full Sun   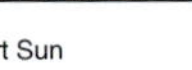 Part Sun   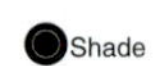 Shade   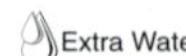 Extra Water   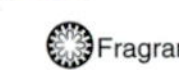 Fragrant   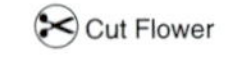 Cut Flower   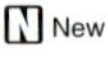 New

BRANCHER

A unique plumeria because of its multi-branching habit. Instead of the usual 2, 3 or 4 branches at each branch tip following flowering, there are 4, 5, 6 or 7 or more branches. This habit results in a very thick plant that is dense with branches, foliage and flowers. Flowers are a nice size (2"-2 1/2") with a small yellow center and a fragrance of frangipani. A must for plumeria collectors.
51031 Rooting Cutting........................$31.95

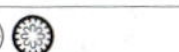

CANARY

A great new variety. Sure to be popular because of its large outstanding flower. A bright yellow with a pale yellow backing. Flower 3"-3 1/2". Slight sweet fragrance.
51251 Rooting Cutting $39.95

E-mail us: info@stokestropicals.com

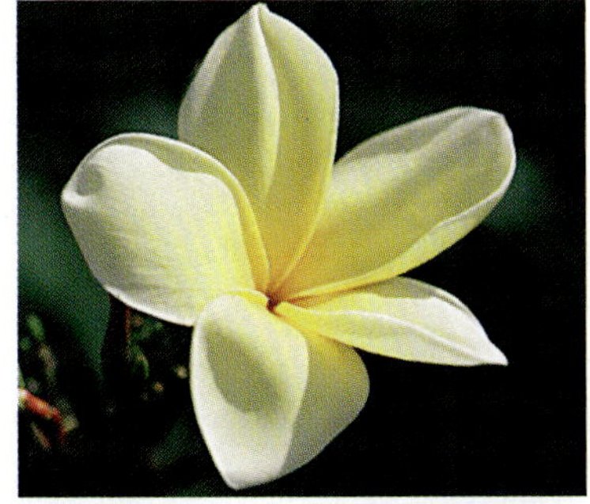

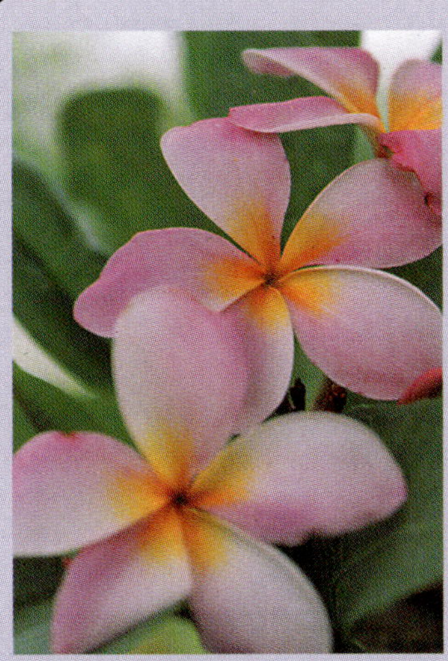

CANCUN PINK ™

A great-looking flower from Cancun, Mexico. Large pink petals that don't overlap; have noticeable dark, grainy lines radiating from center. Splashes of golden yellow spread from the center. Flower is 3" across and has a nice, sweet fragrance. In very short supply.
51321 Rooting Cutting................$39.95

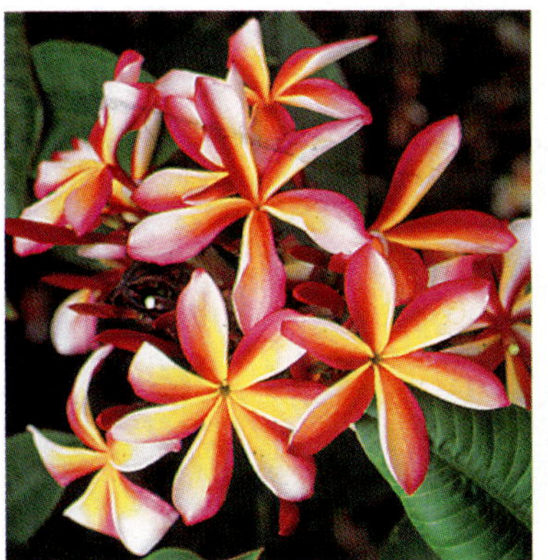

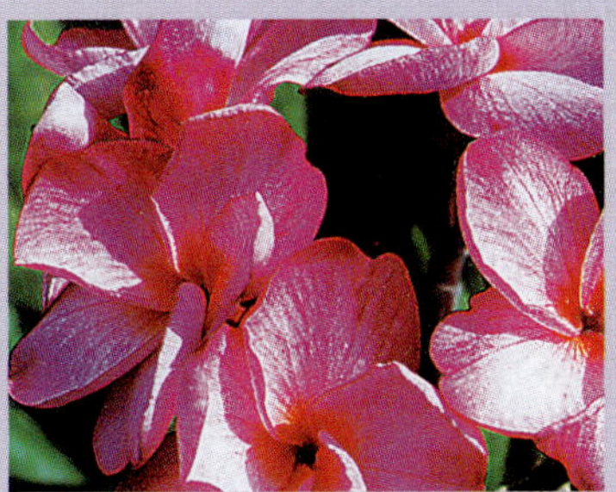

CANDY STRIPE

Has been called Pinwheel, Pinwheel Rainbow, and Barber's Pole. This cultivar is a striking blend of white, red and yellow stripes. Other distinguishing characteristics are its ability to root quickly, its vigor, and a tendency to produce multiple branches. Flower 2 1/2"-3". Sweet fragrance.
51301 Rooting Cutting..................$20.95

CARMEN

Moderate pink and white w/small, brilliant yellow center, wide petals, round tips, moderately overlapping; wide, moderate to strong red band on back, 2 1/2" - 3", slight sweet scent; keeping quality very good.
51261 Rooting Cutting..................$24.95

CAROL ANN™

A striking new seedling of Kimi Moragne. 3" white flower with strong pink edges and a pink blush over most of the flower. Large inflorescenses with up to 10 to 15 blooms at a time. Has sweet rose fragrance. In very limited supply.
51271 Rooting Cutting..................$58.95

Visit our Web Site :
www.stokestropicals.com
E-mail us: info@stokestropicals.com

Plumerias

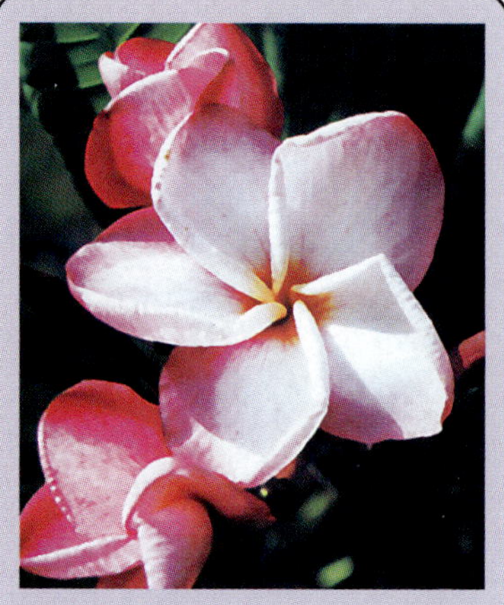

CAROLINE B™

A very special new seedling of Pink Pansy. 4" white flower with a strong pink edge and a gold and pink center with pink rays radiating from the center. Good frangipani fragrance. In very limited supply. Named by Glenn Stokes for his granddaughter.

51281 Rooting Cutting..................$58.95

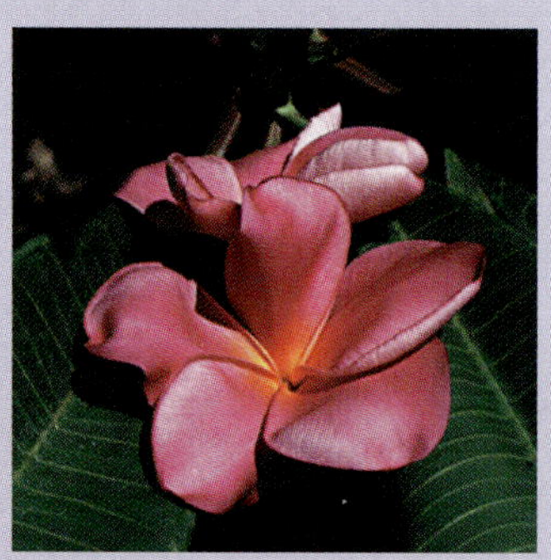

CHARLOTTE EBERT

(Formerly J. L. Giant Pink)
Renamed in honor of Charlotte Ebert for the many contributions she made to preserve the traditions of the Hawaiian culture. A very large soft pastel pink flower with very large (4") petals. A remarkable hybrid.

51451 Rooting Cutting...............$30.95

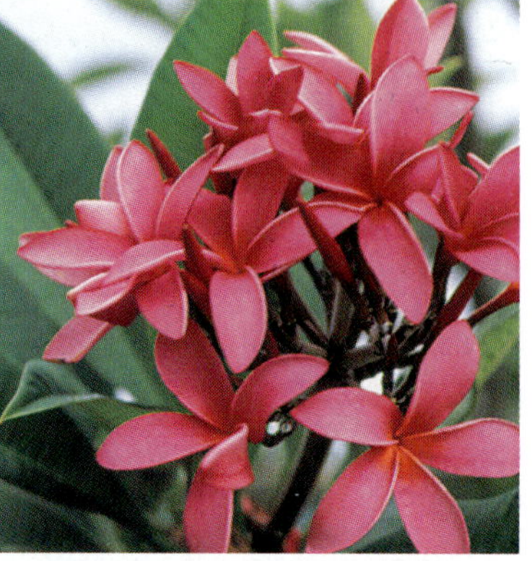

CARTER #2

A marvelous star-shaped 2½" flower with a small yellow center. Flowers have elliptical petals. Flowers are suffused with magenta color and have a mild frangipani fragrance.

51291 Rooting Cutting..................$39.95

Visit our Web Site :
www.stokestropicals.com
E-mail us: info@stokestropicals.com

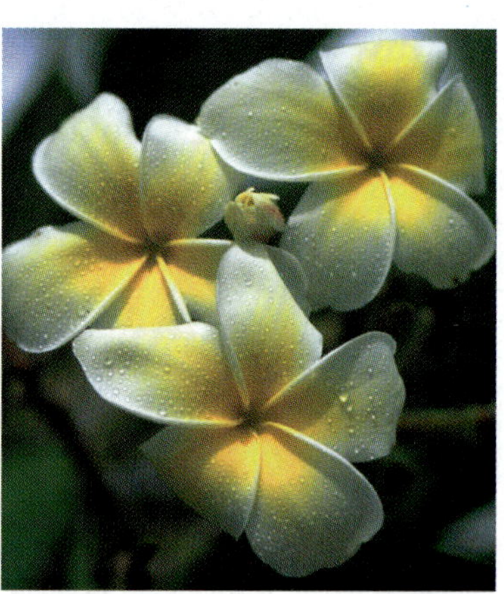

CELADINE

The flowers are medium to large 3½" (8.5cm) and brilliant yellow, with a broad white margin around the firm textured petals. Strong lemon fragrance with good keeping quality.

51351 Rooting Cutting..................$17.95

**Rooting cuttings are shipped from
*March 1st to November 1st.***

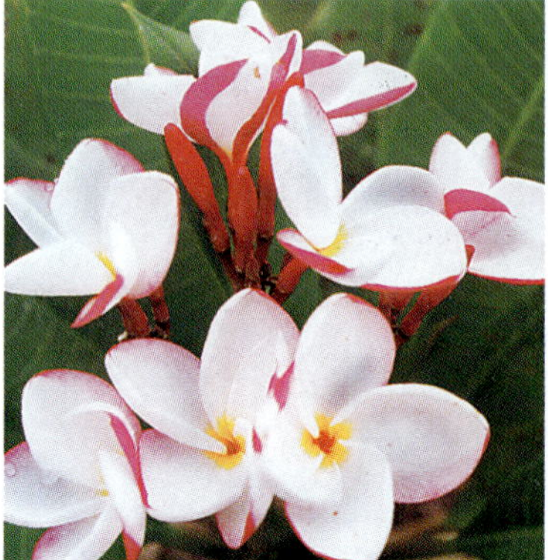

CATHERINE B ™

A delightful new seedling with wonderful pink petals with deep red edges and butter yellow center. Strong red bands on backside of petals. Flowers are of good texture 2½"-3" across. A strong floral fragrance. In very short supply. Named by Glenn Stokes for his granddaughter.

51331 Rooting Cutting..................$49.95

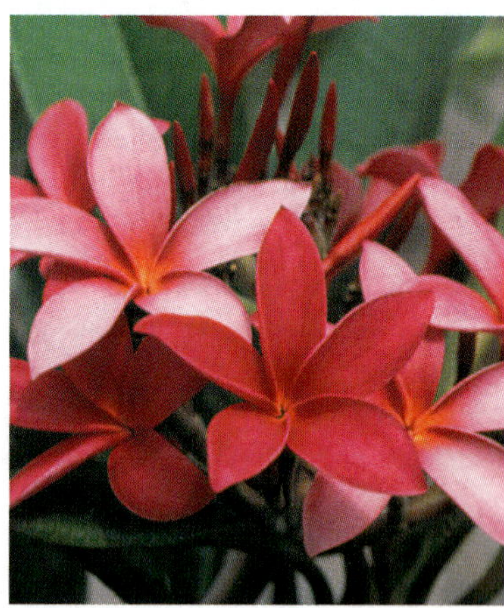

CERISE

Flower is moderate red w/small, brilliant, yellow center; strong red bands on back; narrow petals, elliptical, twisted, pointed tip, slightly overlapping; 3¼" (8cm) diameter; slight sweet fragrance.

51401 Rooting Cutting..................$29.95

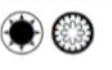

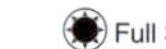 Full Sun   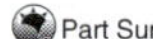 Part Sun   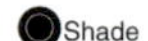 Shade   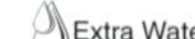 Extra Water   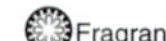 Fragrant    Cut Flower   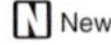 New

TO ORDER CALL **1-800-624-9706**/24 HRS. OR VISIT OUR WEB SITE: www. stokestropicals.com

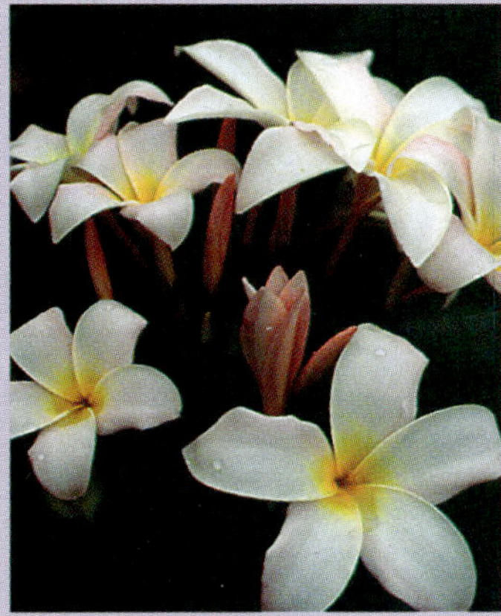

CHRISTINA B™

A spectacular new seedling of Pink Pansy. A 3" medium pink with darker pink edges and tips with a small orange center. Nice dark bands on back. Has good rose fragrance. In very limited supply. Named by Glenn Stokes for his granddaughter.
51461 Rooting Cutting $58.95

CINDY MORAGNE

Flowers are creamy white with large bright yellow center covering three-fourths of flower, top edge of petals curl over; wide petals with rounded tip, highly overlapped; heavy texture; 4" (10cm) diameter; faint scent; keeping quality good.
51551 Rooting Cutting............................$30.95

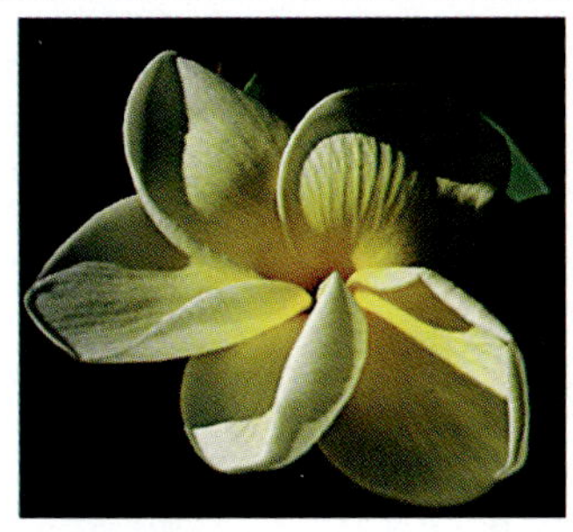

COURTADE PINK

The large (3") flower is light pink with bluish tinge, gold throat and eye, underside medium pink. Petals are rounded, incurved slightly, with slight overlap. Medium lavender fragrance.
51511 Rooting Cutting..............$31.95

CINNAMARK ™

A great-looking flower that is dark pink suffused over white with a barely visible yellow center. Flowers are 2½"-3" in diameter. Nice cinnamon fragrance. Leaves light green color. Plant is compact grower and easy to bloom.
51161 Rooting Cutting $29.95

COZUMEL YELLOW™

A nice yellow flower with a deeper yellow center that spreads to a white edge halfway down the petals. 2½" flowers of moderate texture. Slight sweet fragrance. In very limited supply.
51561 Rooting Cutting............................$39.95

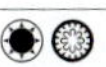

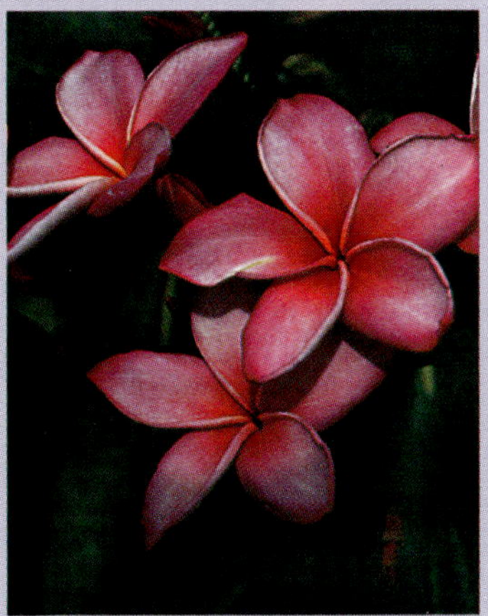

CRANBERRY

A fantastic new variety. A true cranberry color with elliptical petals and slightly pointed flower tips. Slightly scented. Excellent growth characteristics. Large (3"-3½") flower.
51501 Rooting Cutting $39.95

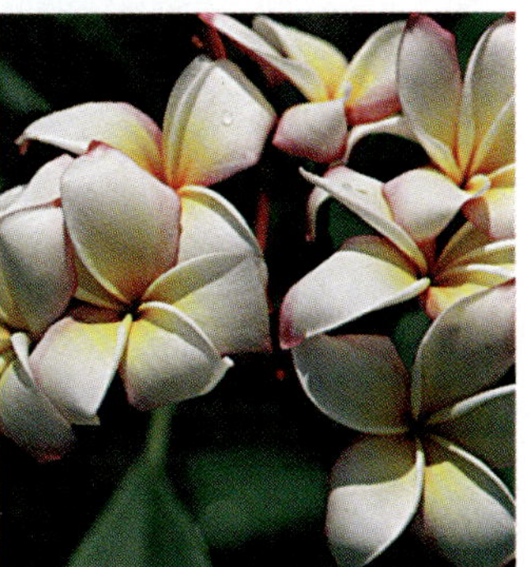

DAISY WILCOX

Very large, creamy-white flowers with prominent yellow center and pale pink buds. Flowers open with a faint pink blush and quickly fade to white. Blossoms measure up to 4½" and have wide, floppy petals, with a light pink band on the reverse of the broad, rounded, heavy-textured petals. Flowers have a spicy fragrance, good keeping quality, and are borne in large, dense clusters.
51601 Rooting Cutting $29.95

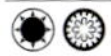

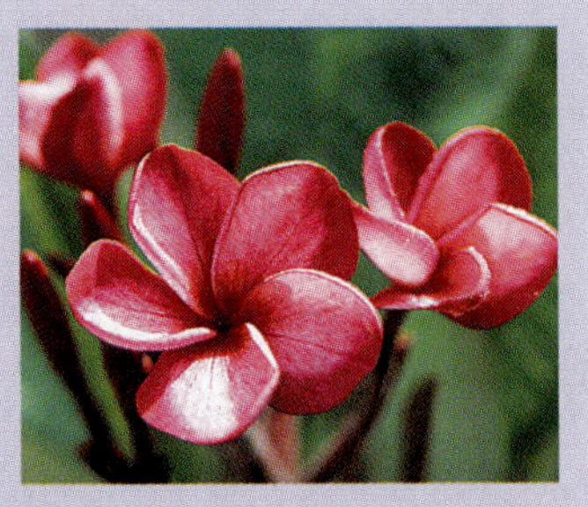

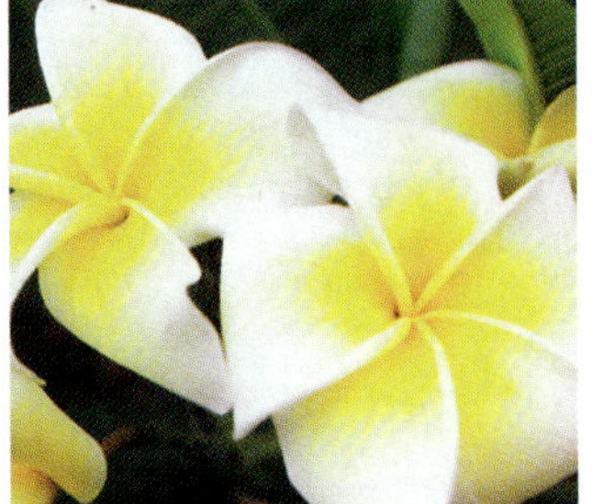

DAN LEIDKE™

A large 3¹/₂"-4" yellow flower with strong texture that is splashed with gold centrally with noticeable, radiating lines. Large overlapping petals that fold back on themselves. A strong frangipani fragrance. New seedling in very short supply.

51621 Rooting Cutting...................$45.95

DORIS YVETTE™

Great new seedling from Pink Pansy. Flowers are medium size 2¹/₂" (6.5cm) and resemble Pink Pansy, however are pinker with red-orange star in center. Petals have dark pink brush stroke edges and numerous white specs. Delightful frangipani fragrance. Very limited supply. Named by Glenn Stokes for his mother-in-law Doris Yvette Cheramie.

51701 Rooting Cutting..............$39.95

DEAN CONKLIN

Flower is salmon colored with large, moderate orange center, reddish margin, light pink tip; moderate red outer band on back; wide petals, long, somewhat elliptical, round tip, twisted, slightly overlapping; medium texture, 3¹/₂" to 4¹/₂" diameter; faint spicy carnation scent.

51651 Rooting Cutting............................$39.95

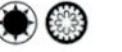

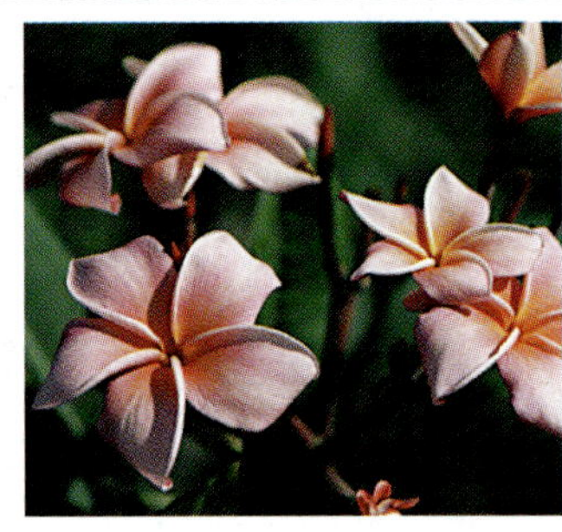

DONALD ANGUS

A brilliant red rainbow flower with burnt orange center and distinct red bands front and back, narrow petals, pointed tip, heavy texture, 3¹/₄" (8cm) diameter, lemon fragrance; keeping quality very good. Named for the famous plant collector of Honolulu, Donald Angus.

51051 Rooting Cutting $30.95

WHAT IS A ROOTING PLUMERIA CUTTING?

It is a cutting that we have specially prepared for you. It takes us 4-10 weeks, depending on time of year and variety, to fully root a cutting. We then simply remove the rooting cutting from its growing medium, gently pack to prevent roots from drying, and ship to you. You should then replant at same level (see band on stem), in a well-drained soil mix either directly into the ground or into a container. Water lightly and fertilize with a half strength fertilizer at sign of first new growth. <u>Don't keep too wet</u> and follow cultural directions that come with plant. We take orders for rooting plumeria cuttings all year. And we ship them from <u>March 1st to November 1st.</u>

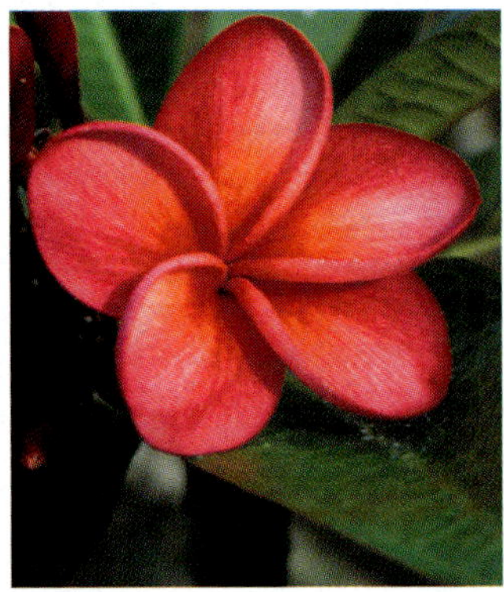

DUKE

Blooms are strong red and pink with small, brilliant yellow center, somewhat grainy pigmentation, radiating dark red lines on front; wide petals, round tip, moderately overlapping, strong red band on front; fair texture, 3¹/₂" (8.5cm) diameter; strong sweet fragrance, becoming stronger on storage; keeping quality fair. Recommended.

51751 Rooting Cutting $39.95

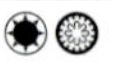

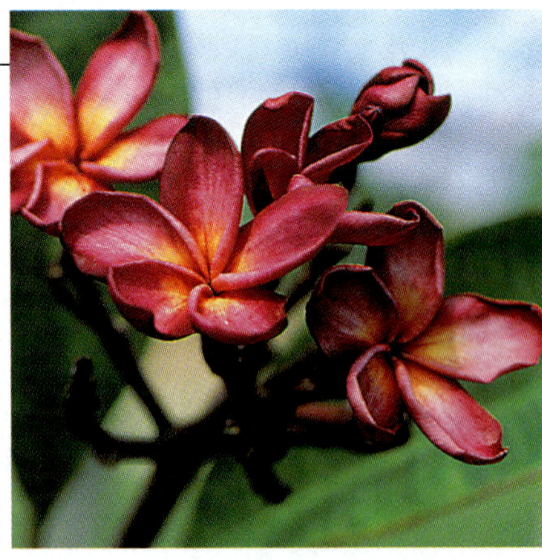

 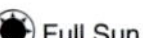 Full Sun 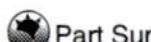 Part Sun 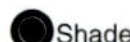 Shade 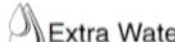 Extra Water 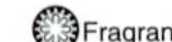 Fragrant 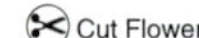 Cut Flower 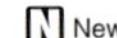 New

DWARF SINGAPORE WHITE

A dwarf form of the famous 'Singapore'. Similar to Dwarf Pink in form and habit with dark green glossy leaves on a many-branched plant. Perfect for small spaces and can even be flowered indoors. Small white slightly cupped flowers borne in tight clusters with a delightful sweet, lemon fragrance. No color bands front or back. Does not lose its leaves in winter. Grows to 6'-7'. Rare.

51901 Rooting Cutting..............................$69.95

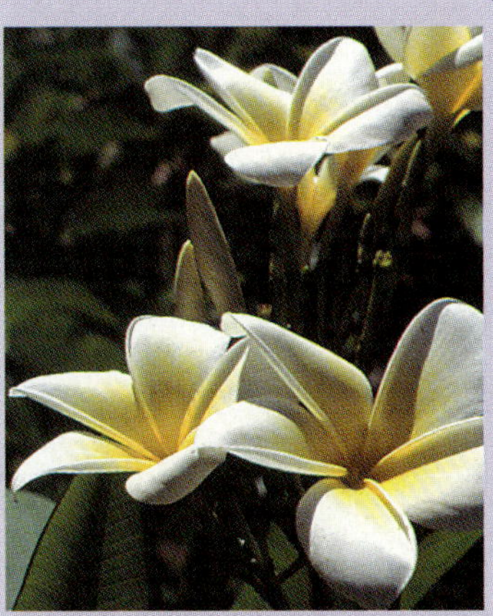

DWARF PINK

Flowers (2"-2½") are a delicate pale pink suffused with pink borders and yellow center. Flower buds are also pink. A true dwarf with dark green glossy leaves on a many-branched plant. Ideal for small spaces. Only dwarf with color. In limited supply. If one could have only one plumeria, this should be the one. Grows only 6" per year—maturing at 6'. Does not lose its leaves in winter and can be flowered indoors. Nice frangipani fragrance. Rare.

51801 Rooting Cutting..............................$69.95

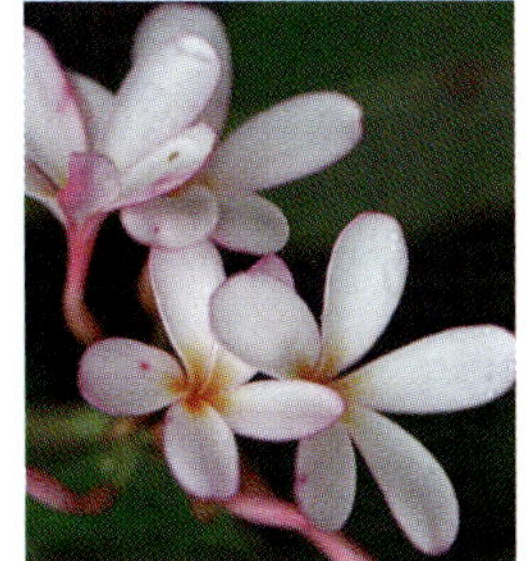

EDIE MORAGNE

White, medium gold throat, gold eye, white underside; petals lifted and incurved, widely overlapped at center, becoming separated, wide, rounded with slight point; large (4") flower, strong jasmine scent.

51911 Rooting Cutting.................$49.95

DWARF DECIDUOUS

Large white flowers with broad oval petals and a golden center. Flowers are about 3" (7.5cm) in diameter. Slightly larger than a Dwarf Singapore. This is a true dwarf, of compact habit and blooms from spring to fall. Very strong citrus fragrance. Rare.

51851 Rooting Cutting.............................$79.95

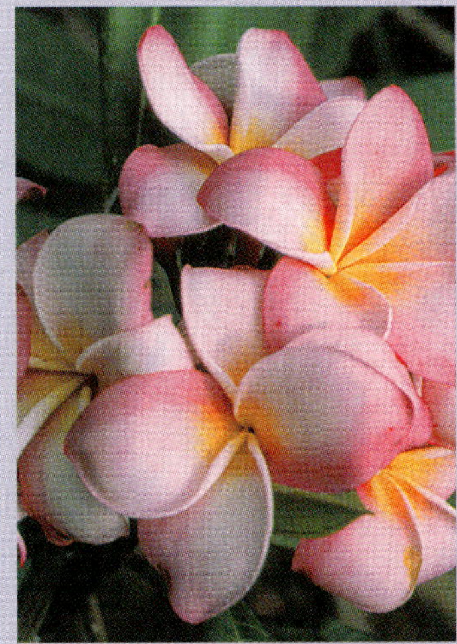

ELENA

Plant has flowers that are white with large, brilliant yellow center, narrow pink band on back; heavy texture, 3¾" (9.5cm) diameter; slight sweet fragrance; keeping quality very good.

51951 Rooting Cutting.............................$32.95

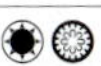

EWC #3

A smashing new introduction. Discovered at the East-West Center of the Pacific at the University of Hawaii, Manoa campus. The flower (4"-4½") is the largest known Cerise with a small yellow eye. The flower is open petaled with an intense color on both sides of the flower. It will become a collector's plant.

51961 Rooting Cutting.............................$39.95

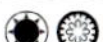

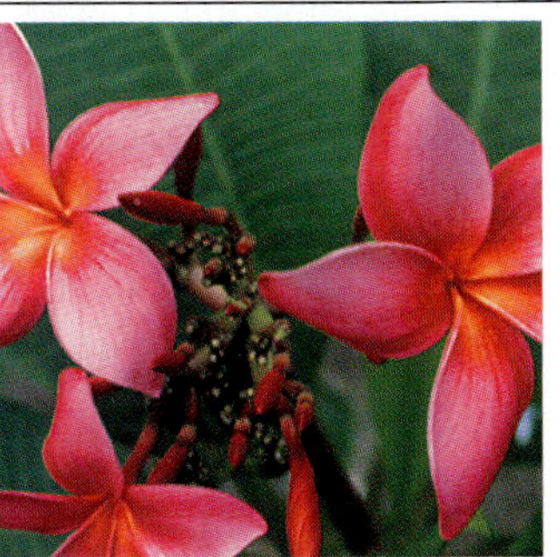

ESPINDA PINK

Moderate pink w/small, brilliant yellow center; wide, oval petal w/round tip, moderately overlapping, deep pink band on back, good texture, 3 1/4" diameter; slight sweet fragrance, good keeping quality.

51921 Rooting Cutting...............$31.95

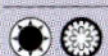

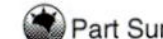 Full Sun   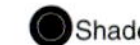 Part Sun   Shade   Extra Water   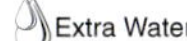 Fragrant   Cut Flower   N New

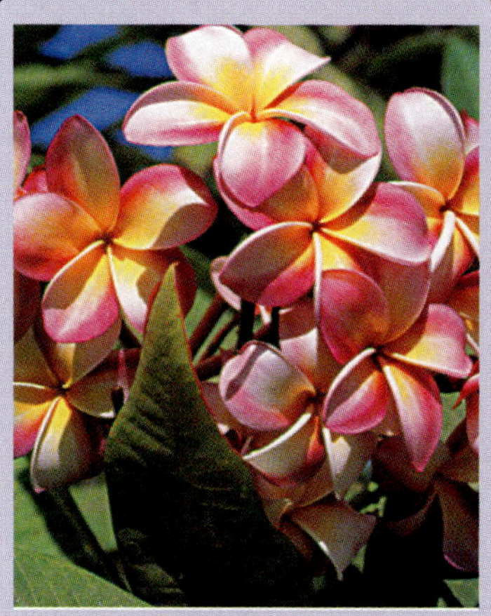

GLORIA SCHMIDT

A lovely new introduction with medium-size rainbow flower that combines the characteristics of Intense Rainbow, Lei Rainbow and Candy Stripe. Its petals have a slight vein appearance with rounded tips. Discovered by Dr. Richard Criley of the University of Hawaii.
52011 Rooting Cutting..............$49.95
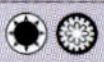

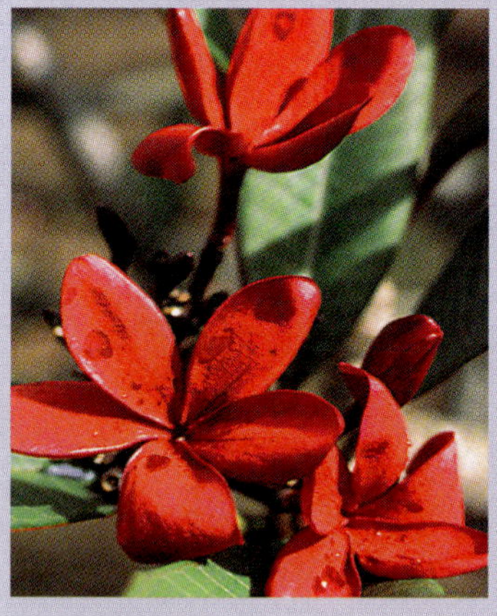

HILO BEAUTY

Flowers are very dark maroon with good texture. Elliptical petals with slightly pointed tips. Flowers are up to 4." Has strong spicy, citrus fragrance. Leaves dark green with reddish tint. A magnificent plant.
52071 Rooting Cutting..................$24.95

GUILLOT SUNSET

A full-color blended rainbow with a spicy scent. It has a cupped shape to the petals that are pinkish fading to a white towards the outer band of the flower petals. (3-3½" flower) Medium texture. A vigorous grower. A very nice new addition.
52041 Rooting Cutting..............$29.95

HAZEL B™

A very pleasing new seedling. A white flower that is splashed with rose pink with a nice cupped appearance. Burnt-orange center offers outstanding contrast. 2 1/2"-3" flower with nice frangipani fragrance. In very limited supply. Glenn Stokes named this seedling after his mother Hazel B. Stokes.
51221 Rooting Cutting..............$49.95

GROVE FARM

Flowers are moderate pink with small, brilliant yellow center; petal wide, elliptical, round tip, highly overlapping, strong red bands on front and back; heavy texture; 4½" (11.5cm) diameter; slight sweet fragrance; good keeping quality. Highly recommended.
52001 Rooting Cutting $30.95

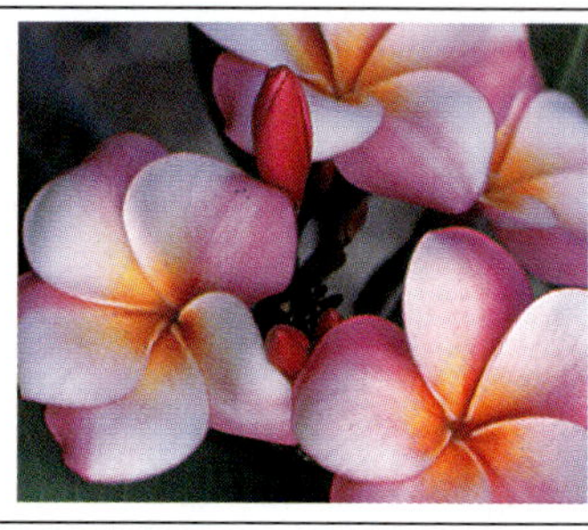

HAUSTEN WHITE

Large white flowers 3½" (8.5cm) to 4 " (10cm) with a small, brilliant yellow center and medium pink bands on the back. Petals are wide with round tips, moderately overlapping with a heavy texture and a sweet fragrance. Upright, densely branching plants with moderate to heavy flower production. Good keeping quality.
52051 Rooting Cutting $21.95

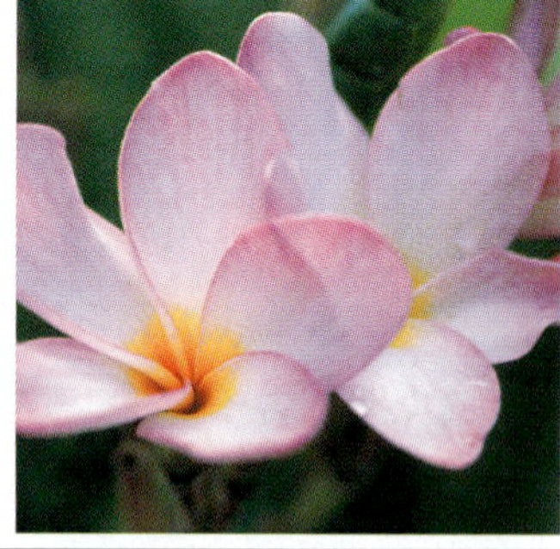

HEIDI

Brilliant yellow covering entire blossom, top of petals curl over showing white edge on reverse, no distinctive eye; rounded petals with rounded tips, moderately overlapped; heavy texture; 2" diameter; faint peachy scent; keeping quality very good.
52061 Rooting Cutting $24.95
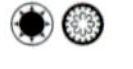

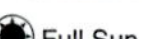 Full Sun 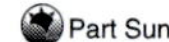 Part Sun 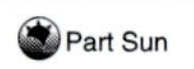 Shade Extra Water 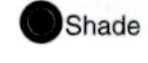 Fragrant 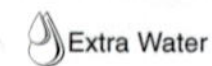 Cut Flower  New

INDIA

A very large (3¹/₂"-4") strongly textured rounded flower that is a beautiful soft yellow orange grainy flower with heavy veining. A knockout flower. Nice frangipani fragrance.

52151 Rooting Cutting $49.95

INTENSE RAINBOW

Vibrant pink edges fading to lighter pink, intense gold inner edge; elliptical petals with rounded tip, moderately overlapped; heavy texture; 3 1/2" dia.; slight sweet scent.

52161 Rooting Cutting $34.95

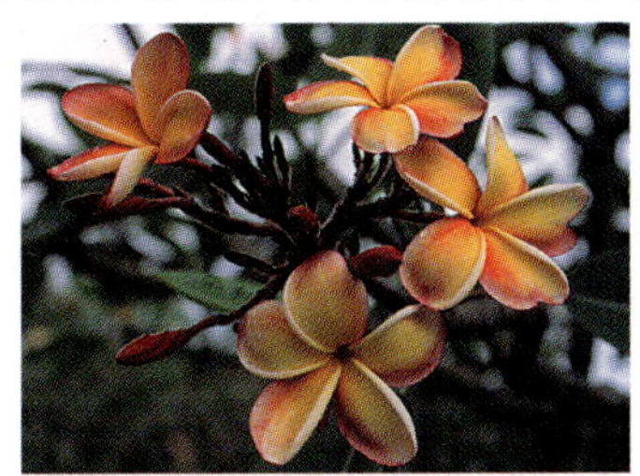

IRMA BRYAN

Flowers are moderate strong red with small pale orange-yellow center; petals wide, elliptical, pointed tip, moderately overlapping, slightly wavy edges, moderate reddish-brown bands on front and back; fair texture, 2¹/₂" (6.5cm) diameter; slight spicy scent becoming stronger on storage.

52201 Rooting Cutting $30.95

J. L. HAWAIIAN SUNSET

A "Moragne" seedling cultivated by Jim Little. Red-orange with a red velvet shine on the backside. Round petals with flower 4" (10cm) wide. A sweet fragrance. A real knockout.

52251 Rooting Cutting $49.95

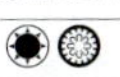

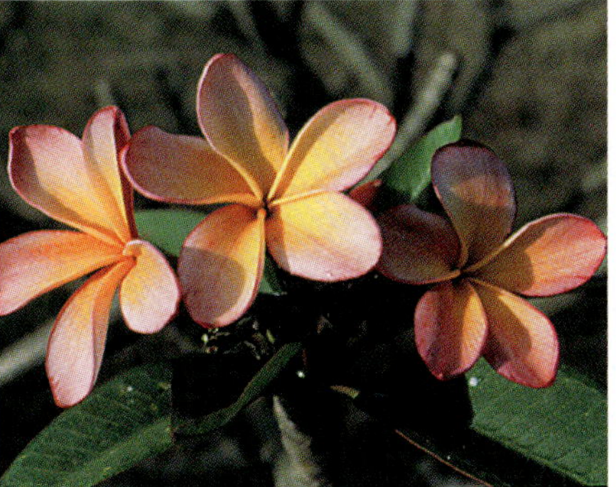

HORACE CLAY

An interesting new variety with large 4" (10cm) waxy flowers in a rainbow combination of peach, yellow and pink suffused with lavender. Large clusters of flowers with rounded overlapping petals. A vigorous grower and a prolific flower producer. In limited supply.

52951 Rooting Cutting ...$37.95

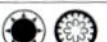

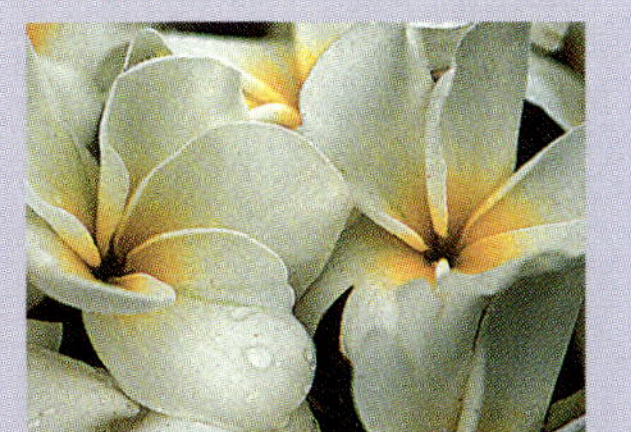

J.L. BRIDAL WHITE

A snow white flower with a bright yellow center and round, overlapping petals. Has a penetrating sweet fragrance. Plant has a close branching form making it bushy. Flower clusters are very large.

51201 Rooting Cutting $39.95

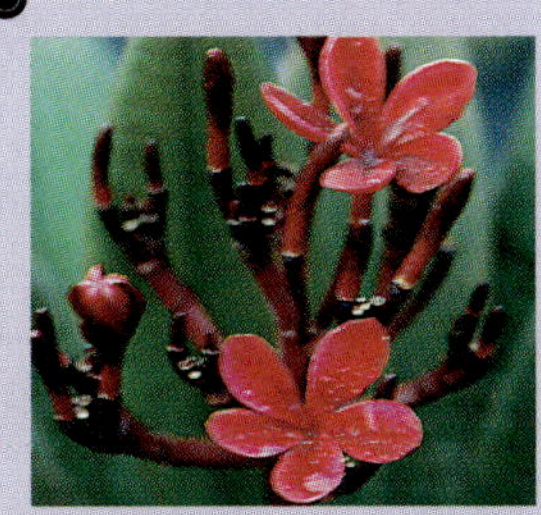

J.L. RED/ORANGE

A stunning deep red with a muted splash of orange radiating from the center out to the edge of the petals. Slightly scented with medium texture. A velvet red-pinkish under-petal. This is a open-pollinated seedling from Irma Bryan.

52101 Rooting Cutting.................$39.95

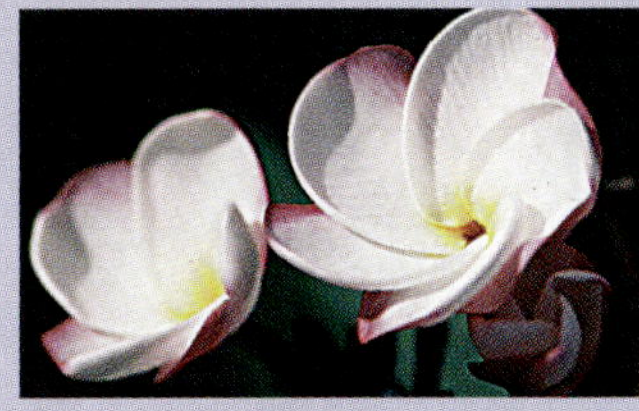

J. L. PINK PANSY

A striking flower reminding one of a pansy. An exquisite light lavender-pink color with violet pink edges and violet lines running through the rounded overlapping petals. Flower has a small yellow throat and is very sweet scented. A favorite.

52301 Rooting Cutting...............$29.95

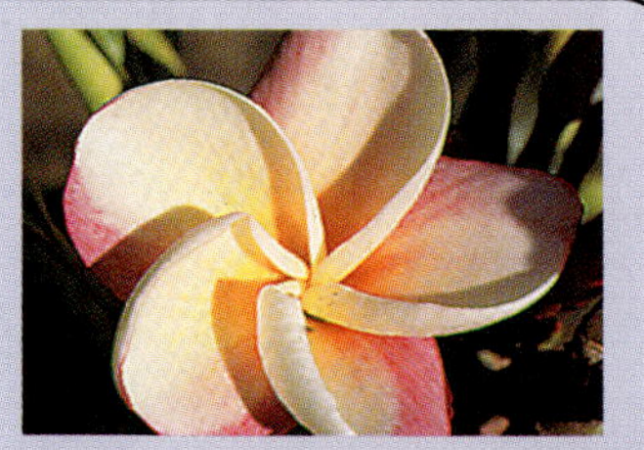

J.L. WHITE/PINK RAINBOW

A spectacular Hawaiian hybrid. Flowers (3"- 3 1/2") have wide overlapping petals that are a soft white fusing into a pink-reddish rainbow then into a golden yellow center. Flowers have very good texture with an excellent blooming habit and are sweetly fragrant.

52321 Rooting Cutting................*$49.95*

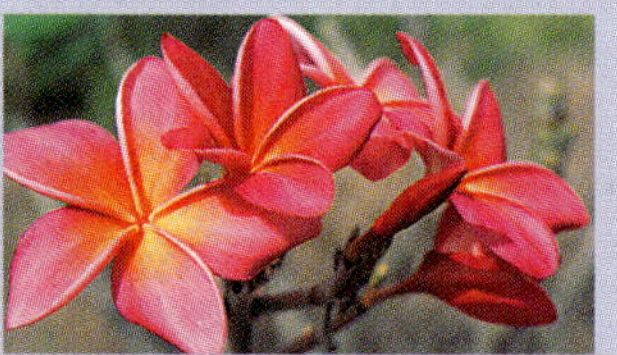

KANEOHE SUNBURST

Deep pink w/large, brilliant-yellow center, dark-red radiating lines; narrow, elliptical petal, pointed tip, slightly overlapping, narrow strong red band on back; good texture; 3"-3 1/4" diameter; mild sweet fragrance.

52661 Rooting Cutting...................*$24.95*

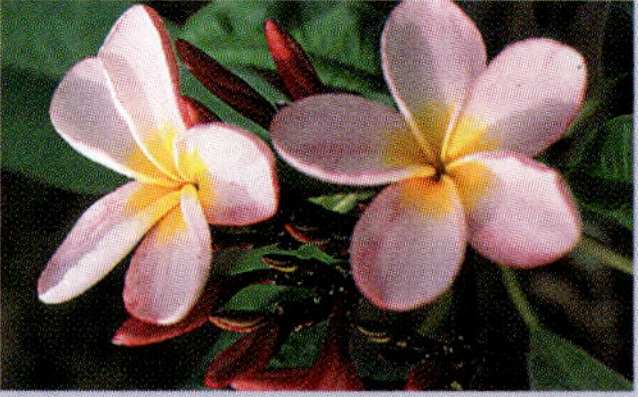

JULIE MORAGNE

Another of the rare 'Moragne' hybrids. Large 3" (7.5cm) flower, pink with half white rounded petals and a large brilliant gold center. Inside of petals dark pink veins on petals. Extremely nice. In limited supply.

52601 Rooting Cutting................*$48.95*

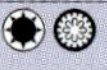

J. L. TRUMPET

A beautiful variety with a small 2" flower shaped like a trumpet, and a severely dark red-maroon striped line under the back side of a brilliant white flower.

52401 Rooting Cutting.............................*$49.95*

Save $30 on rooting cuttings off listed prices by purchasing an entire collection.
See pages 107 - 109

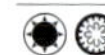

J. L. STARLIGHT

This beauty has huge 4" (10cm) flowers, white with large yellow center. Red band on backside of petals visible from the front. Petals are oblong with rounded tips. A Hawaiian beauty. In limited supply.

52351 Rooting Cutting..........................*$39.95*

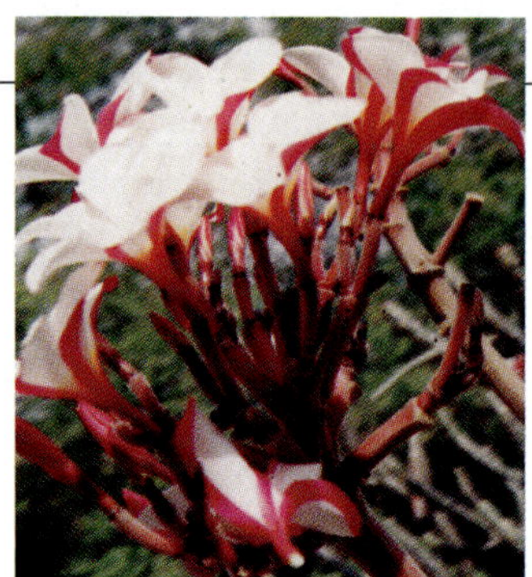

JAPANESE LANTERN

('Flower Basket') The plant has flowers that are moderate strong red with small, brilliant yellow center; petals narrow, elliptical, pointed tip twisting downward, narrow, strong red band on back; poor texture; 3" (7.5cm) diameter; slight sweet scent. Flower clusters hang like red lanterns. Very distinctive even from a distance.

52451 Rooting Cutting...................................*$39.95*

JEAN MORAGNE JR.

One of the rare 'Moragne' hybrids. Very large up to 5 1/2" flowers that appear orange upon opening, then changing to pink at the edges. Tight pinwheel shape. Petals are slightly pointed giving a star shape. Very showy with red veins in petals. A hybrid of 'Scott Pratt' and 'Daisy Wilcox.' Strong rose fragrance.

52501 Rooting Cutting...........................*$48.95*

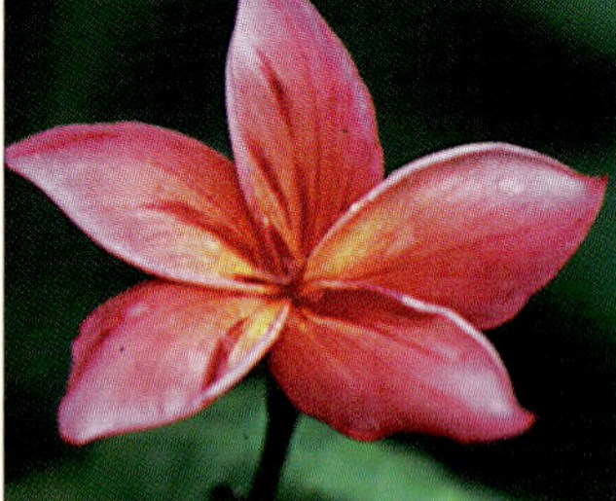

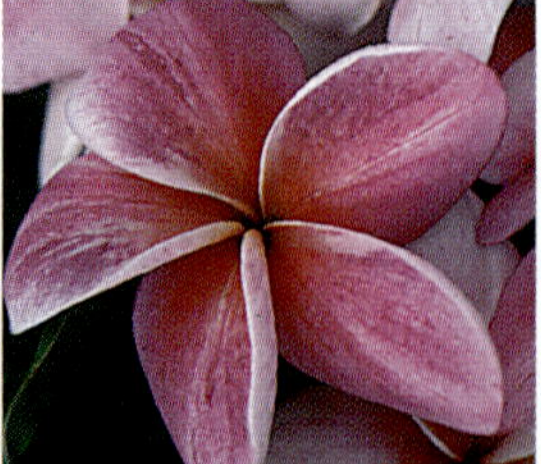

JEAN MORAGNE SR.

Has been called Morangne #9. A smashing hybrid 'Moragne' with a large (4/2"-5/2") floppy pink flower with reddish-orange streaks from the center to the edge. Full rounded elliptical petals.

53651 Rooting Cutting...................................*$60.95*

KATIE MORAGNE

Plant makes flowers that are vibrant brick red contrasted with soft white of the rolled inner edge of each petal, radiating with yellow shading from center. Elliptical petals with rounded tip, moderately overlapped; heavy texture; 4" (10cm) diameter; strong sweet scent.

52651 Rooting Cutting...........................$39.95

KAULANANI

A combination color scheme of Kimo and Paul Weissich, but more goldish in color. The flower is of good texture with average diameter of around 3". Slightly scented with a slight orangish band gracing the front side of the petals. There is a slight pinkish band on the backside. Discovered by Dr. Richard Criley of the University of Hawaii.

52671 Rooting Cutting..$49.95

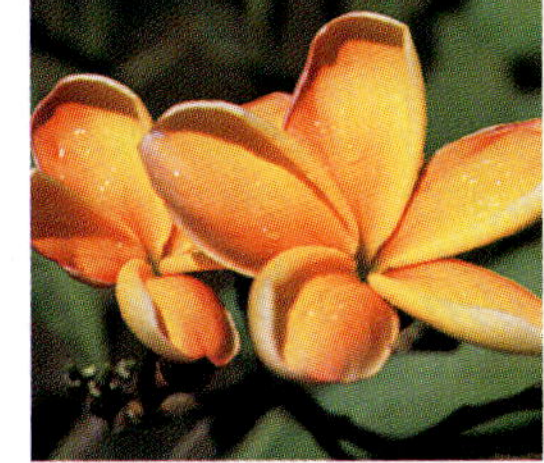

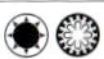

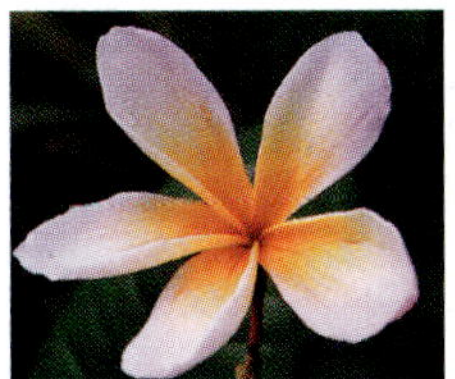

KEY WEST ELIZABETH

A magnificent specimen from a cutting of a mature tree on Elizabeth St. in Key West, Florida. Medium flowers 2" (5cm) that are slightly overlapping and highly angled. Flowers have pinkish rose background with flashes of yellow in center of petals. Petals have dark rose tips and dark pink throat. Faint frangipani fragrance. Very strong grower.

52751 Rooting Cutting $49.95

KEY WEST RED

This beauty has dark red 3" (7.5cm) flowers. Petals are slightly overlapping and slightly pointed giving a star shape. Flowers are borne on a long dark red pedicel. Low growing tree excellent for container growing. Strong frangipani fragrance.

52801 Rooting Cutting $28.95

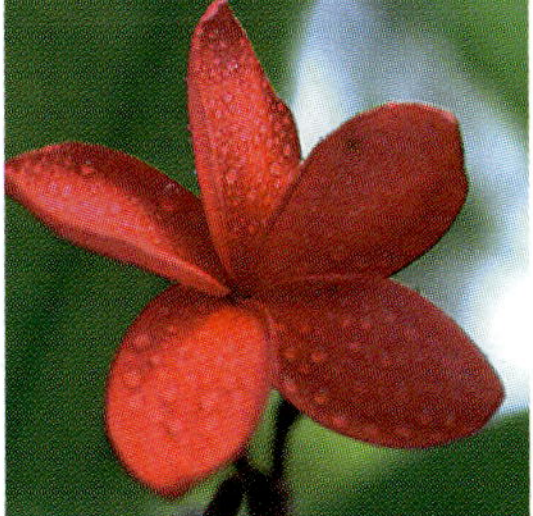

KIMI MORAGNE

Another of the rare 'Moragne' hybrids. Very large, 4¹/₂" (11.5cm), sweetly fragrant, intense rose-pink flowers shading to lighter pink at the extreme edge of each petal and a golden-orange center. Petals are round and overlapping. Clusters are large and dense with many flowers open at one time. A cross of 'Daisy Wilcox' and 'Scott Pratt'.

52851 Rooting Cutting............................$39.95

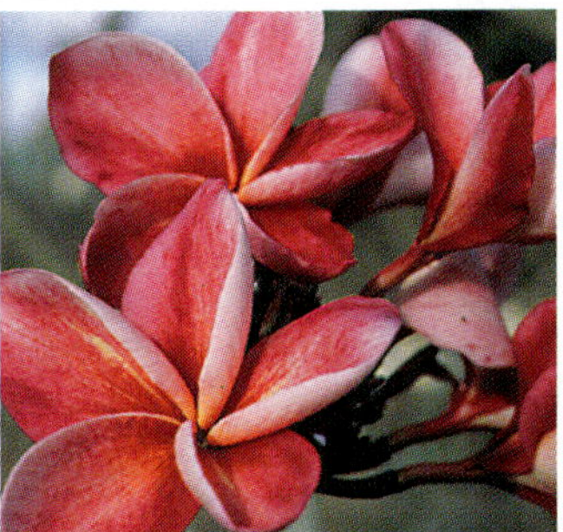

KAUKA WILDER

A remarkable star-shaped flower 3" (7.5cm) with a breathtaking combination of yellow and red that gives the appearance of a fiery orange blossom. Petals are wide and slightly overlapping with a pointed tips. Has a very strong sweet fragrance and is early and easy to bloom.

52701 Rooting Cutting $21.95

KIMO

The glowing apricot-orange blossoms have a strong pink band on the reverse showing through on front and the wide, rounded, heavily overlapping petals nearly form a complete circle. Flowers average 3" (7.5cm), have a very heavy texture, good keeping quality and a sweet, fruity fragrance.

52901 Rooting Cutting............$35.95

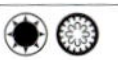 Full Sun   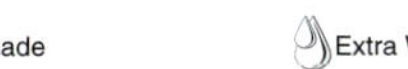 Part Sun   Shade   Extra Water   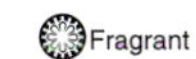 Fragrant   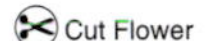 Cut Flower   N New

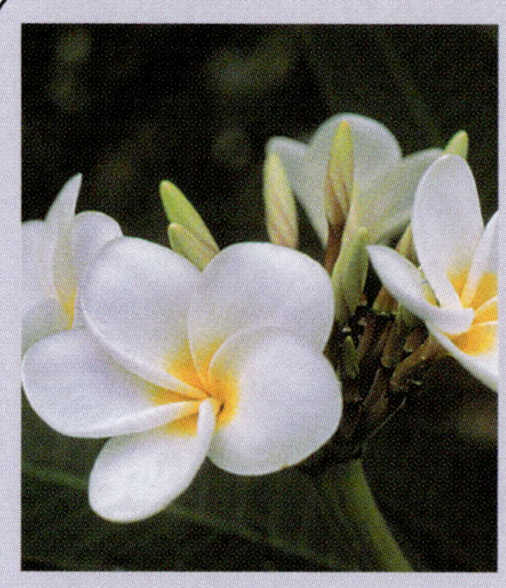

KING KALAKAUA
'Minature White'

White with small, brilliant-yellow center; petal wide, pointed tip, moderately overlapping; medium texture; 1¹/₂" diameter; scent similar to gardenia; keeping quality good.
52871 Rooting Cutting..............$44.95

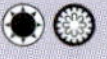

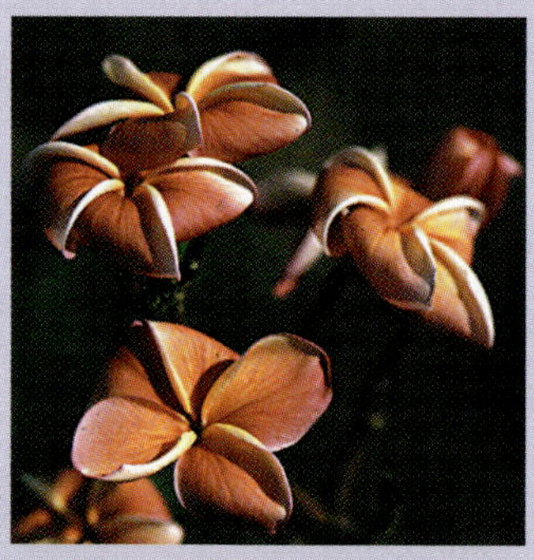

LURLINE

A striking combination of bright red-orange on yellow with a orange star at the center. The tips of the petals and outer margins are purplish-red. The heavily textured flowers are large to 4" (10cm), and have a spicy fragrance. Flower production is heavy and continues for many months. Good keeping quality.
53201 Rooting Cutting $34.95

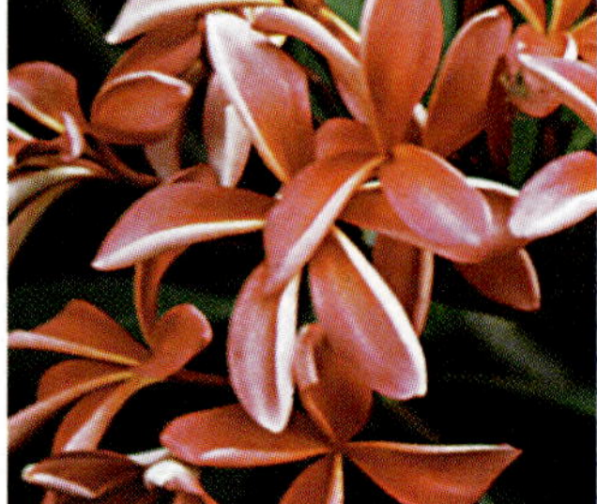

LA JOLLA SUNSET ™

An extremely nice variety with dark green leaves. Stem is somewhat willowy. Flowers are outstanding rose color fading to orange in center. Scent is delicate but exquisite like an expensive French perfume. Flower color does not fade.
53001 Rooting Cutting $40.95

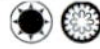

LAGUNA PINK ™

Vigorous grower. Foliage has bronze cast. Flowers are very interesting; pink with a little orange in center and subtle mottling on the petals. Nice frangipani fragrance. Cuttings root very quickly. Plant is erect with good symmetry.
53051 Rooting Cutting $40.95

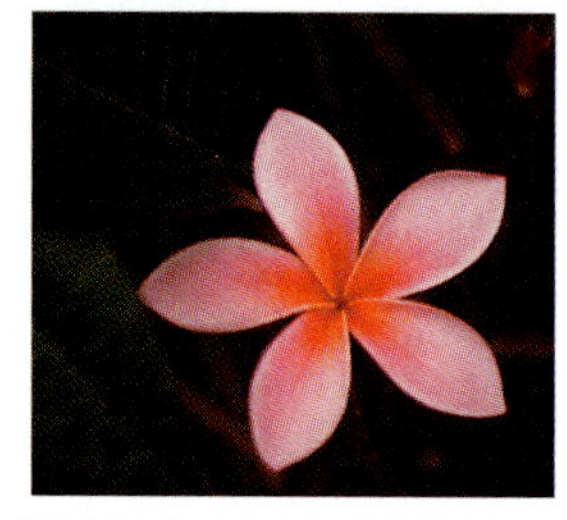

LORETTA

The blooms are moderate pink and white with moderate red spot in small, brilliant yellow center; grainy pigmentation; petal wide and oval with round tip, moderately overlapping; deep pink grainy band on back; good texture; 2¹/₂" (6.5cm) to 3" (7.5cm) diameter; slight sweet scent; keeping quality good.
53151 Rooting Cutting $30.95

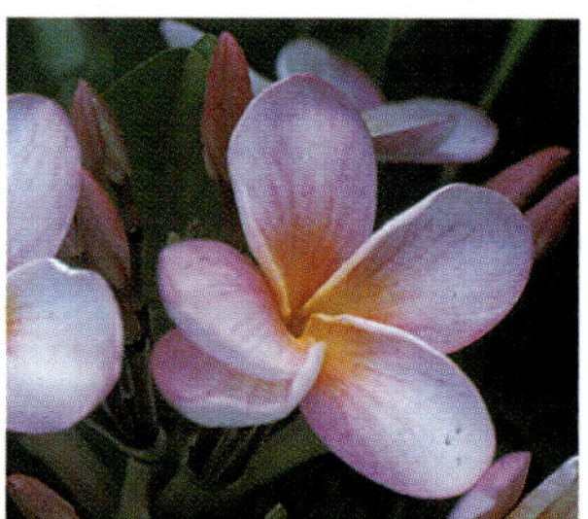

LURLINE MATSAMOTA

A great new addition to our Hawaiian plumerias. Flowers (1¹/₂"- 2¹/₂") are white with a small yellow eye. A continuous bloomer from spring to fall. Tree has a pleasing symmetrical branching pattern. Flower has a nice mild, sweet fragrance.
52311 Rooting Cutting............................$49.95

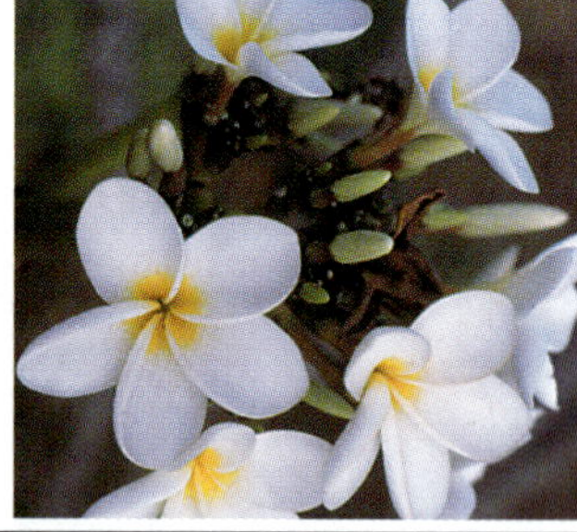

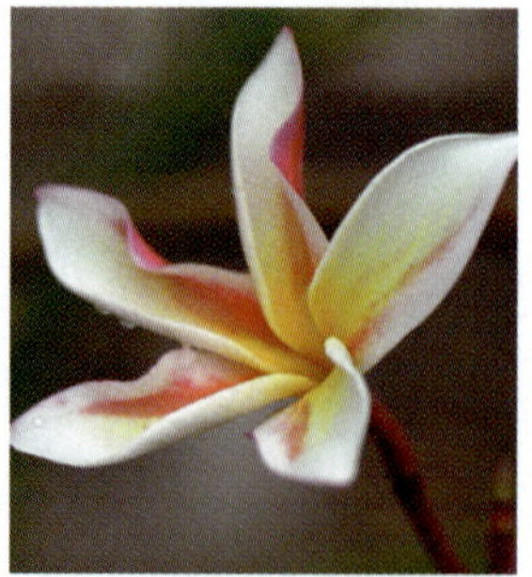

MADAME PONI

A challenge to categorize, one of the most incredible of all plumerias. Flowers are large to 3¹/₂" (8.5cm), with narrow, curved and fluted petals,that are white with a greenish-yellow band that extends down the middle of each petal and sienna-red stripes within the bands. Petals are widely separated and have strong red bands on the back. Good texture, good keeping quality, and sweet fragrance. *53251 Rooting Cutting.......$25.95*

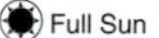
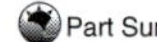
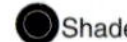

Full Sun   Part Sun   Shade   Extra Water   Fragrant   Cut Flower   New

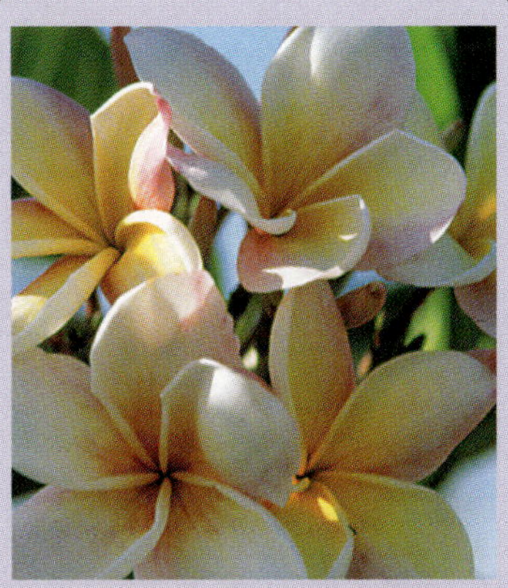

MADAME YVONNE™

A wonderful new seedling with medium size flowers 2½" (6.25m); white flower with yellow center. Very good bloomer with nice compact and symmetrical growth habit. Nice frangipani fragrance. Highly recommended for beautiful glossy leaves. Named by Glenn Stokes for his wife Yvonne. *See page 109 for picture of plant.*
53301 Rooting Cutting *$49.95*

MARION B.™

A smashing new seedling of 'Pink Pansy'. A striking rainbow of pink, white and yellow colors. Has good frangipani fragrance. Compact grower. In very limited supply. Named by Glenn Stokes for his granddaughter.
53361 Rooting Cutting *$59.95*

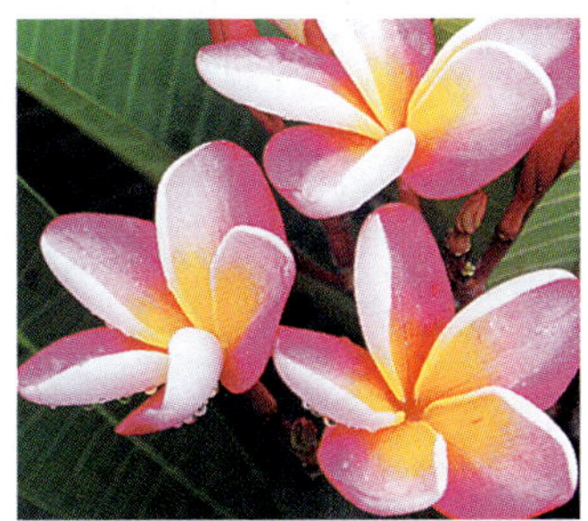

MARINO'S RAINBOW ™

A wonderful new seedling variety from Aztec Gold. Large 3½" (8.5cm) flower with widely separated petals suffused with pink front and back. A burnt yellow center with indications of reddish pink veins showing through. Wonderful fresh peach fragrance. Limited supply.
53351 Rooting Cutting *$49.95*

MARY MORAGNE

An outstanding 'Moragne' hybrid. Creamy pale pink petals shaded darker on one edge with a golden orange center, oval petals, moderately overlapped; heavy texture; large 4" (10cm) flower; spicy sweet scent, good keeping quality.
53401 Rooting Cutting...................*$48.95*

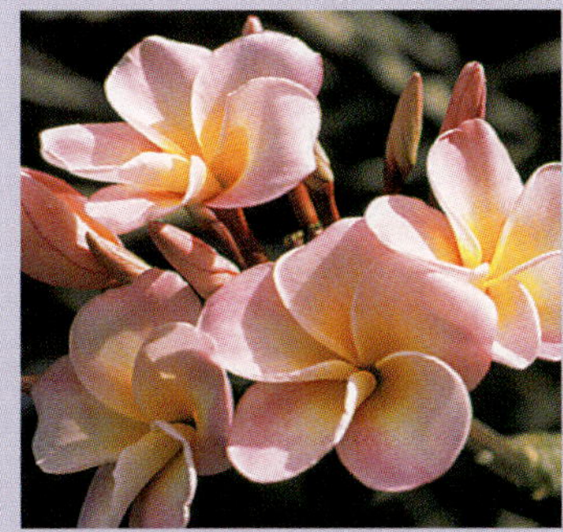

MARY PUKUI (PAT BACON)

A great looking yellow flower with a pleasant sweet fragrance. Flowers measure 3" across. Very nice round petals that is slightly overlapping. Heavy texture, good keeping quality. New.
53471 Rooting Cutting *$49.95*

MAUI BEAUTY

Abundant clusters of brilliant 3¼" (8.5cm) flowers are pink with a yellow center and wide, rounded petals. Broad, strong pink bands on the reverse create a striking contrast between flowers and buds. Heavy texture and very good keeping quality further distinguish this cultivar. Slight lemon scent.
53451 Rooting Cutting................*$28.95*

MAUI PICOTEE

A wonderful new plumeria with 2" flowers that are whitish with red bands and a yellow center. Flowers have heavy waxy texture with slight fragrance. New.
53421 Rooting Cutting...................*$49.95*

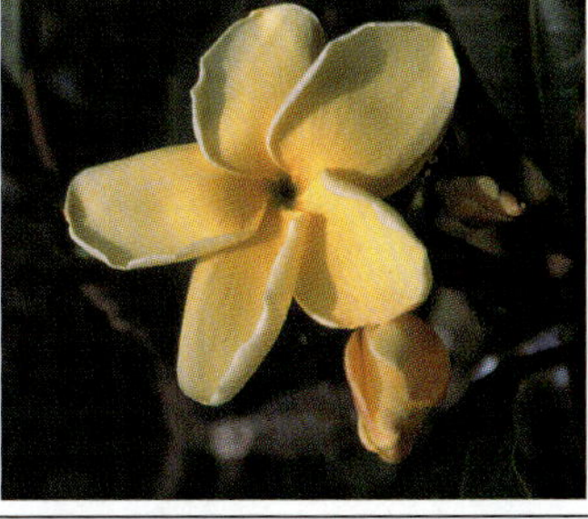

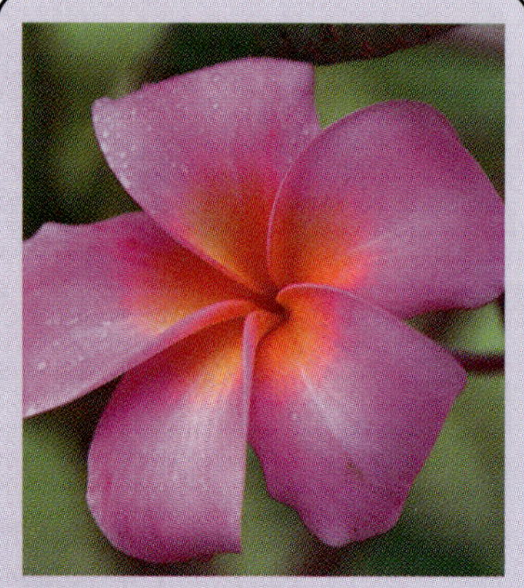

MELE MATSON

Produces abundant clusters of large, medium pink flowers 3" (7.5cm) with a brilliant yellow center and rounded overlapping petals exquisitely shaped. Dark pink band on back. Has a delightfully sweet, lemon fragrance. Blooms over a long period. Good keeping quality.

53501 Rooting Cutting..................*$30.95*

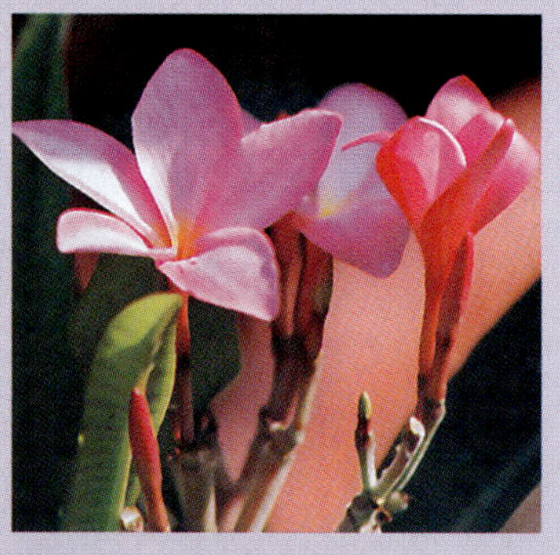

METAIRIE PINK™

A wonderful seedling whose flower is a delicate pink with radiating darker pink lines and a slight yellow center. Strongly overlapping petals makes flower resemble a lily flower. Dark pink band on the reverse of petals. A very nice, sweet fragrance. Very limited supply.

52191 Rooting Cutting..................*$49.95*

Visit our Web Site:
www.stokestropicals.com

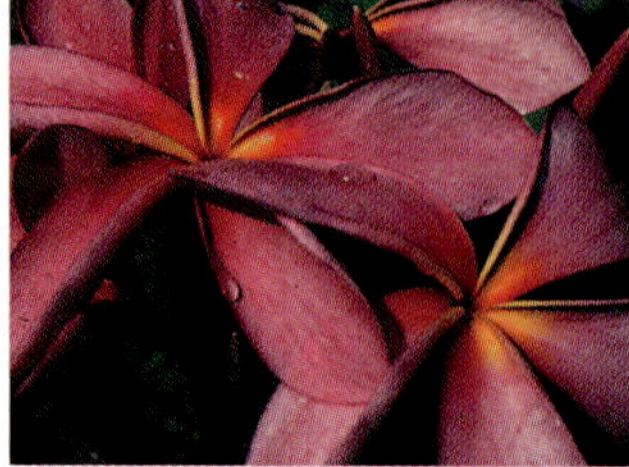

MELE PA BOWMAN

('Evergreen Singapore Yellow') Large highly fragrant yellow blossoms edged in white; obovate petals with rounded tips, no overlap; moderate texture; 4" (10cm) diameter; strong citrus scent. A magnificent plant.

53526 Rooting Cutting *$41.95*

MOIR

Moderate pink with small, brilliant yellow center; petal wide and elliptical with pointed tip, moderately overlapping; wide, deep pink band on back; fair texture; 3 1/4" diameter; mild lemon scent; keeping quality good.

53611 Rooting Cutting *$24.95*

MAUVE

The flowers are borne in large clusters. The pale lilac-tinted flowers with widely separated petals and a golden yellow center are very large. The flower (4-4 1/2") has a sweet fragrance.

54851 Rooting Cutting *$49.95*

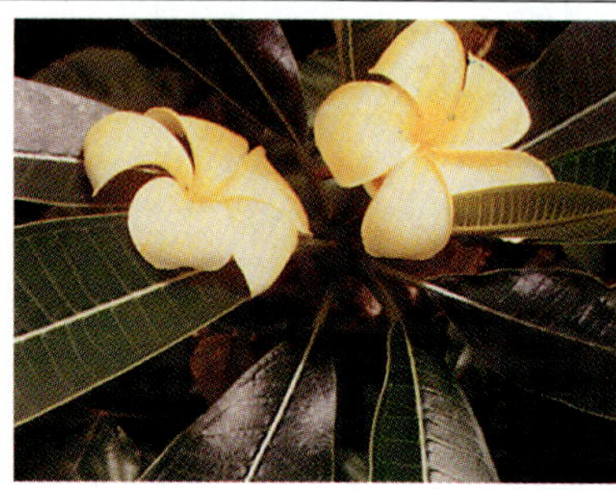

MIAMI ROSE

Medium (2 1/2") flower with rose pink background and wide light pink bands. Petals are round with small golden yellow throat. The strongest and most commonly grown plumeria in the Miami area. Will grow to 30' (9m) high in the Florida Keys. Very strong fragrance of coconut oil.

53551 Rooting Cutting *$28.95*

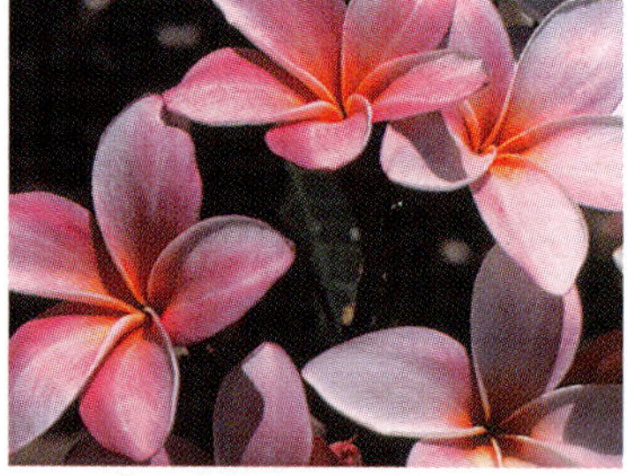

MONTEGO BAY™

A wonderful new white-flowered plumeria seedling. Flowers are a pure white with bright yellow center. Petals are broadly overlapping. Medium size flower 2"-3" with a nice frangipani fragrance.

53631 Rooting Cutting *$39.95*

**MEMBERSHIP INFORMATION
ON THE PLUMERIA SOCIETY OF
AMERICA, INC.**
See page 135

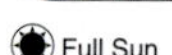 Full Sun 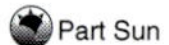 Part Sun 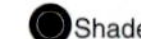 Shade 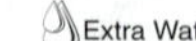 Extra Water 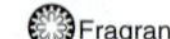 Fragrant 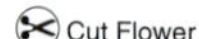 Cut Flower 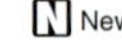 New

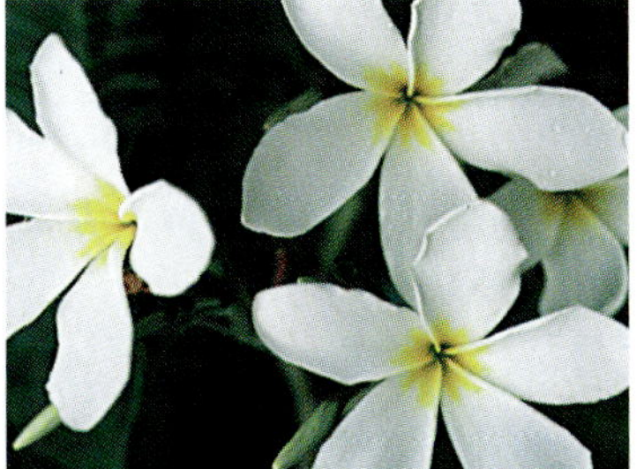

MOONLIGHT

Small 2" (5cm) white flower with a distinct yellow center. A very strong growing tree. The most prolific bloomer in South Florida. Will frequently produce seed pods. A very nice fragrance of citrus.

53601 Rooting Cutting $35.95

MORAGNE # 23

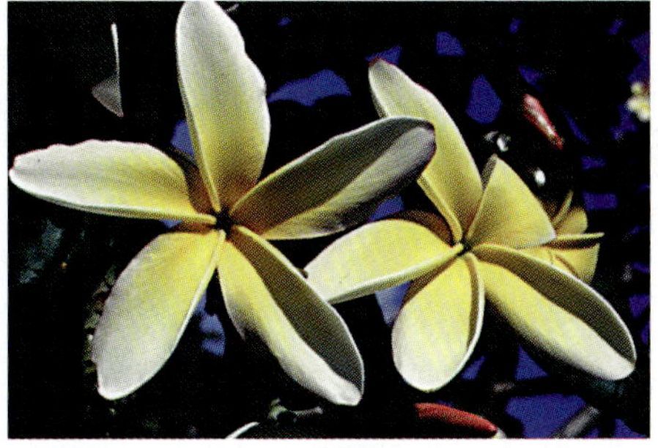

One of the largest flowers in the 'Moragne' group at 5" (12.5cm) to 6" (15cm) in diameter. The flowers are soft-textured, creamy white shaded from the center with a rich gold and suffused with pink from the pink band along the back edge of each petal. Petals are broad and slightly recurved. The center of the flower is marked by a tiny red spot. The buds are pink and the flowers are in dense clusters. This plant is a cross of Daisy Wilcox and Scott Pratt.

53751 Rooting Cutting $60.95

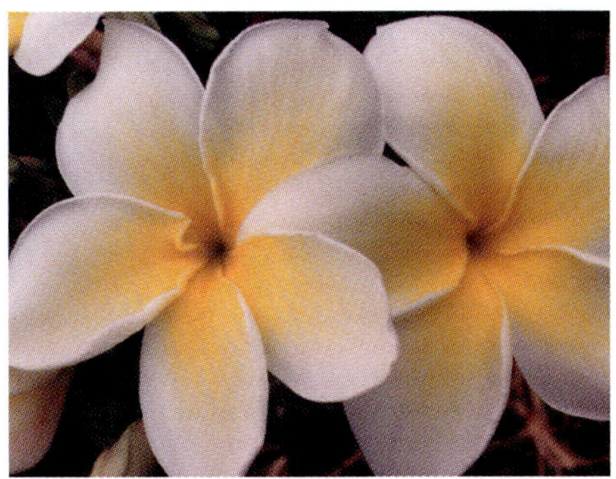

MORAGNE # 27

Another outstanding 'Moragne' hybrid with a typical large (4-5") Moragne flower. Full bodied with good texture and scent with lemon-colored center fading to a white border. Full elliptical petals pointed tip and slightly overlapped.

53801 Rooting Cutting $69.95

MORAGNE #93 (Reddish Moragne)

One of the famous Moragne hybrids. The variety is still unnamed and referred to by its original designation. Large $4^1/2$"-5" flower is reddish pink on white; center is yellow overlaid with grainy reddish purple, resulting in orange appearance. Wide, elliptical, delicate petals with round tips. Mild, sweet, floral fragrance. Light-green colored leaves. Resulted from cross of Scott Pratt and Daisy Wilcox.

54401 Rooting Cutting $59.95

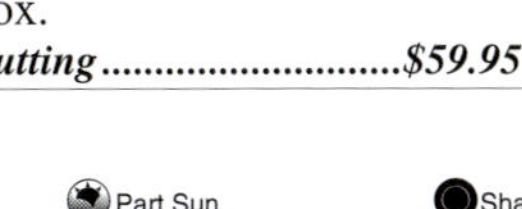

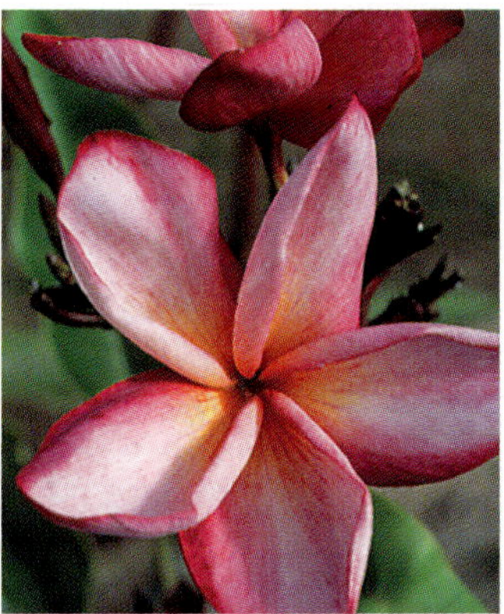

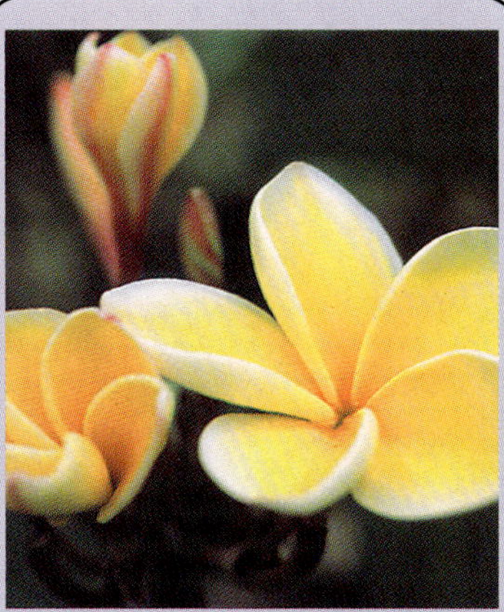

NEBEL'S GOLD

An often-overlooked flower very popular in Hawaii. Similar to Nebel's Rainbow except has more yellow with no pink on front of flower. 3" flowers are yellow with reddish bands on reverse. Texture is good. Petals are elliptical to obovate with rounded tips. Strong frangipani fragrance.

53911 Rooting Cutting $29.95

FOR CUSTOMER SERVICE:
337-365-6998 - Mon.–Fri.,
8:30 am-4:00 pm C.T.

STOKES TROPICALS' PLUMERIA BLEND

Controlled Release Fertilizer
(3-Month Formula)

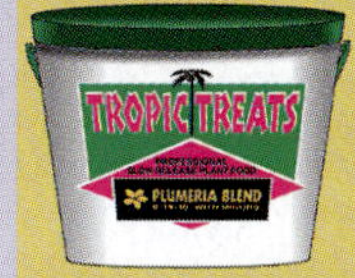

ANALYSIS 8-14-10 w/minors.

Uniquely formulated for best growth of Plumerias. This total nutrient formula provides a complete balance of all major and minor elements.

6040 (1 lb. Bucket) $6.00
6041 (4 lb. Bucket) $17.00

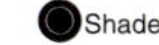 Full Sun    Part Sun   Shade   Extra Water   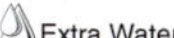 Fragrant   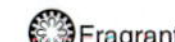 Cut Flower   N New

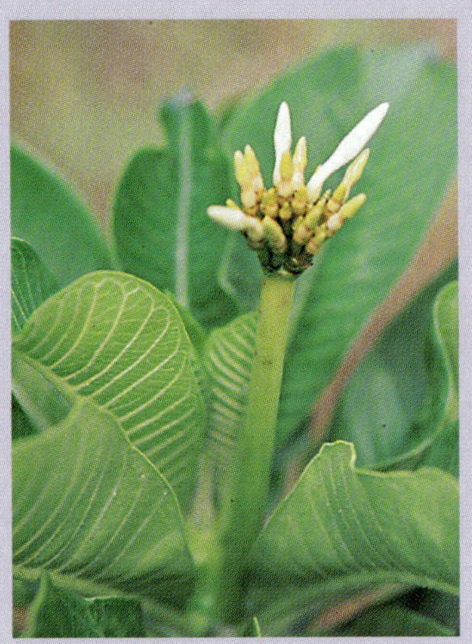

OBTUSA 'Isabella'™

A very interesting Plumeria that comes from Columbia, S.A., by way of Key West. The main attraction is the large, very wavy leaves. Flowers 2¹/2"-3" are white with yellow center. Nice frangipani fragrance. In very limited supply.
52181 Rooting Cutting $59.95

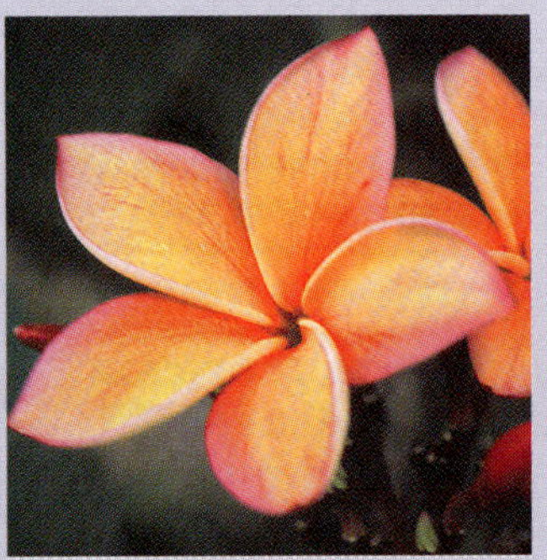

PAUAHI ALII (Formerly Angus Gold Selection)

A wonderful deep-yellow flower streaked with grainy, red markings. 3 1/2" flowers with good texture. Petals are elliptical with pointed tips and dark red stripes on back. Nice mild frangipani fragrance. Leaf color is light-green.
54111 Rooting Cutting $41.95

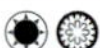

NOVELTY

A real novelty with a star-shaped cream and yellow flower with good texture; has mild fragrance. Has narrow twisted petals that slightly overlap. A 2¹/2"- 3" flower.
53925 Rooting Cutting........$49.95

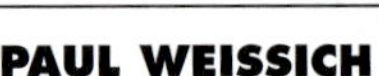

NEBEL'S RAINBOW

Has been called Lei Rainbow. Large 3" (7.5cm) yellow flower with a moderate red band on front and back. Petals are very wide with rounded tips and moderately overlap. Mild sweet fragrance. Flowers have excellent keeping quality. Flower production heavy on strong branches.
53901 Rooting Cutting $29.95

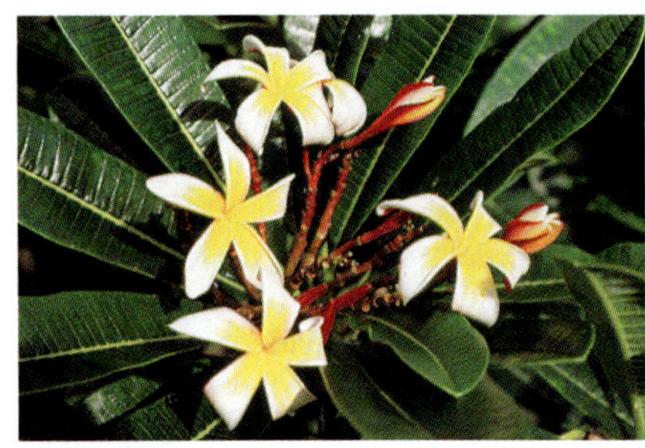

OBTUSA 'Fairchild'

A species that was originally obtained from one of the obtusa trees growing in Fairchild Tropical Gardens in Miami, Florida. Flowers are 2¹/2"-3", slightly overlapping white with small yellow center. Petals are wavy and floppy. Fragrance is slight. Leaves are ovate and dark green. In very short supply.
54281 Rooting Cutting $49.95

PAUL WEISSICH

Large golden yellow flower with an orange center. Petals have radiating orange-pink lines. Flowers are up to 3-4" and have large rounded, overlapping petals. Faint peach fragrance. Vigorous plant that was named in honor of the director of Foster Botanic Garden in Hawaii. Keeping quality is good.
54001 Rooting Cutting $40.95

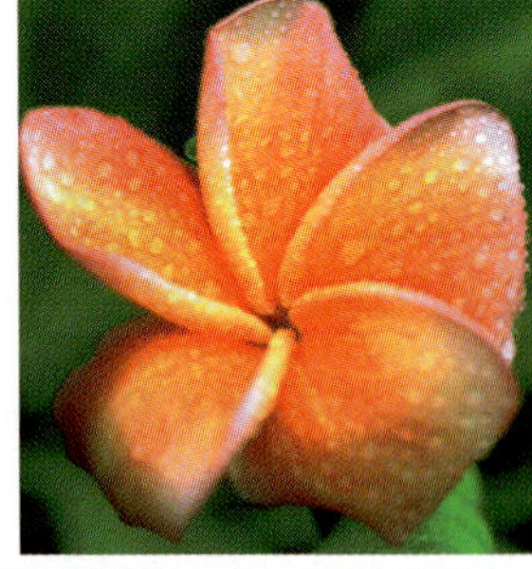

PENANG PEACH

Apricot-peach, yellow-colored flower with round petals. A smashing looking flower. Very limited supply. Without a doubt it will become very popular.
54051 Rooting Cutting $60.95

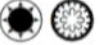

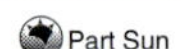 Full Sun 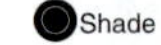 Part Sun ● Shade ◊ Extra Water 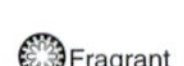 Fragrant 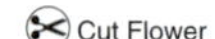 Cut Flower Ⓝ New

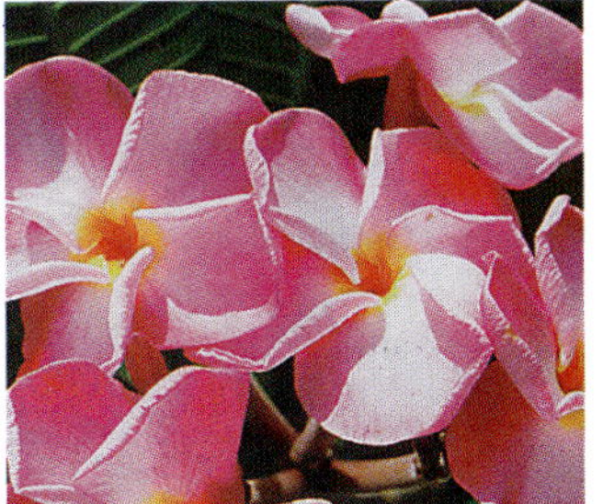

PINK RUFFLES™

An amazing seedling from J.L. Pink Pansy with light-pink petals that are suffused with rose-pink grainy lines. Petal tips are distinctly ruffled. Slightly yellow cup. Dark-green leaves add to its appeal. Nice frangipani fragrance. Flowers measure 3" across. In very short supply.
54171 Rooting Cutting $69.95

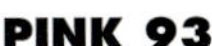

PINK 93

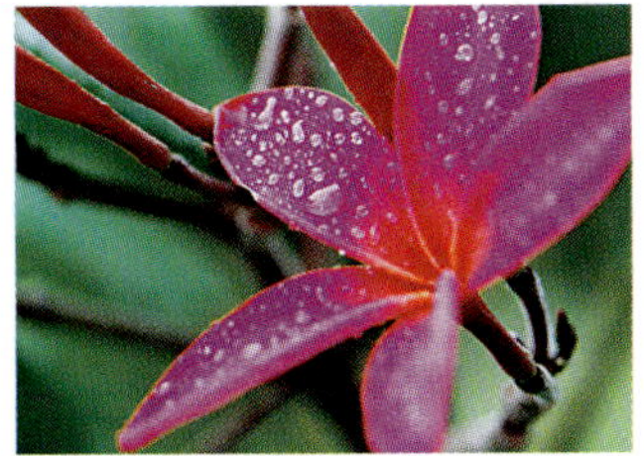

A very nice pink hybrid. Medium 2¹/₂" (6.25cm) pink flower with narrow petals and a nice yellow center. Good frangipani fragrance.
54101 Rooting Cutting $25.95

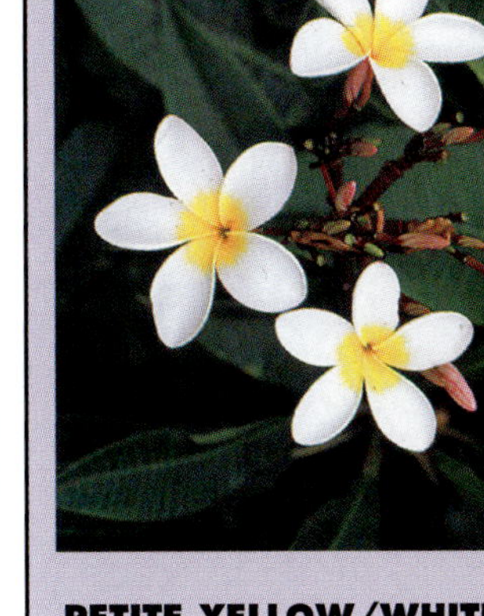

PETITE YELLOW/WHITE

A beautiful new plumeria with a small white flower (2''- 2.5'') with a yellow eye. Fair texture with a sweet scent. Semi-compact growth makes this an excellent landscape tree and great for container culture. New.
54061 Rooting Cutting...........$39.95

PINK SHELL

A pink and white flower that looks like a curled shell before fully opening. Noted primarily for it's novelty. Slightly scented.
54151 Rooting Cutting.......$35.95

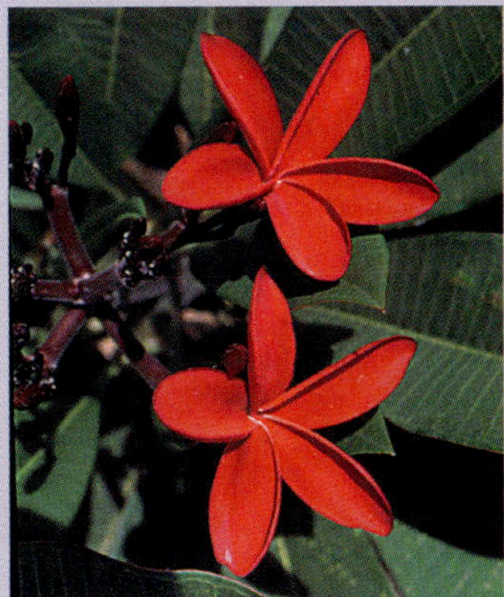

PLASTIC PINK

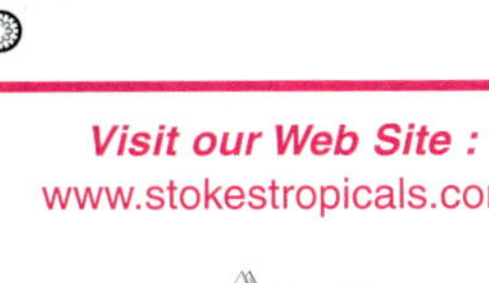

Intense pink flowers 3" (7.5cm) have brilliant yellow centers and a red band on the reverse. Petals are wide, with round tips and overlap slightly. Good keeping quality and flowers profusely. Mild lemon fragrance. Highly recommended. In limited supply.
54251 Rooting Cutting $25.95

POMPANO DARK PINK

Large, dark pinkish-red flowers up to 3¹/₂" (8.5cm) with stiff petals with slight white markings. Inflorescence always upright. A strong compact grower. Nice frangipani fragrance. In limited supply.
54301 Rooting Cutting.................$28.95

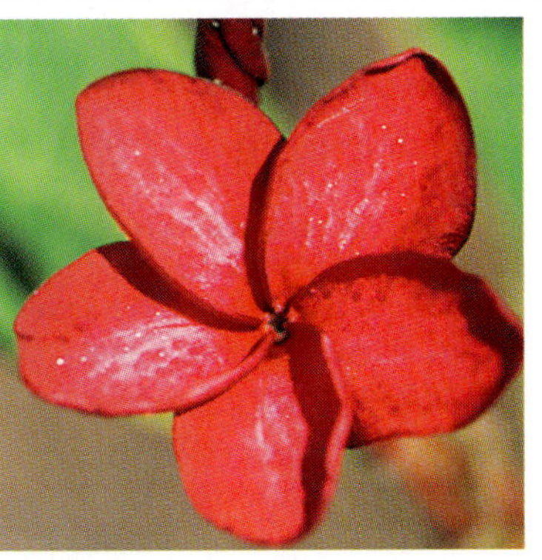

POPS

A new prize plumeria with one of the best red flowers yet. The flower is 3¹/₂"x 4" in Diameter. Flower texture, flower habit and lei quality is outstanding. Fragrance is mild. Rated as #1 flower by Jim Little Nursery. New.
54311 Rooting Cutting $49.95

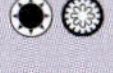

Visit our Web Site :
www.stokestropicals.com

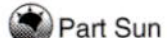

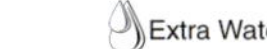

Full Sun   Part Sun   Shade   Extra Water   Fragrant   Cut Flower   N New

Plumerias

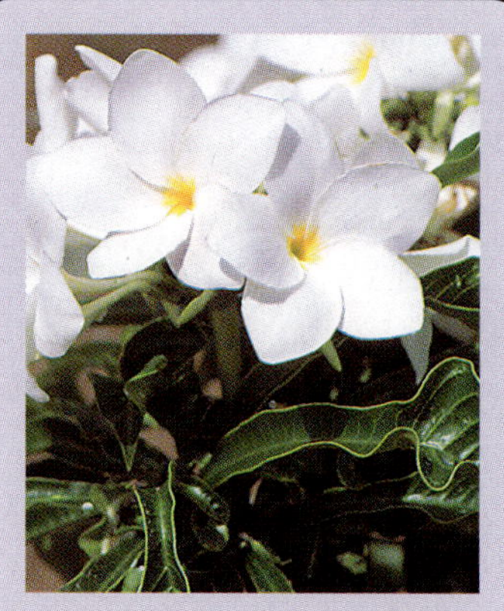

PUDICA 'BRIDAL BOUQUET'

An unusual Plumeria from Puerto Rico with dark-green spatula-like leaves. Has very different branching habits. Fast growing, rather narrow stems. Bears small white flowers with yellow centers. Main interest is leaves and unusual branching habits. Branches from middle of stem without need to flower first. A must plant for the Plumeria collector. Also flowers 2-3 times per year on same growth axis without branching.

54271 Rooting Cutting..................*$19.95*

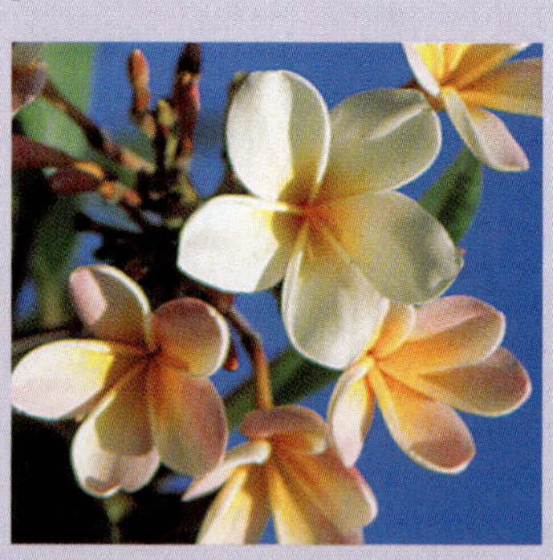

RAINBOW'S END™

A very charming new rainbow-flowered plumeria seedling. Flowers have a light rainbow pattern of color that blush (become lighter in color) as they age. Petals are slightly overlapping. Flower is 3"-3¹/₄" across. Plant is a very upright grower. Flower has a nice gardenia fragrance.

54380 Rooting Cutting................*$39.95*

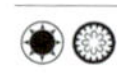

Photo by Joey Rosselli

PUU KAHEA

(*O'Sullivan, Fiesta*) Flowers are brilliant yellow w/strong red bands; petal long, narrow, pointed tip, slightly overlapping; narrow strong red bands on front and back; 4¹/₂" (11.5cm) diameter; mild lemon fragrance; keeping quality good.

54351 Rooting Cutting............................*$30.95*

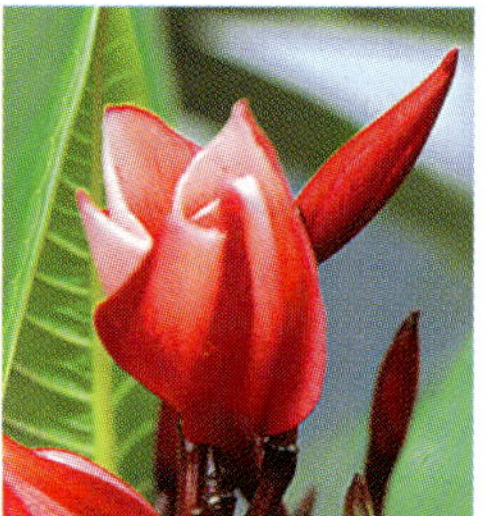

RED SHELL

A marvelous plumeria with rosebud-like flowers. Flowers stay tightly closed and display dark rose pink bands on underside of petals. A mild fragrance. A must for collectors.

54321 Rooting Cutting *$29.95*

RUFFLES

Moderate pink w/large brilliant-yellow center; petal wide, round tip, moderately overlapping; strong pink bands on front and back; margins very wavy; fair texture; 2" diameter; slight sweet scent; keeping quality fair.

54331 Rooting Cutting.............................*$24.95*

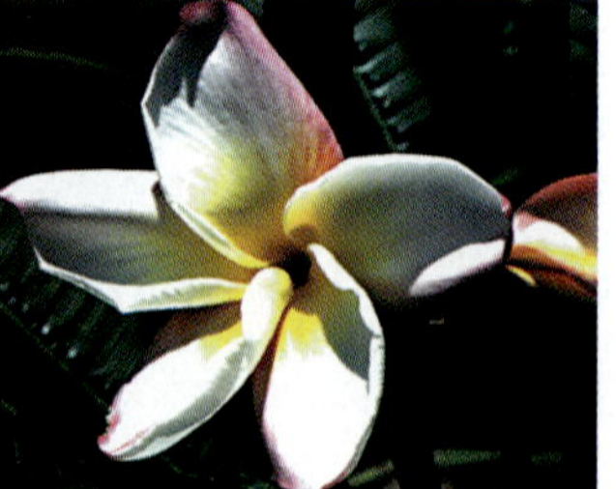

PRINCESS VICTORIA™

The most beautiful plumeria that we have seen. A seedling from Metairie Pink. Large (3"-3¹/₂") spectacular red and white splotched flowers with butter yellow centers. Good gardenia fragrance. Keeping quality good. Extemely short supply. Named by Joey Rosselli for his new bride. New.

55161 Rooting Cutting *$299.95**

**Available in 2001*

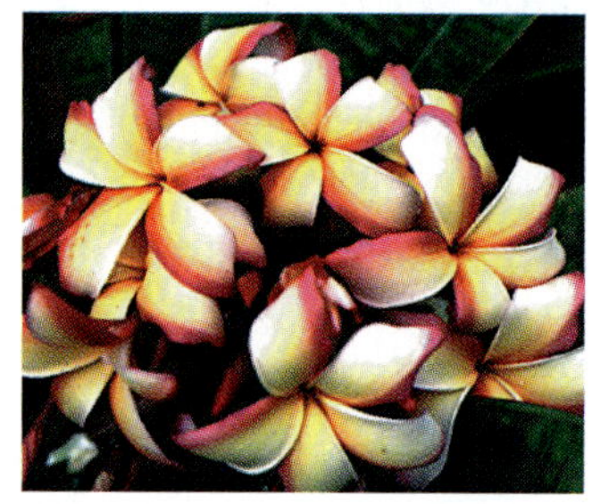

SALLY MORAGNE

Large, light peachy pink with a golden center and pink shading at the edge of petal, distinctive red veining radiating to the outer edge; wide petals with rounded tip, highly overlapped; heavy texture; 4¹/₂" (11.5cm) to 5" (12.5cm) diameter; strong sweet fragrance; keeping quality good.

54451 Rooting Cutting...............................*$39.95*

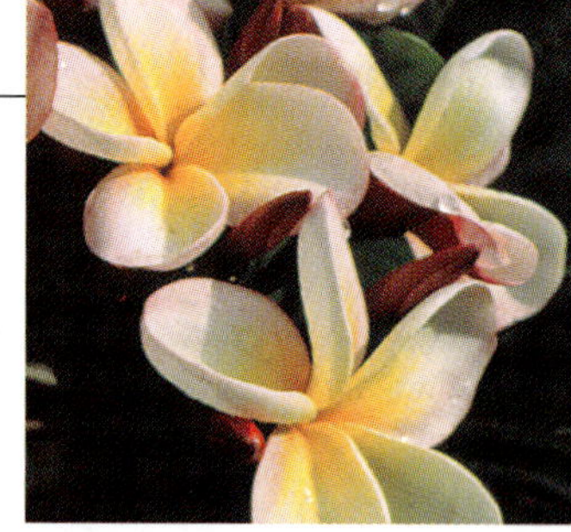

 Full Sun 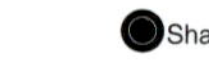 Part Sun 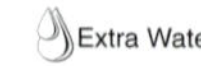 Shade 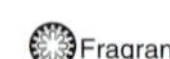 Extra Water 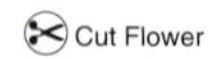 Fragrant Cut Flower New

TO ORDER CALL **1-800-624-9706**/24 HRS. OR VISIT OUR WEB SITE: www. stokestropicals.com

SAMOAN FLUFF

The striking, round, full petals are white with a small, brilliant, greenish-yellow center and medium pink bands on the reverse. Petals are overlapping and of good texture. Flowers are 3 1/2" (8.5cm), have very good keeping quality, with a slight sweet fragrance.

54501 Rooting Cutting *$35.95*

SAN GERMAIN

One of the most outstanding plumerias from Hawaii. In extremely short supply. Large white flowers (4"-4 1/2") with hint of pink and large yellow centers. Good sweet fragrance. Heavy texture. Presently one of the most sought after plumerias.

54521 Rooting Cutting *$59.95*

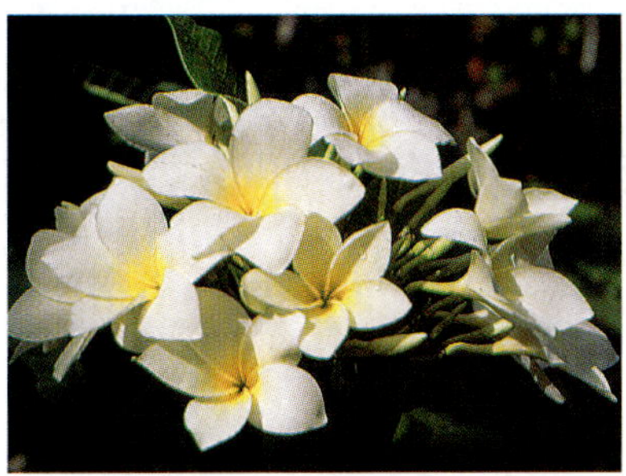

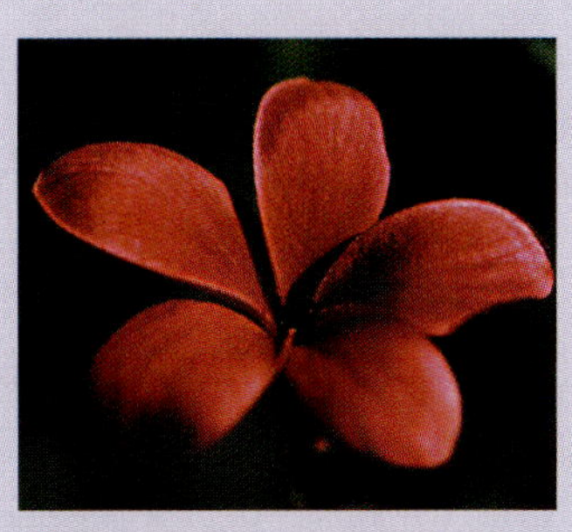

SCOTT PRATT

Dark velvety red flowers 2 1/2" (6.5cm) that have fine purple-black veins radiating from the center and a reddish-brown band on the reverse side. A very long blooming variety. Slight spicy or coconut scent increases after picking. Easy to grow.

54651 Rooting Cutting..............*$28.95*

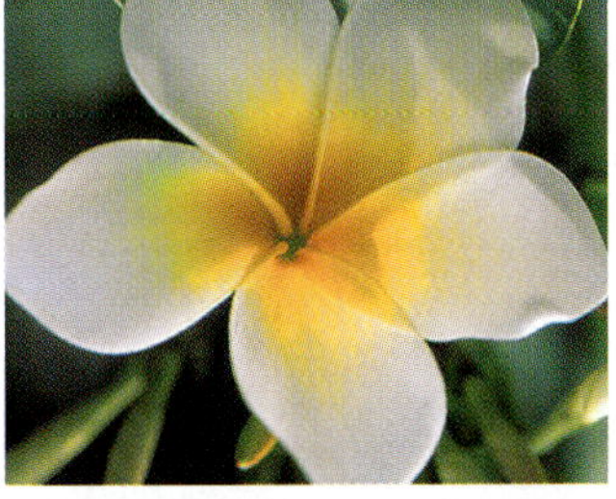

SAN PEDRO DULAC™

An interesting variety from Guatemala with a moderate-size (3") white flower with a dark-yellow center that spreads about 1/3 down the petals. A moderate spicy fragrance. In very limited supply.

54511 Rooting Cutting *$39.95*

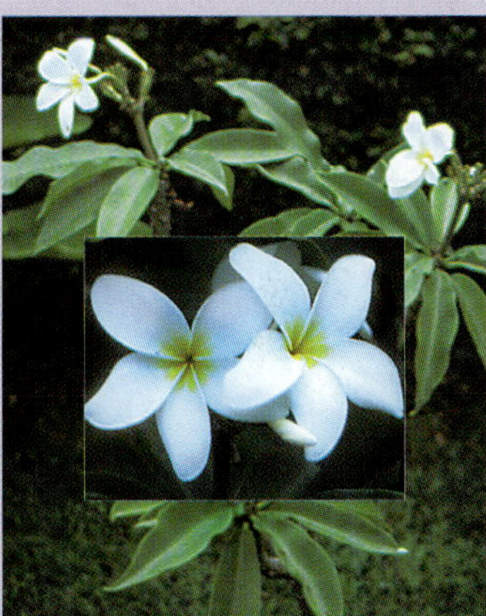

SANTA BARBARA CLASSIC WHITE ™

Outstanding variety with clean, erect, symmetrical growth. Vigorous grower. Cuttings easy to root. Lush green foliage. Classic white flower with yellow center and frangipani fragrance. Flowers are held erect above foliage.

54551 Rooting Cutting *$40.95*

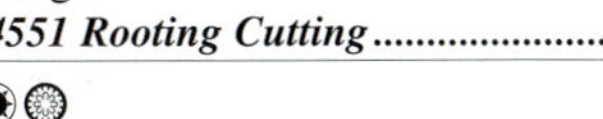

SHERMAN 'Polynesian White'

Beautiful large sweet-scented 4 1/2" (11.5cm) white flowers with brilliant golden center. No color bands, petals are wide, round tipped, and overlap slightly. Very nice. Plants make large symmetrical trees with dense branches.

54701 Rooting Cutting *$25.95*

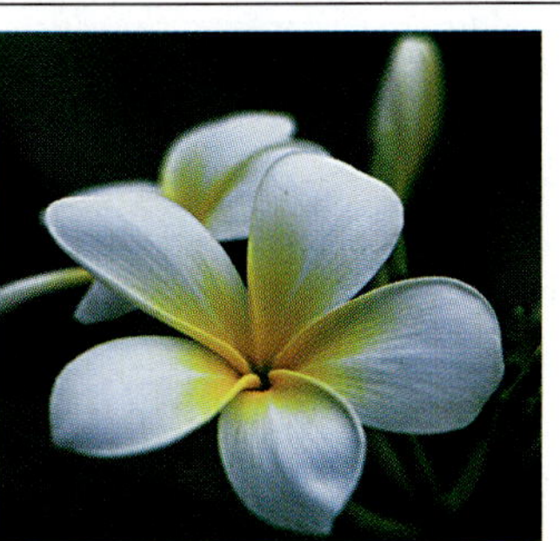

'SIERRA MADRE' PLUMERIA SP.

A horticultural first: a Plumeria that is cold hardy. Almost certainly a new species. Probably world's rarest plumeria and for certain world's toughest. Plant is slow growing, with silvery green leaves, slender stems with a swollen, knobby base. Lends itself to bonsai culture. Flowers are white with yellow center and have classic frangipani fragrance. In very short supply.

54291 Rooting Cutting *$149.95*

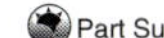 Full Sun   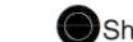 Part Sun   Shade   Extra Water   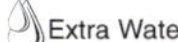 Fragrant   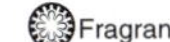 Cut Flower   New

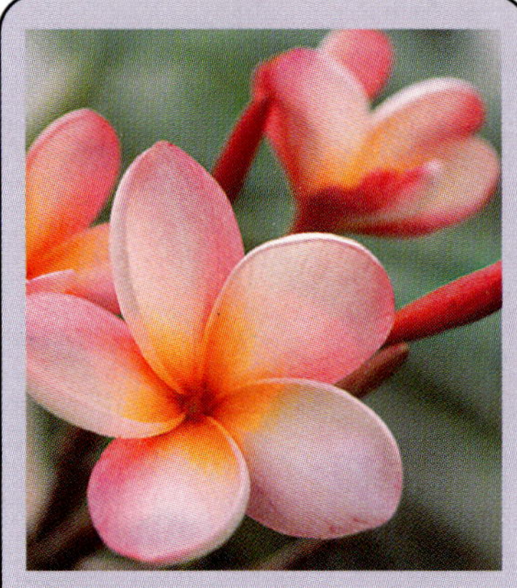

SONDRA B™

A new, very distinctive seedling. Large overlapping petals are white with slight pinkish bands on front. On reverse, petals have deep rose-pink bands. Yellow seems to bleed from the center. Good texture with a 3"-3 1/2" flower. A strong gardenia fragrance. In very short supply. Named for Glenn Stokes' daughter.
54761 Rooting Cutting $49.95

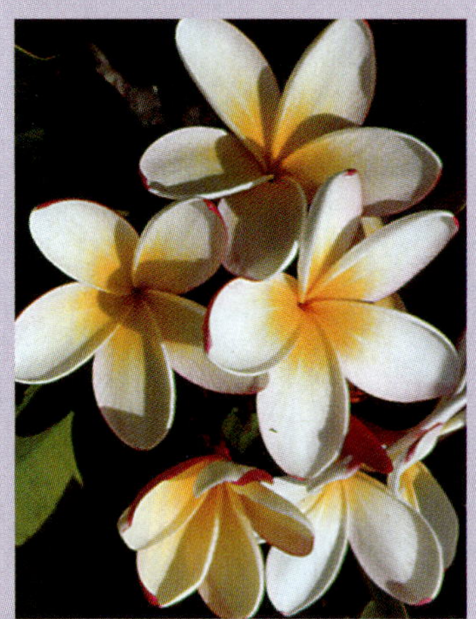

TILLIE HUGHES

Pale pink w/small, brilliant-yellow center; petal narrow, round tip, moderately overlapping; wide, moderate pink band on back; good texture; 3 1/4" dia.; slight sweet fragrance; keeping quality fair.
54911 Rooting Cutting...............$24.95

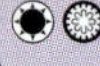

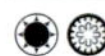

SINGAPORE WHITE

Plant has flowers that are white with small, brilliant yellow center; no pink or red bands on front or back; petal wide, round tip, no overlapping, or color bands; moderate texture; 3½" (8.75cm) diameter; strong lemon fragrance; keeping quality poor. Possesses shiny evergreen leaves. Common plumeria of the South Pacific and Southeast Asia.
54751 Rooting Cutting............................$20.95

STENOPHYLLUS

This is a species form. Leaves are a wonderful bright shiny green and curly. It would be worthwhile growing for its foliage alone. Nice small white flowers are an added attraction. Flowers have no scent. A standout plant that is easy to distinguish from other plumerias.
54771 Rooting Cutting.................$37.95

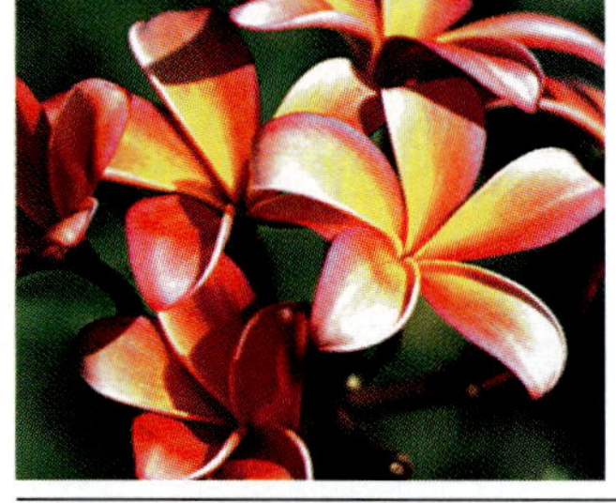

TEXAS SUNSHINE

An outstanding plant with a full size medium deep yellow flower that fades into a creamy white toward the outside. The tree has a good growth habit with balanced branching and full blooming flower heads.
54821 Rooting Cutting.............................$39.95

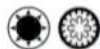

SINGAPORE WHITE

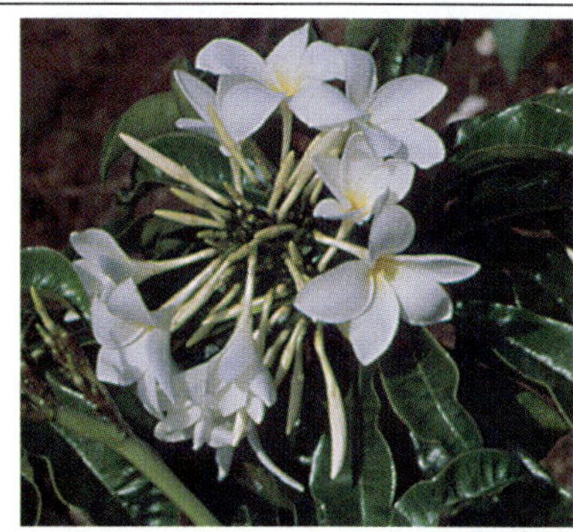

TERESA WILDER

Rediscovered by Jim Little in Hawaii after being missing for over 30 years. Related to Kauka Wilder. One of the brightest rainbow colors in the plumeria world. A heavy bloomer with very large (3½") flower heads. A show stopper.
54801 Rooting Cutting $39.95

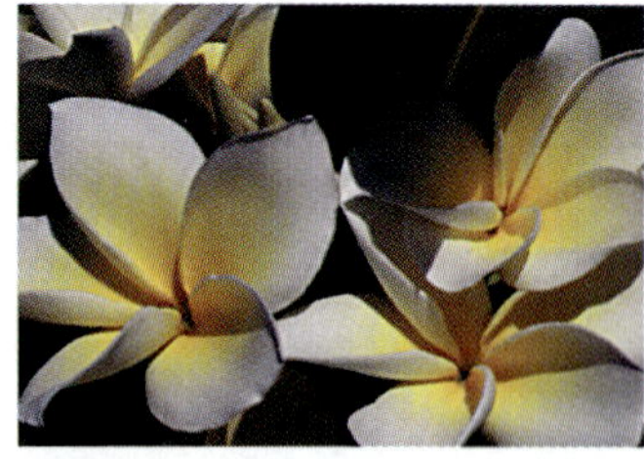

THORNTON LEMON

(*Courtade Lemon*) The flowers are pale yellow spreading to white. Flowers are about 5½" (13.5cm) across. This lemon scented variety produces large clusters of massive blooms like the Courtade.
54901 Rooting Cutting $49.95

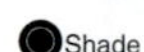 Full Sun   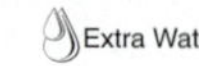 Part Sun   Shade   Extra Water   Fragrant   Cut Flower   New

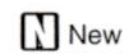

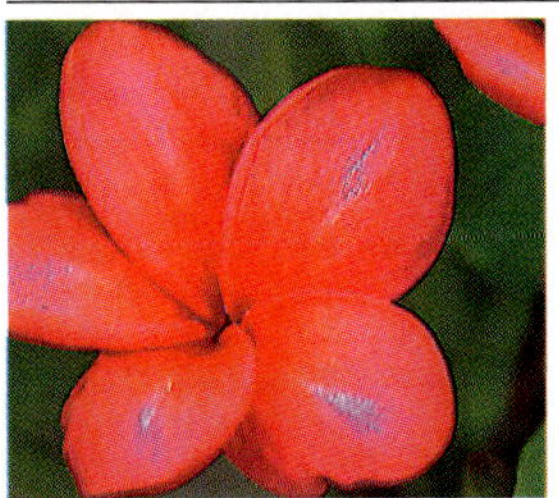

TINA ™

An outstanding new seedling variety. Has medium (2") white flower with a small yellow center and a very attractive pink edge. Great frangipani fragrance. Compact grower. In very limited supply.
54951 Rooting Cutting $49.95

TOMLINSON PINK

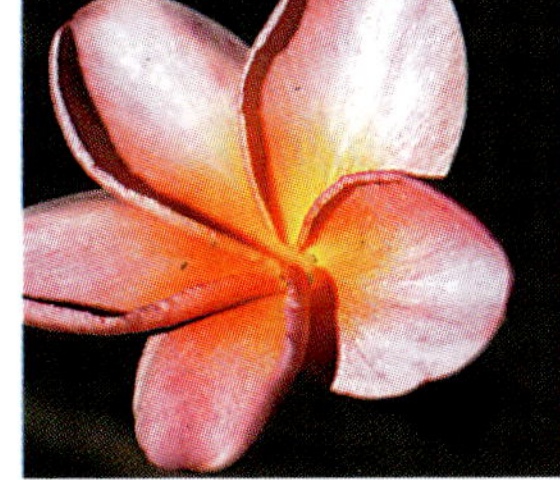

Flowers are a moderate, grainy pink and white with small, brilliant yellow center; petals wide, round tip, moderately overlapping; deep pink margin around tip, distinctive white venation in center, deep pink band on back; fair texture; 3" (7.5cm) diameter; keeping quality very good.
55001 Rooting Cutting...................$29.95

UNIVERSITY CHERRY PINK

Plant has 3" (7.5cm) cherry pink flowers with a slight yellow cast in the center of petals. Petals have specks of white. Upright grower. Produces strong perfume of frangipani. In limited supply.
55051 Rooting Cutting $25.95

WATANABE #3

A great new plumeria with a 4" pink windmill flower with nicely pointed petals, a gold center and darker pink bands on back. Good frangipani fragrance. Numerous inflorescences on a low growing tree. Produces many large seed pods.
55071 Rooting Cutting $49.95

WHITE 93

The plant has 2½" (6.5cm) subdued white flower with a small intense yellow center. The throat of the flower turns dark orange the second day. Petals are slightly overlapping with rounded tips. In limited supply.
55101 Rooting Cutting.............................$25.95

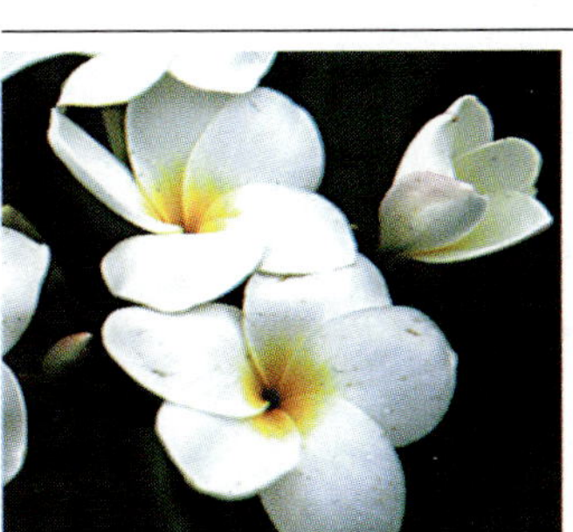

Rooting cuttings are ship ped from *March 1st to November 1st.*

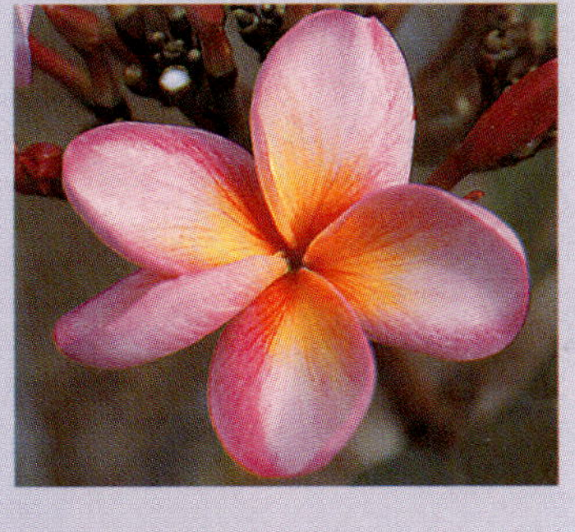

VANDA RUFFLES

Very nice wavy petals like a Vanda orchid. Medium size flower that is symmetrical. Pink color with a large brilliant yellow center and strong pink bands on the front and back. Plant has compact growth form. Easy flowering.
55061 Rooting Cutting $29.95

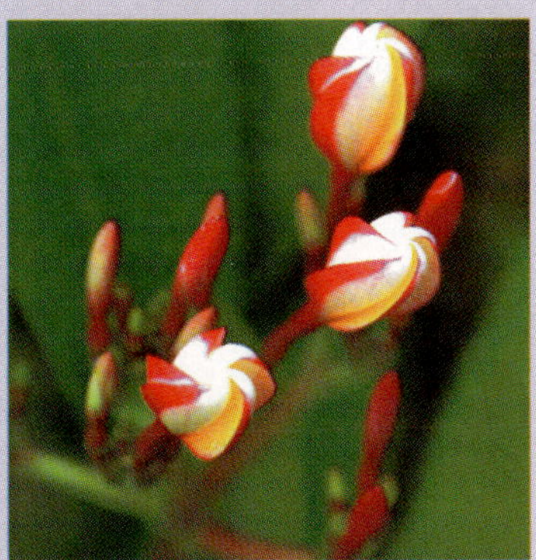

WHITE SHELL

A very unusual cultivar with white flowers banded red on one edge of the reverse of the petals. Flowers 1" (2.5cm) have a golden-yellow center, but in cooler weather only open partially and resemble seashells. Texture is good and keeping quality is very good. Fragrance is strong and sweet. A must for collectors.
55151 Rooting Cutting..............$20.95

Orders Placed Through Our Web Site Receive a 15% Discount

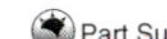
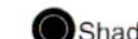
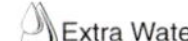
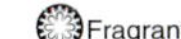
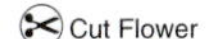

Full Sun   Part Sun   Shade   Extra Water   Fragrant   Cut Flower   N New

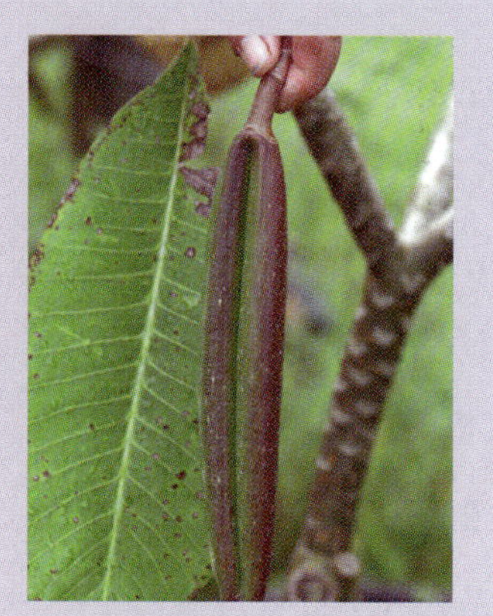

Green Plumeria Seed Pod
(not expanded)

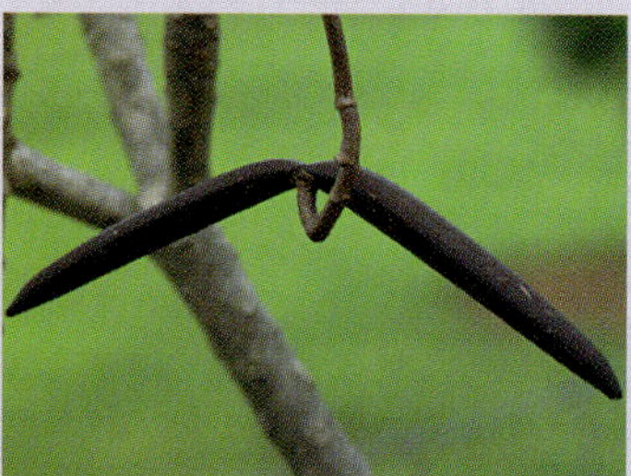

Ripe Plumeria Seed Pod

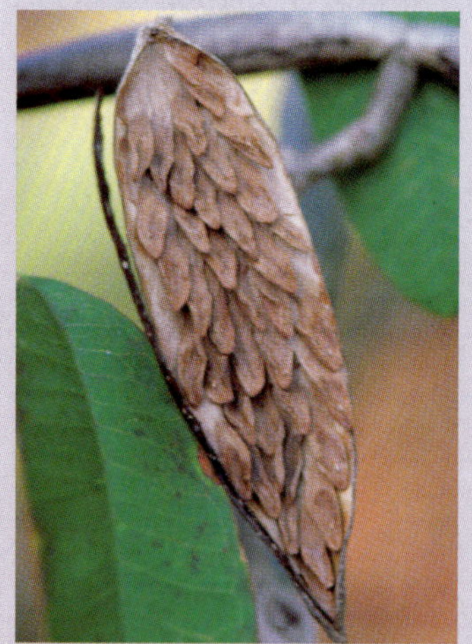

Open Plumeria Seed Pod with seeds
exposed.

**Membership Information
on The Plumeria Society of
America, Inc. See page 135.**

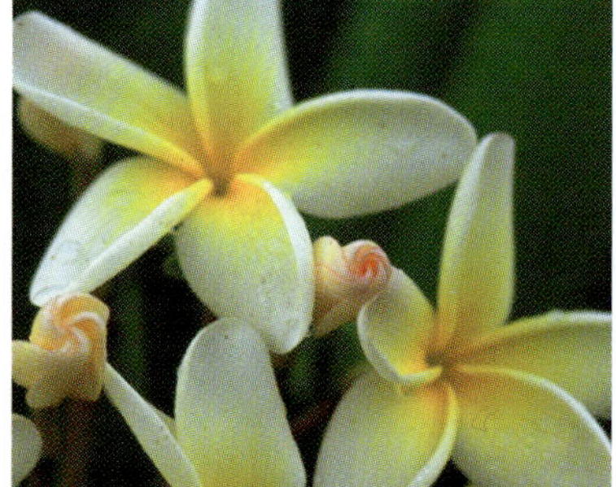

YELLOW JACK

A large 3¹/₂" (8.5cm) yellow flower with wide white margin. Excellent bloomer. Makes a very strong, compact tree. Good seed producer. Very sweet delicate fragrance.
55251 Rooting Cutting $14.95

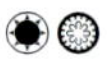

**Rooting cuttings are shipped from
*March 1st to November 1st.***

YELLOW SHELL

Flowers are a bright lemon-yellow that pales toward petal tips. Flowers have good texture up to 3" in width. Mild frangipani fragrance. Good branching habit on an upright, compact plant.
52261 Rooting Cutting.....$15.95

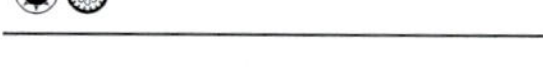

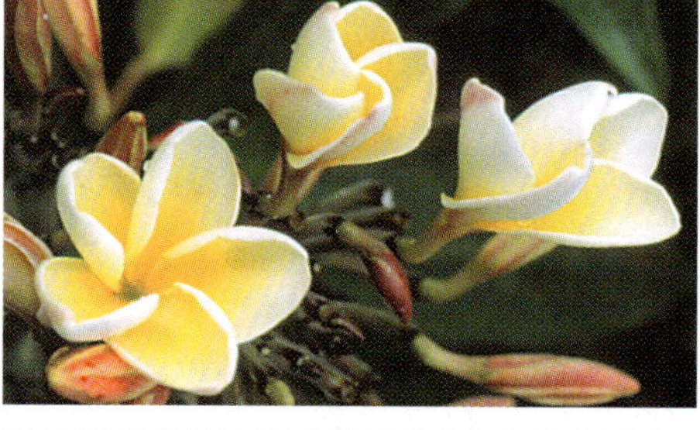

COMING IN 2001
Call about availability and price.

Visit our Web Site :
www.stokestropicals.com

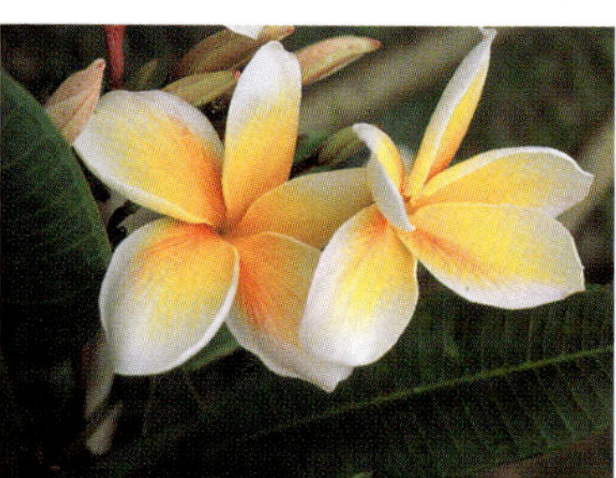

ELLEN #15

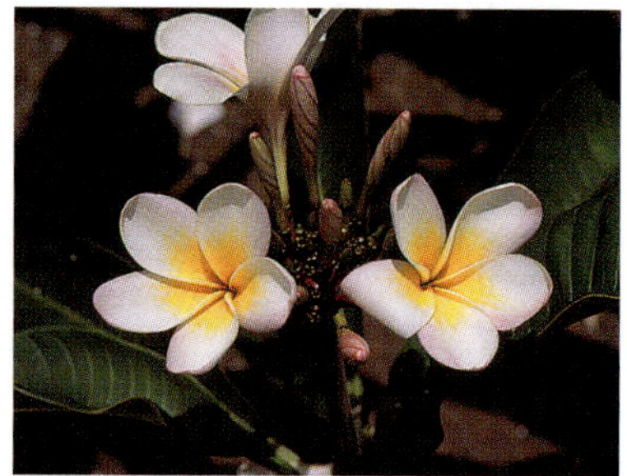

GARDENIA

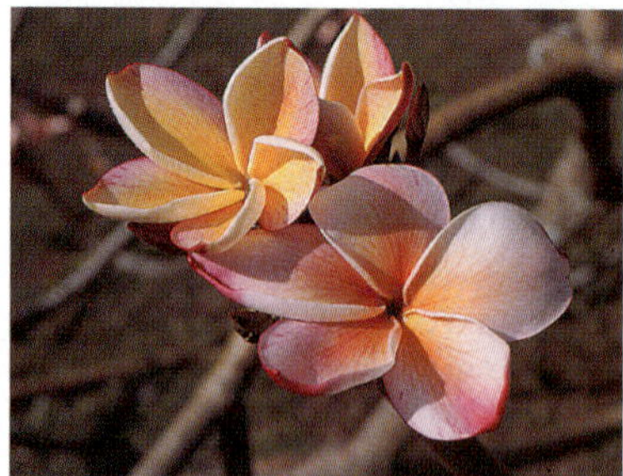

INDONESIA ROSE

THE EXOTIC PLUMERIA
(FRANGIPANI)

By Elizabeth H. Thornton, and Sharon H. Thornton

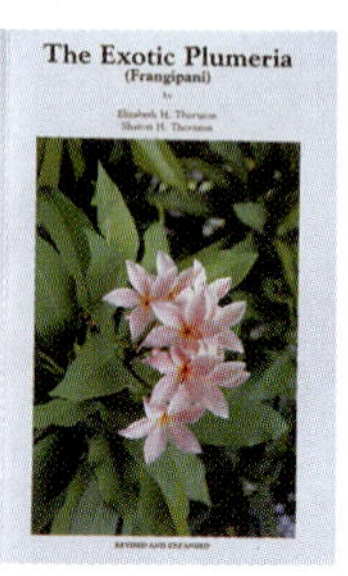

77500........$12.00

See page 125 for more information on this book and others.

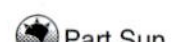 Full Sun   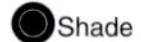 Part Sun   Shade   Extra Water   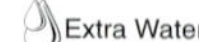Fragrant   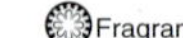Cut Flower   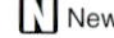 New

PLUMERIA COLLECTIONS

(Save $30 on rooting cuttings off listed prices by purchasing collection)

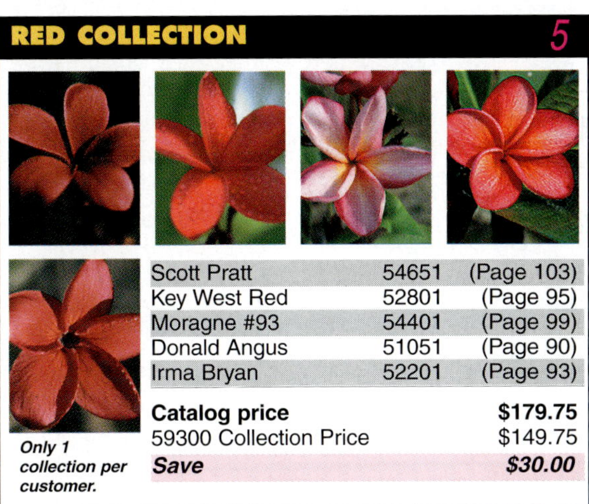

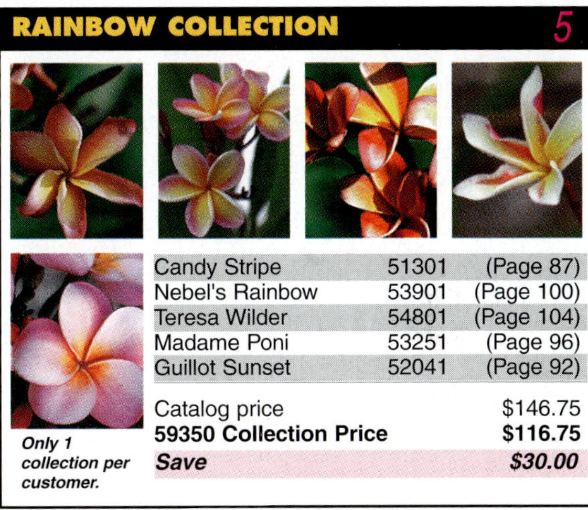

1999 BEST-SELLERS COLLECTION 5

Candy Stripe	51301	(Page 87)
Key West Red	52801	(Page 95)
Celadine	51351	(Page 88)
Kaneohe Sunburst	52661	(Page 94)
Mele Matson	53501	(Page 98)
Catalog price		$123.75
59030 Collection Price		**$93.75**
Save		*$30.00*

Only 1 collection per customer.

SPECIAL VARIETIES COLLECTION 5

Penang Peach	54051	(Page 100)
Bali Whirl	51151	(Page 86)
Charlotte Ebert	51451	(Page 88)
J.L. Trumpet	52401	(Page 94)
Tomlinson Pink	55001	(Page 105)
Catalog price		$221.75
59250 Collection Price		**$191.75**
Save		*$30.00*

Only 1 collection per customer.

RED COLLECTION 5

Scott Pratt	54651	(Page 103)
Key West Red	52801	(Page 95)
Moragne #93	54401	(Page 99)
Donald Angus	51051	(Page 90)
Irma Bryan	52201	(Page 93)
Catalog price		**$179.75**
59300 Collection Price		$149.75
Save		*$30.00*

Only 1 collection per customer.

RAINBOW COLLECTION 5

Candy Stripe	51301	(Page 87)
Nebel's Rainbow	53901	(Page 100)
Teresa Wilder	54801	(Page 104)
Madame Poni	53251	(Page 96)
Guillot Sunset	52041	(Page 92)
Catalog price		$146.75
59350 Collection Price		**$116.75**
Save		*$30.00*

Only 1 collection per customer.

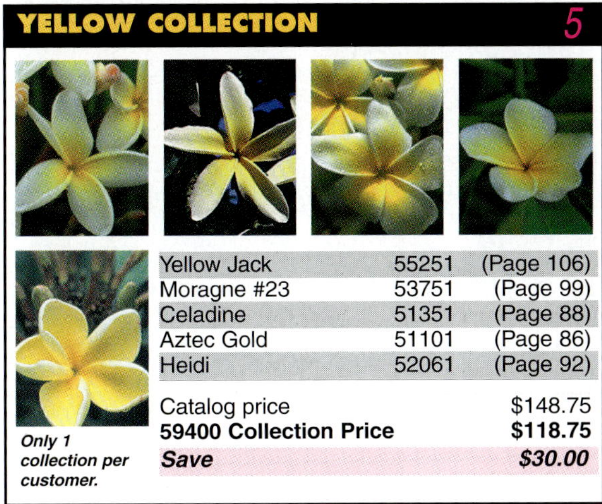

YELLOW COLLECTION 5

Yellow Jack	55251	(Page 106)
Moragne #23	53751	(Page 99)
Celadine	51351	(Page 88)
Aztec Gold	51101	(Page 86)
Heidi	52061	(Page 92)
Catalog price		$148.75
59400 Collection Price		**$118.75**
Save		*$30.00*

Only 1 collection per customer.

PINK COLLECTION 5

Charlotte Ebert	51451	(Page 88)
Tomlinson Pink	55001	(Page 105)
Pink 93	54101	(Page 101)
Maui Beauty	53451	(Page 97)
Laguna Pink	53051	(Page 96)
Catalog price		$156.75
59450 Collection Price		**$126.75**
Save		*$30.00*

Only 1 collection per customer.

TO ORDER CALL **1-800-624-9706**/24 HRS. OR VISIT OUR WEB SITE: www. stokestropicals.com

Plumerias

CONNOISSEURS COLLECTION 5

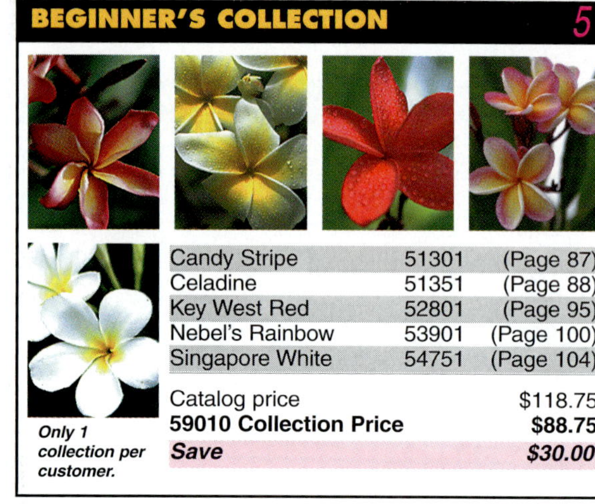

Bali Whirl	51151	(Page 86)
Dwarf Deciduous	51851	(Page 91)
Dwarf Singapore White	51901	(Page 91)
Jean Moragne Jr.	52501	(Page 94)
Penang Peach	54051	(Page 100)
Catalog price		$309.75
59500 Collection Price		**$279.75**
Save		***$30.00***

Only 1 collection per customer.

BEGINNER'S COLLECTION 5

Candy Stripe	51301	(Page 87)
Celadine	51351	(Page 88)
Key West Red	52801	(Page 95)
Nebel's Rainbow	53901	(Page 100)
Singapore White	54751	(Page 104)
Catalog price		$118.75
59010 Collection Price		**$88.75**
Save		***$30.00***

Only 1 collection per customer.

WHITE COLLECTION 5

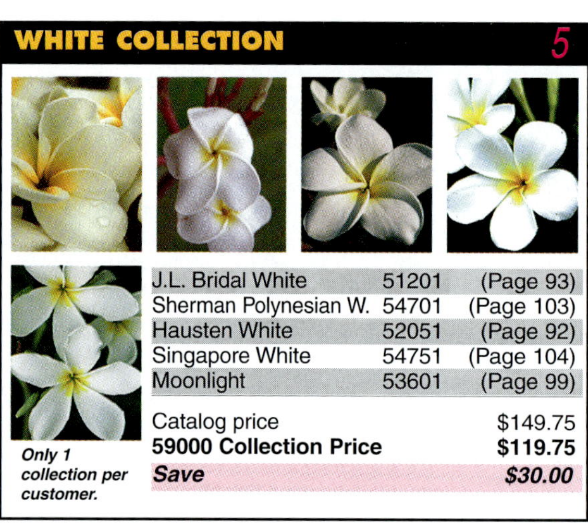

J.L. Bridal White	51201	(Page 93)
Sherman Polynesian W.	54701	(Page 103)
Hausten White	52051	(Page 92)
Singapore White	54751	(Page 104)
Moonlight	53601	(Page 99)
Catalog price		$149.75
59000 Collection Price		**$119.75**
Save		***$30.00***

Only 1 collection per customer.

EXCLUSIVE VARIETIES COLLECTION 5

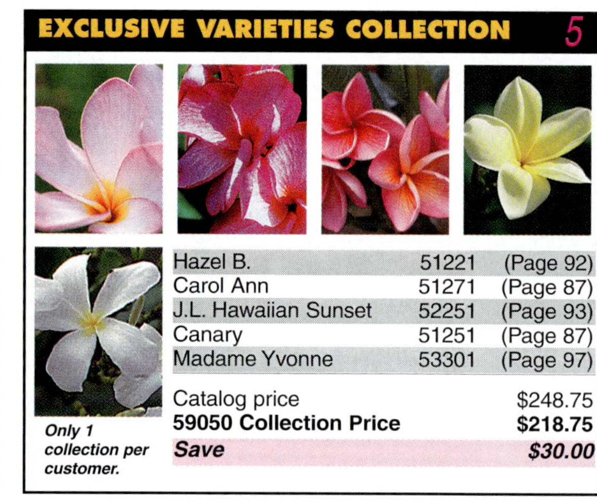

Hazel B.	51221	(Page 92)
Carol Ann	51271	(Page 87)
J.L. Hawaiian Sunset	52251	(Page 93)
Canary	51251	(Page 87)
Madame Yvonne	53301	(Page 97)
Catalog price		$248.75
59050 Collection Price		**$218.75**
Save		***$30.00***

Only 1 collection per customer.

MORAGNE COLLECTION 5

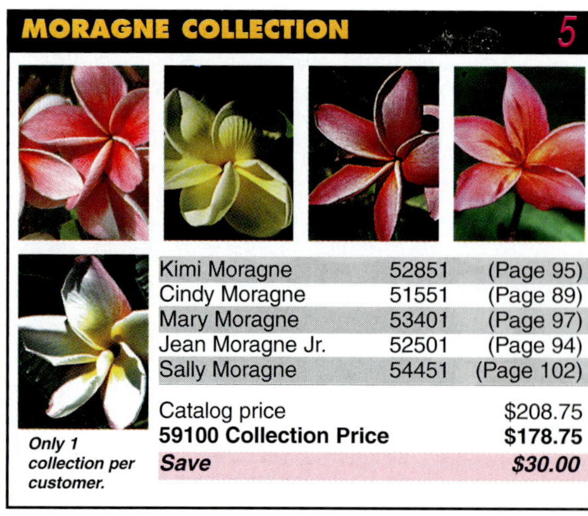

Kimi Moragne	52851	(Page 95)
Cindy Moragne	51551	(Page 89)
Mary Moragne	53401	(Page 97)
Jean Moragne Jr.	52501	(Page 94)
Sally Moragne	54451	(Page 102)
Catalog price		$208.75
59100 Collection Price		**$178.75**
Save		***$30.00***

Only 1 collection per customer.

RARE MORAGNE COLLECTION 5

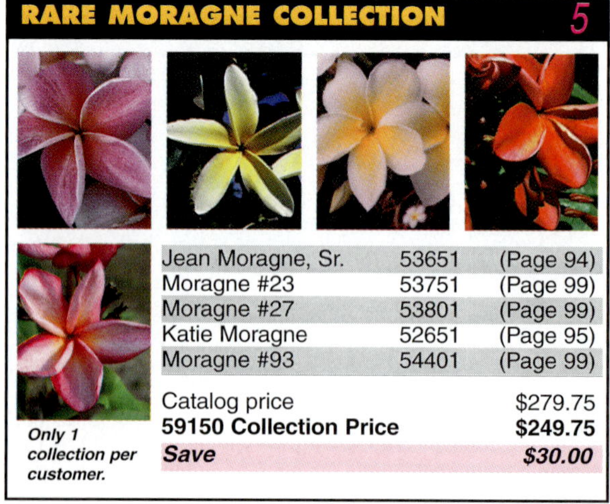

Jean Moragne, Sr.	53651	(Page 94)
Moragne #23	53751	(Page 99)
Moragne #27	53801	(Page 99)
Katie Moragne	52651	(Page 95)
Moragne #93	54401	(Page 99)
Catalog price		$279.75
59150 Collection Price		**$249.75**
Save		***$30.00***

Only 1 collection per customer.

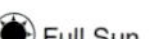 Full Sun   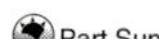 Part Sun   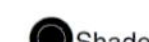 Shade   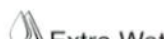 Extra Water   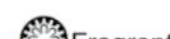 Fragrant   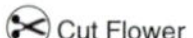 Cut Flower   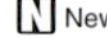 New

TO ORDER CALL **1-800-624-9706**/24 HRS. OR VISIT OUR WEB SITE: www. stokestropicals.com

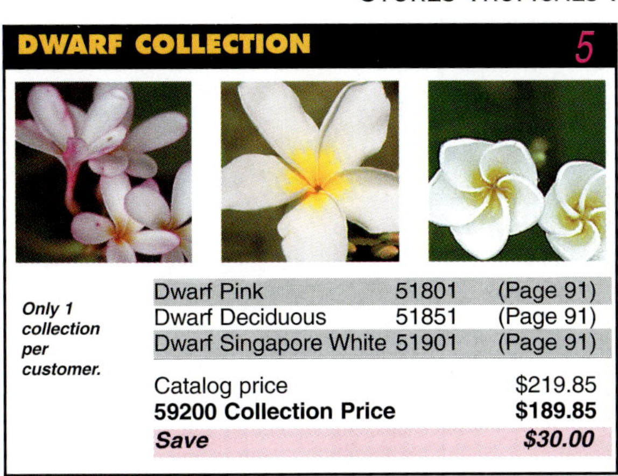

Only 1 collection per customer.

Dwarf Pink	51801	(Page 91)
Dwarf Deciduous	51851	(Page 91)
Dwarf Singapore White	51901	(Page 91)

Catalog price	$219.85
59200 Collection Price	**$189.85**
Save	**$30.00**

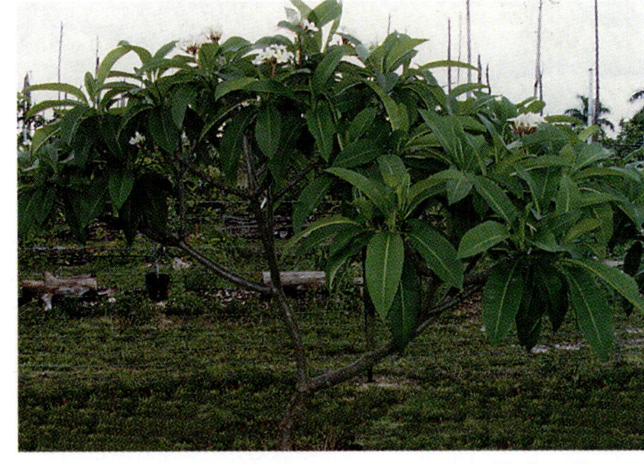

▲ *Madame Yvonne*

PLUMERIA CARE CHART

Month	Weeks			
	1	2	3	4
January	dormant	dormant	dormant	dormant
February	dormant	dormant	dormant	dormant
March	dormant	dormant	rp/r-w-f	rp/r-w-f-es
April	rp/r-w-f-es	F or SPh-BD	f	F-es
May	f	F-FL	f	F-es
June	f	F	f	F-es
July	f	F	f	F
August	f	F	f	F
September	f	f	f	f
October	f	f	Store	Store
November	dormant	dormant	dormant	dormant
December	dormant	dormant	dormant	dormant

Key

w = Water. Soak root-ball thoroughly to promote vigorous growth. Keep well watered April through September.

rp/r = Root prune & Repot. Topdress those not repotted with composted manure to enhance growth.

F = Feed with **Stokes Tropicals Plumeria Blend (8-14-10)** (Or substitute SPh once or twice during entire year)

SPh = Feed 1/4 cup each Super Phosphate & Bone Meal for 5-7 gal. container.

es = Feed Epsom salt (MgSO4.xH2O). Magnesium(Mg) is the core element of chlorophyll which makes plants green. Epsom salt may also help prevent leaf sunburn and promote feeder root growth. Apply at a rate of approximately 1 teaspoon per gallon pot size.

f = Optional feeding, or light application (Some people do not recommend feeding after mid-August). One may substitute a balanced (20-20-20) fertilizer with trace elements for the light feedings to round out the nutrient menu for your plumeria through the month of July.

BD = Flower buds begin to appear on many plumeria.

FL = Flowering season begins.

Notes:

1. This is only a rough guideline. Many people are able to have flowers on some plants as early as March.

2. Be cautious about bringing plants out of dormancy before the last frost. This may be as late as the end of March in Texas, Louisiana, and Florida.

3. Be on the lookout for pests and disease ALL year. Infestations of spider mites have been found on dormant plants during winter storage in a garage.

4. The blooming season is dependent upon many factors. For example:

    a. Variety of plant and age.
    b. Soil mix.
    c. Fertilization schedule.
    d. Light intensity.
    e. Winter storage methodology

TO ORDER CALL **1-800-624-9706**/24 HRS. OR VISIT OUR WEB SITE: www. stokestropicals.com

FAQ

What is a rooting plumeria cutting?

It is a cutting that we are rooting for you. It takes us 4-16 weeks, depending on time of year and variety, to fully root a cutting. We then simply remove the rooting cutting from its growing medium, gently pack to prevent roots or callus from drying, and ship to you. You should then replant at same level (see band on stem), in a well-drained soil mix either directly into the ground or into a container. Water lightly and fertilize with a half strength fertilizer at sign of first new growth. Don't keep too wet and follow cultural directions that come with plant. We take orders for rooted plumeria cuttings all year. And we ship them from March 1st to November 1st.

What is the most fragrant plumeria?

This is hard to say because nearly all of the hybrid plumerias are fragrant. One of the most fragrant is the Dwarf Deciduous. And all the Moragnes are very fragrant. What you really need to do is pick out the fragrance you like the most such as coconut, frangipani, lemon, citrus, or other and make your choice accordingly.

If I could get only one kind of plumeria, which one would you recommend?

This is a pretty easy question to answer. The Dwarf Pink would be our choice because it is a true dwarf never getting any taller than 6 feet. It is evergreen, that is, doesn't lose its leaves. It flowers all year if not exposed to freezing temperatures. And it can even flower indoors in high light. Plus because of its slow growth, 6" or so per year, it lends itself to being containerized.

What is the easiest way to start growing a particular group of tropical plants, such as, gingers, bananas, heliconias, plumerias, hibiscus, bougainvilleas, or cannas?

That's easy to answer. We have chosen collections in each of these groups. In some of the larger groups of plants, we have selected a "beginner's collection". A collection will not only save you money but will give you a nice variety to get started with. If you do well with your initial collection, then you can expand to more plants of the same group or you could try your luck with other groups.

Why won't my plumeria bloom?

My first question is, do you have it growing in full sun? Plumerias need full sun. Then I ask, are you fertilizing it with a high phosphorus (P) fertilizer? To encourage blooming, a fertilizer such as, Stokes Tropicals' Plumeria Blend (8-14-10), is ideal. Rooted plumeria cuttings can bloom the first year if they are terminal and contain enough plant auxin. And all plumeria cuttings should flower in the 2nd or 3rd year with proper sunlight, fertilizer, and care.

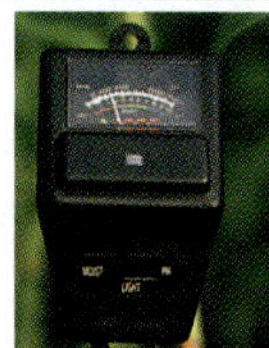

MULTI METER

Test light, moisture and pH for indoors & out.

80100 ....*$19.95*

MAKE YOUR PLUMERIAS BLOOM!

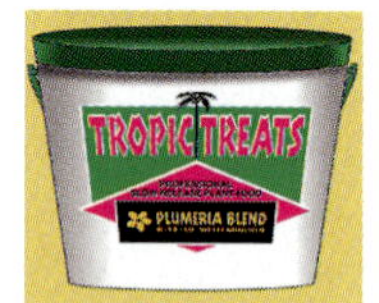

TROPIC TREATS PLUMERIA BLEND FERTILIZER
(8-14-10)

6040 1 lb. Bucket *$6.00*
6041 4 lb. Bucket *$17.00*

STOKES TROPICALS GIFT CERTIFICATE SEE PAGE 134

SPECIAL PLANTS

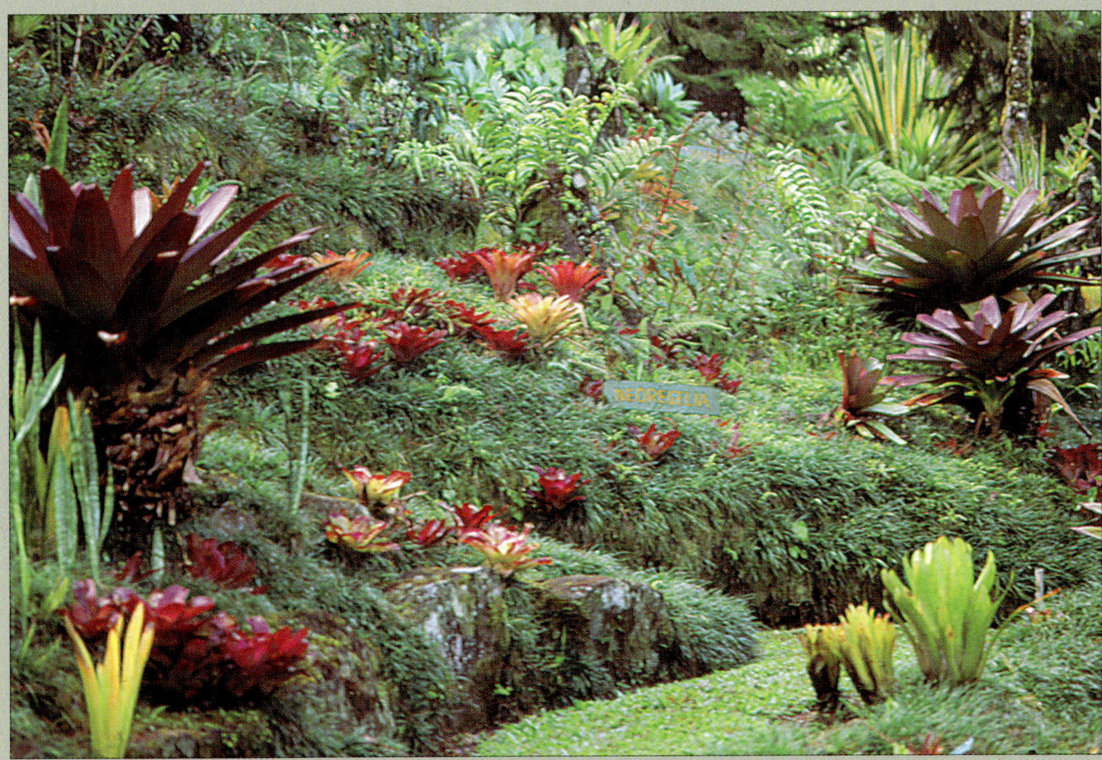

Bromeliad planting at Wilson Gardens, Costa Rica.

Special Plants are those that we think are unique and interesting. We offer them to the adventurous gardeners who would like to add more tropical interest and color to their garden or home.

Included in this section are bromeliads, euphorbs, calatheas, clivias, aglaeonemas, and many other distinctive plants not usually available to catalog customers.

Stokes Tropicals has carefully chosen a wide range of exciting tropical plants that are easy-to-grow, that are not commonly available, that have some unusual horticultural interest, and can be successfully grown in containers. We are constantly searching for new and exciting plants, particularly tropicals—from Europe, Asia, Africa, Australia, North America, and South America. We import regularly and test new plants for possible introduction in our Guide/Catalog. At any one time, we might have 20-30 "new" plants undergoing trials. If a plant passes our rigorous standards of testing, we will put it into production and offer it to our customers as soon as possible. Several of our "special plants" proved so popular that their collections were increased and they now have their own sections, e.g., bougainvilleas, cannas, and hibiscus. Enjoy our selection of Special Plants.

Bromeliads

BROMELIADS have a tremendous will to survive and can offer infinite variety, challenge, and exciting plant forms and color combinations. The most common genera in cultivation are: Aechmea, Billbergia, Cryptanthus, Dyckia, Guzmania, Neoregelia, Nidularium, Tillandsia and Vriesea. All make good house plants if given a reasonable amount of care. The roots of most potted bromeliads like to be moist, but never soggy. Bright, diffused light is needed by most bromeliads. No bromeliad likes a dark environment. Bromeliads will be comfortable when you are. Generally, they prosper at temperatures between 50 and 90 degrees F. They are not winter hardy except in subtropical and tropical regions. In nature many bromeliads grow on trees as epiphytes or air plants. Their roots are used mainly for support; they are not parasites. Some bromeliads grow on rocks and cliff faces. They are remarkably versatile and form one of the most adaptable plant families in the world. Try Stokes Tropicals Bromeliad Blend Fertilizer (10-14-14 with minors) for best results.

Bromeliad varieties are available as growing plants in pots with the pot diameter indicated in inches and centimeters. Detailed cultural directions are supplied with each order.

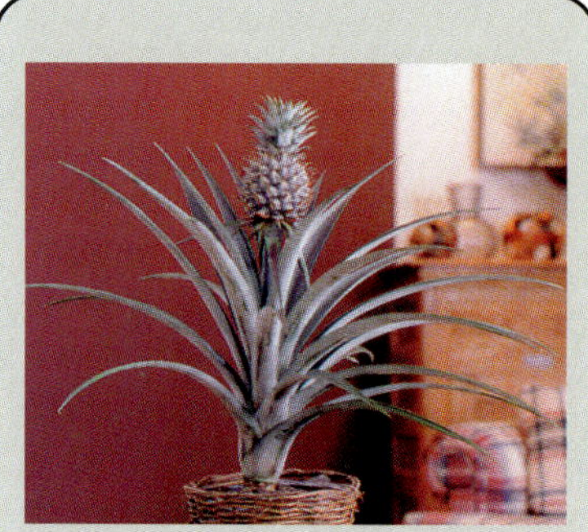

ANANAS COMOSUS
'Smoothe Cayenne'
Edible pineapple

Easy to grow. Delivered to you in fruit, which will ripen in 4-6 months. Average plant height is 25". Can be enjoyed as an indoor plant, patio plant, or even an outdoor plant (in frost free areas). Provides tropical accent along with delicious tropical taste. Full sun to 30% shade. Zone 10.
89600 Container size–6 1/2".........*$34.95*

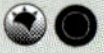

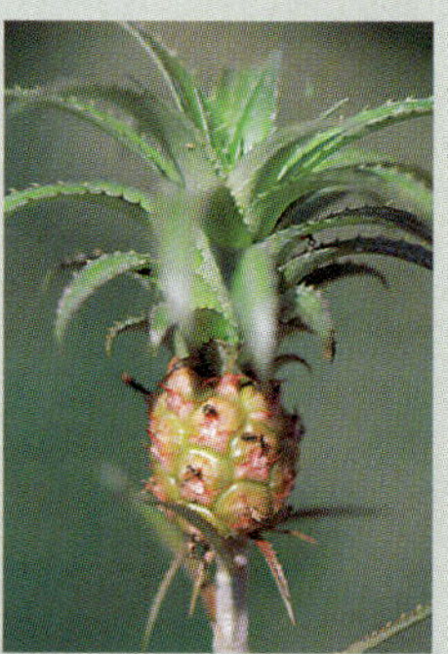

ANANAS NANA -
Ornamental pineapple

Fantastic looking dwarf ornamental pineapple. Comes in brightly colored fruit that will last for months. Easy to care for requiring little water and fertilizer. Average plant height is 15". Indoor plant, patio plant, or outdoor plant (in frost free areas.) 30% shade (strong indirect light). Zone 10.
89700 Container size–4"...........*$14.95*

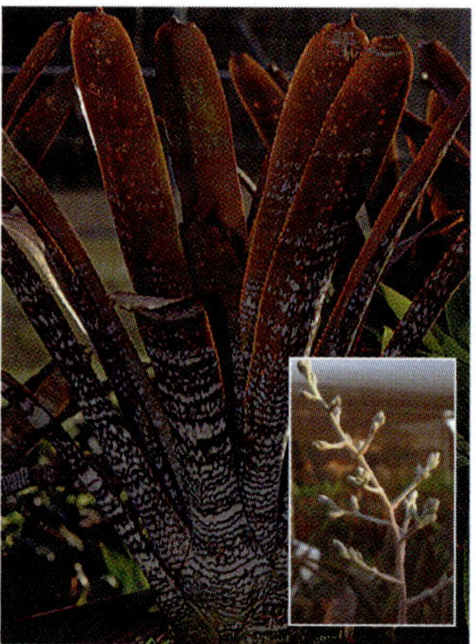

HOHENBERGIA CORREIA-ARAUJEI 'Fudge Ripple'

Hohenbergia correia-araujei is from Brazil. From an offset it will grow to full size in about two years. The plant has dark chocolate-brown foliage with silver banding, grows to almost 4' (1.2m) tall and the branching inflorescence can exceed 5' (1.5m). The bloom is frosted pink with gray clusters at the end of each branch and is long lasting (up to 5 months in good light). Can be mounted in trees or grown in a pot.
21050 Container size–10"....................*$45.00*

NEOREGELIA CONCENTRICA X ? 'Medium Rare'

Grows to almost 30" (75cm) across with green to bronze foliage and a large reddish pink center when blooming.
21100 Container size–8".............*$35.00*

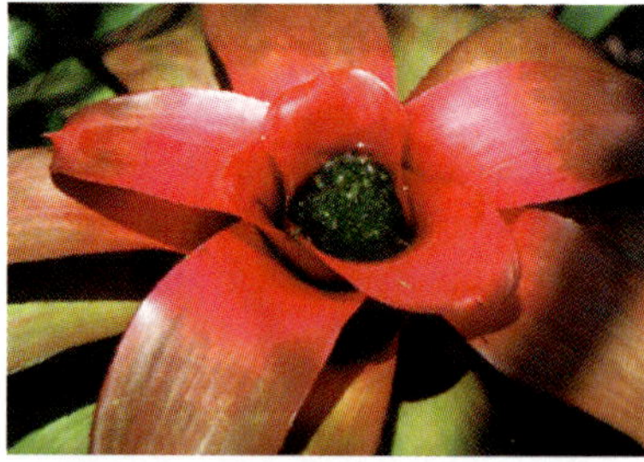

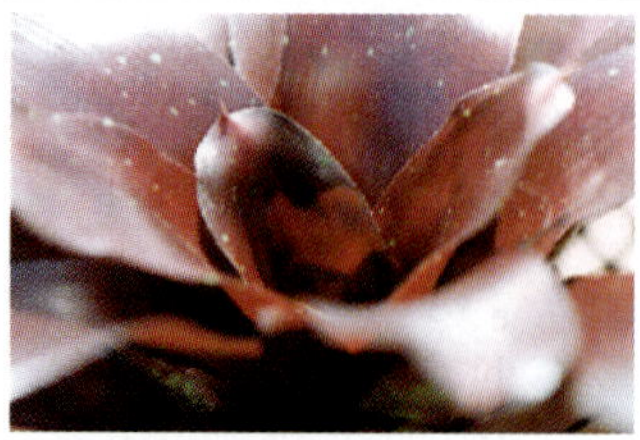

NEOREGELIA X 'Royal Burgundy'

Grows to 15" (38cm) across with dark burgundy foliage with few green spots. It tolerates stronger light. In good light this plant will be an attractive conversation piece for over a year.
21250 Container size–5½"....................*$15.00*

Full Sun   Part Sun   Shade   Extra Water   Fragrant   Cut Flower   N New

TO ORDER CALL **1-800-624-9706**/24 HRS. OR VISIT OUR WEB SITE: www. stokestropicals.com

VRIESEA GIGANTEA
'Gigantea Nova'

Has patterned green and white foliage and can reach an impressive size of 4' (1.2m) wide and can live for many years before blooming. Foliage appears to be hand painted. Outstanding plant.

21350 Container size–6" $25.00
21351 Container size–10" $60.00

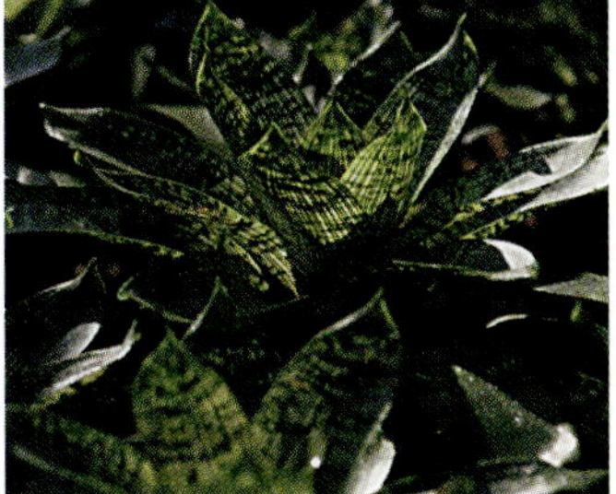

VRIESEA INTERMEDIA X 'Mint Julep'

Striking leaves patterned dark and light green with white. Foliage appears to be hand painted with horizontal squiggly green lines. Requires over two years to reach maximum size of 30" (75cm) wide and 24" (60cm) tall. Beautiful purple feather-shaped bloom approximately 4' (1.2m) tall.

21400 Container size–10" $60.00

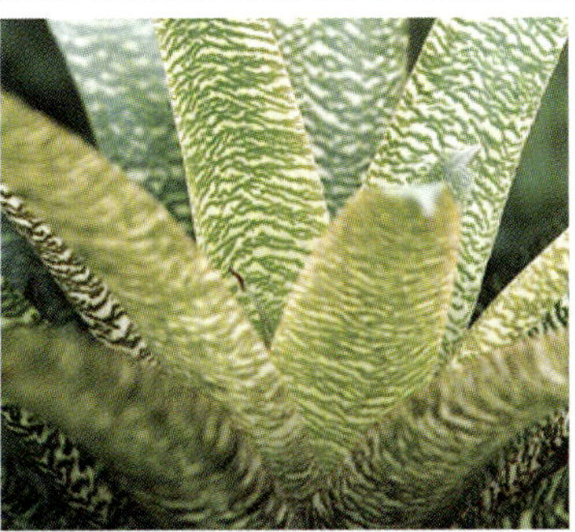

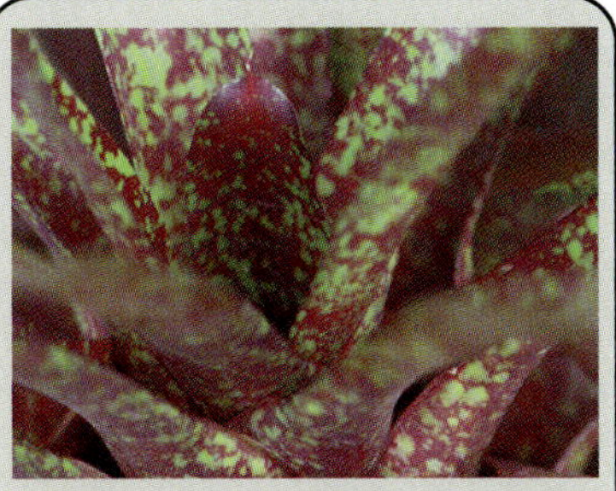

NEOREGELIA X 'Mocha Mint'

Grows to 15" (38cm) across. The foliage is dark reddish-brown and the leaves grow more upright with numerous yellow-green specks. This plant grows to full size in fifteen to eighteen months.

21200 Container size–5¹/₂" $15.00

Euphorbia 'Chinese Lucky Plants'

These are wonderful new Thai *Euphorbia milii* hybrids that are considered to be lucky plants by the Thais in Bangkok, Thailand. There are literally hundreds of these fantastic hybrids--each with different flower bracts, flowers, and /or leaves. They are traded and sold in the markets of Bangkok. There are several full-color books in Thai covering the many cultivars of these amazing plants. Having one of these exquisite easy-to-care for plants is believed to confer good luck on the plant owner and their home. Since they are a cactus-like succulent, they require little care, little water, and little food. They prefer strong light and soil on the dry side. And they don't require a lot of growing space. They thrive and flower in a small pot and can be shaped by judicious pruning. Each year we will introduce more of these fantastic easy-to-grow, easy-to-care-for plants. We are now growing over 200 different cultivars. Next year we will introduce several more cultivars. Try one or more of our Siamese Lucky Plants—maybe they'll make you lucky. We have also introducing 3 cultivars of *Euphorbia milii* that are dwarfs and are self-mounding in growth habit.

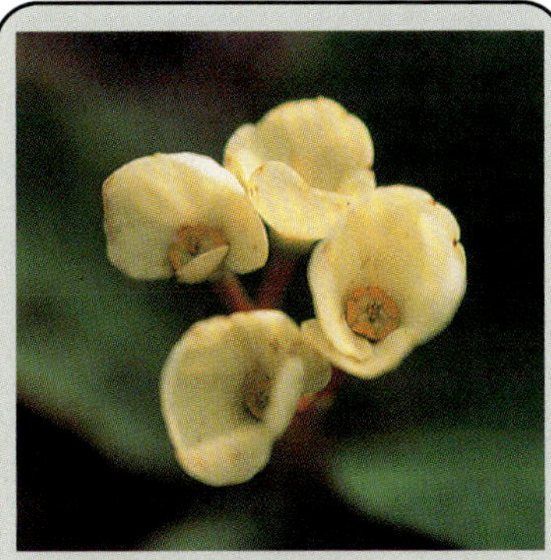

EUPHORBIA MILII
'Jingle Bells'

A very special lucky plant with an extraordinary inflorescence. Bracts appear to be hand painted by Santa's workers with shades of pink, red and green. Nice big, oblong green leaves. Great houseplant. Zone 10 and higher. Full sun or high light. Ever bloomer.

85030 Growing Plant (4" pot)...$9.95

EUPHORBIA MILII
'Fall Song'

A very interesting new hybrid from Thailand with solid cream-colored bracts that are cupped rather than flat. Only Siamese Lucky Plant that we offer with cupped flowers. Large beautiful leaves. Same growing requirements as other Siamese Lucky Plants. Good houseplant. Ever-bloomer. Zone 10 and higher.

85065 Growing Plant (4" pot)..$10.95

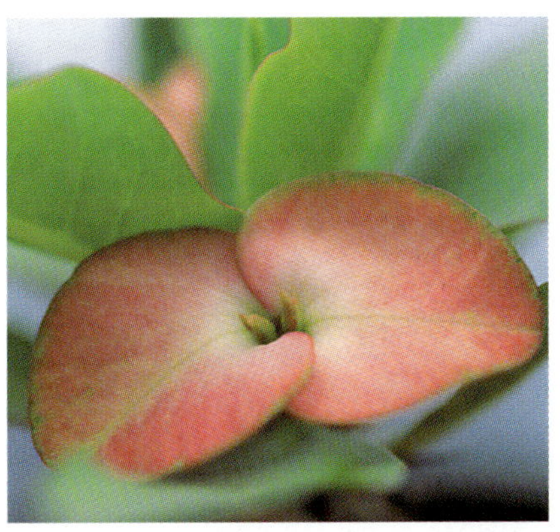

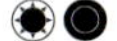

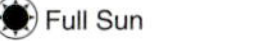 Full Sun   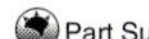 Part Sun   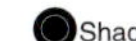 Shade   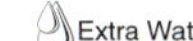 Extra Water   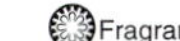 Fragrant   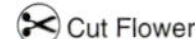 Cut Flower   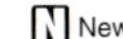 New

TO ORDER CALL **1-800-624-9706**/24 HRS. OR VISIT OUR WEB SITE: www. stokestropicals.com

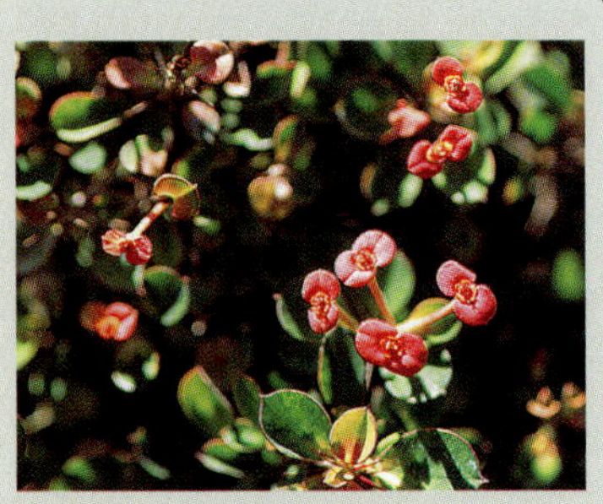

EUPHORBIA MILII 'Mini Bells'

An exquisite dwarf E. milii that has small oval leaves and small red flowers (bells). As it grows it stays round in a similar fashion to 'Short & Sweet' and 'Salmon Dome'. Makes a great houseplant. Full sun or strong light. Zone 10 or higher. Ever bloomer.

85031 Growing Plant (4" pot)....$6.95

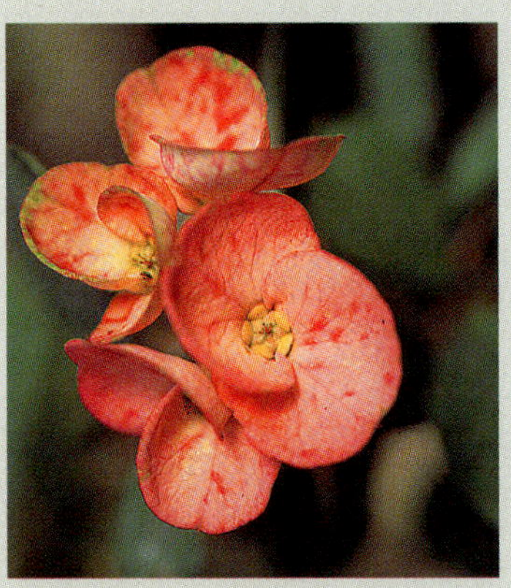

EUPHORBIA MILII 'Rosy Yellow'

A fantastic new hybrid from Thailand. Small waxy yellow flowers are embedded in large rosy pink bracts with dark rose spot and veination. Like other Siamese lucky plants, needs high light, little fertilizer, little water, and mild temperatures. Great houseplant; blooms all year. New.

85045 Growing Plant (4" pot)..$10.95

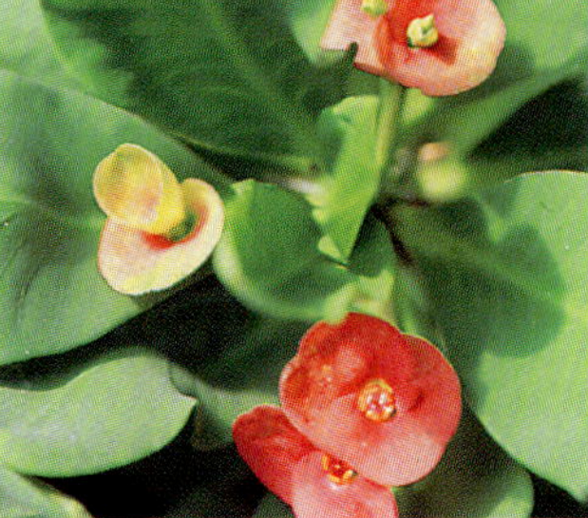

EUPHORBIA MILII 'New Year'

A great looking lucky plant that undergoes color change in flowering. Early flowers are cream color, becoming intense red with age. Large oblong leaves that are flushed with burgundy underneath. Full sun or strong light. Zone 10 or higher. Great houseplant. Blooms all year.

85050 Growing Plant (4" pot) $9.95

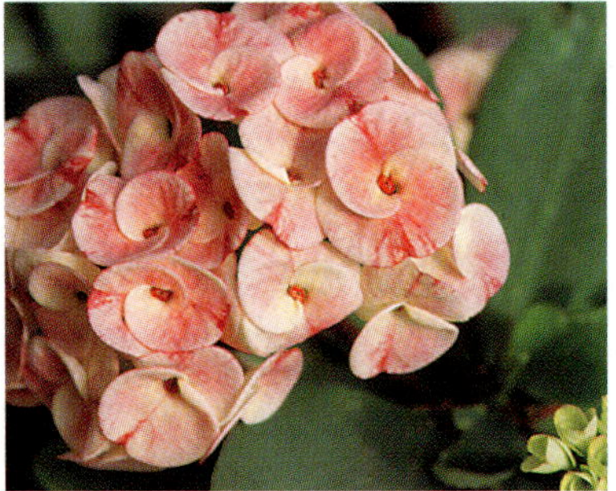

EUPHORBIA MILII 'Pink Christmas'

A magnificent hybrid cultivar with a huge pink floral bouquet. Peachy pink bracts that start creamy colored. Nice oblong green leaves. Great houseplant. Full sun or high light. Zone 10 and higher. Ever bloomer.

85040 Growing Plant (4" pot)........$9.95

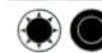

EUPHORBIA MILII 'Spring Song'

A magically colored lucky plant with huge oblong leaves up to 6" long and 1 1/2" wide. A creamy-bracted inflorescence with buttercup-gold centered flowers. Produces a large 6" x 8" globe of flowers. Full sun or strong light. Pinch to make bushier. Great houseplant. Blooms all year.

85070 Growing Plant (4" pot) $9.95

EUPHORBIA MILII 'Salmon Dome'

A semi-dwarf variety that has wonderful salmon pink flowers with dark oblong green leaves. Like "Short and Sweet" has a self-mounding growth habit. Makes a great pot plant. Great houseplant. Needs absolutely no pruning, just high light, a little fertilizer, a little water and non-freezing temperatures. After 6 years growth with no pruning, plant will be about 2' high and about 4' in diameter. Zone 10 and higher outside.

85210 Growing Plant (4" pot) $6.95

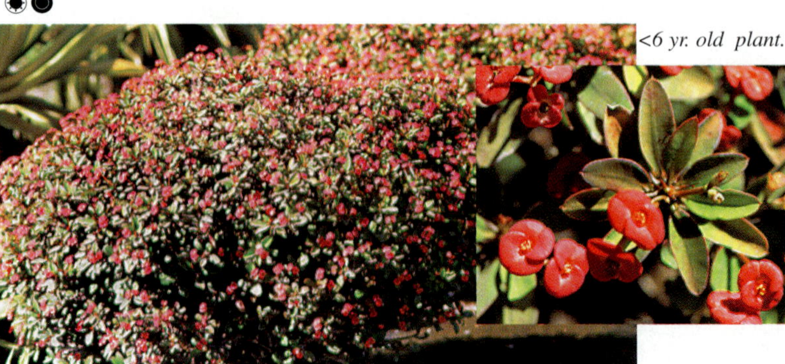
<6 yr. old plant.

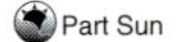 Full Sun 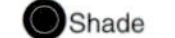 Part Sun 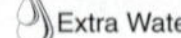 Shade 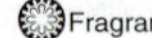 Extra Water 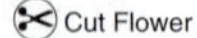 Fragrant 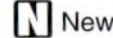 Cut Flower N New

TO ORDER CALL **1-800-624-9706**/24 HRS. OR VISIT OUR WEB SITE: www. stokestropicals.com

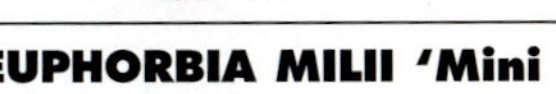

EUPHORBIA MILII 'Short & Sweet'

A true dwarf variety that has small bright red flowers with small oblong leaves. Plant has a wonderful mounding growth habit. Makes an excellent pot plant and does very well in a hanging basket. Likes full sun but can take some shade. Should be kept on the dry side. Does not need a lot of attention and care. Zone 10 and higher.

85200 Growing Plant (4" pot)..............................$5.95

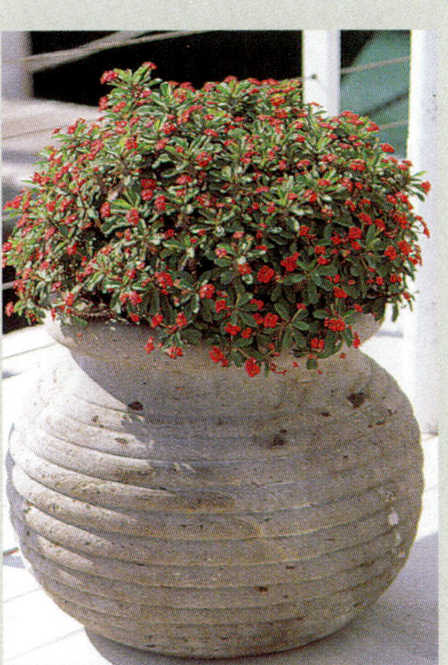

"Short & Sweet" growing in a landscaping urn.

EUPHORBIA MILII 'Mini Spring Song'

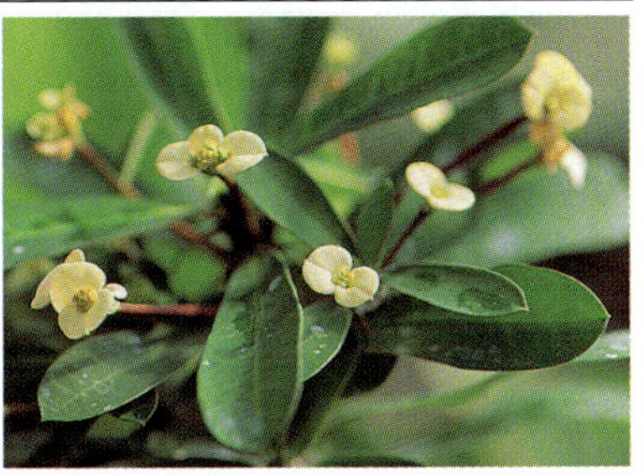

A miniature flowered version of 'Spring Song'; flowers are only 1/3 size. Also, leaves are slightly smaller. Same light, water and fertilizer requirements. Same outstanding growing characteristics. New.

85095 Growing Plant (4" pot)....$9.95

EUPHORBIA MILII 'Summer Song'

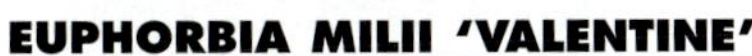

A striking new hybrid from Thailand. Flower bracts are cream with green marginal markings giving it a camouflaged look among the wonderful large green leaves. All the same growth characteristics and requirements. Sure to become one of our most popular 'Siamese Lucky Plants'. New

85075 Growing Plant (4" pot)................$10.95

EUPHORBIA MILII 'VALENTINE'

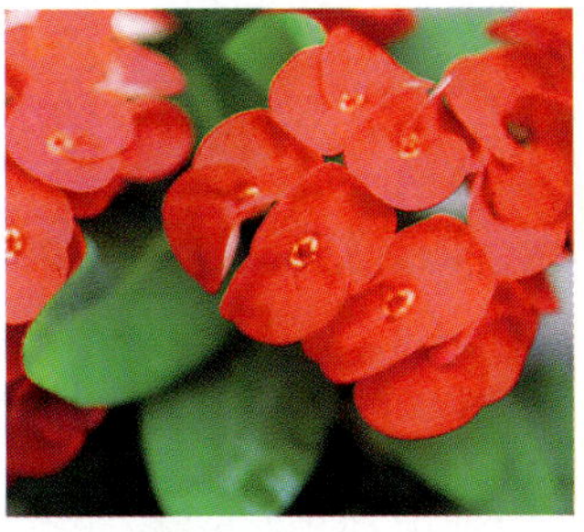

An amazing hybrid cultivar that is reminiscent of a valentine with a large bouquet of valentine-red flowers topping a dark green-leafed plant. Great houseplant. Zone 10 and higher. Full sun or some shade.

85080 Growing Plant (4" pot) $9.95

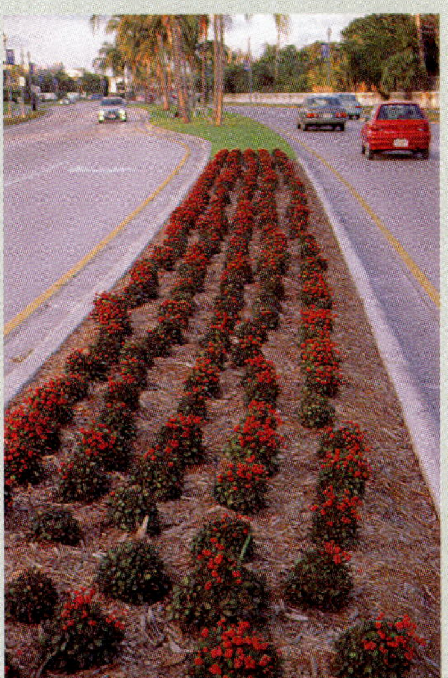

Euphorbia 'Short & Sweet' used in landscaping (Key Biscayne, Florida).

EUPHORBIA MILII 'Winter Song'

Another new hybrid from Thailand. Flower bracts are pale yellow with pink edges. And leaves tend to be larger. Similar growing habits and requirements. Makes a great houseplant; everbloomer. New.

85085 Growing Plant (4" pot)................$10.95

Please inquire about other new Euphorbia milii hybrids for names, descriptions and prices.

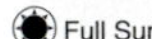 Full Sun   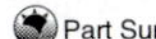 Part Sun   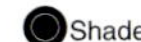 Shade   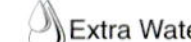 Extra Water   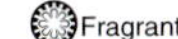 Fragrant   Cut Flower   N New

115

Special Selections

Special Plants

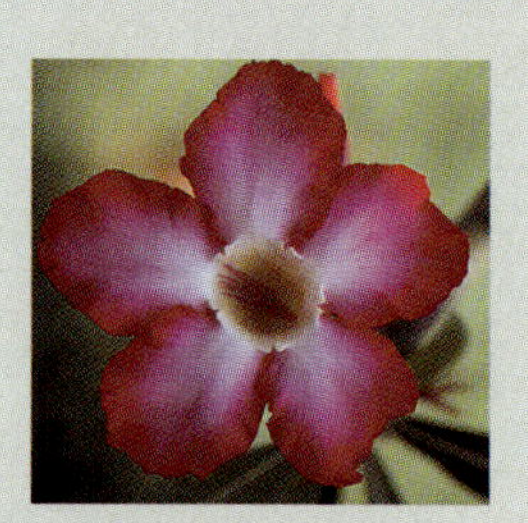

ADENIUM OBESUM
'Desert Rose'

An easy plant to grow, that makes beautiful flowers. Can be grown inside or outside. A member of the dogbane family (Apocynaceae) which includes plumeria, mandevillea, oleander, alamanda and many other plants. Prefers full sun, likes to be on dry side and require little fertilizer. Flowers are hot rose with white throats that splash out on 5 petals of trumpet shaped flowers, Zone 10 and higher. Please note we are growing 12 new hybrids of this species–including a pure white, a ruby red, and a fragrant, pure white flowered form. We will be introducing several of these next year.
89091 Growing Plant (6" pot)....$10.95

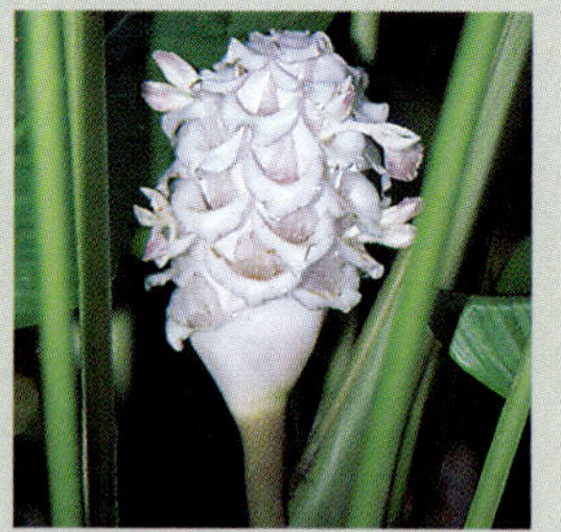

CALATHEA BURLE-MARXII
'Blue Ice'

A dynamite plant growing 3'-4' high. Requires shade. Has big, pure-green leaves. Produces a shiny bluish-white bracted inflorescence down in plant with delicate flowers. Zone 10 and higher.
83200 Rhizome $10.95
83201 Growing Plant (6" pot) ..$17.95

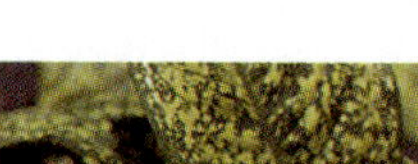
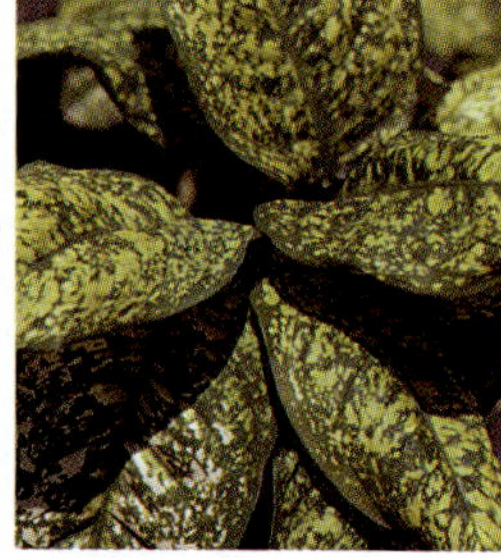

AGLAEONEMA SP.
'Margarita'

A striking plant with silver streaked leaves, that resembles 'Stripes' but with stems that are ivory pink. Zone 10 and higher. Easy to grow.
89051 Growing Plant
(6" pot).......................$9.95
(12"-15" plant w2/3 stalks)

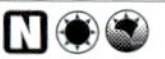

AGLAEONEMA SP.
'MoeMoe'

Striking leaves speckled with yellow. Has all the same great indoor growing characteristics as the other aglaeonemas Zone 10 and higher.
89061 Growing Plant
(6" pot).......................$9.95
(12"-15" plant w2/3 stalks)

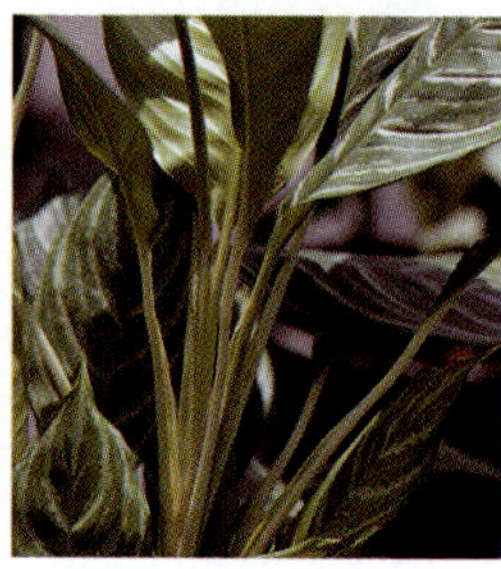

AGLAEONEMA SP.
'Stripes'

A perfect interior plant with silver striped leaves, requiring little water, fertilizer, and thriving in low light. Does well outside, in low light, during warm periods. Zone 10 and higher.
89041 Growing Plant
(6" pot) $9.95
(12"-15" plant w2/3 stalks)

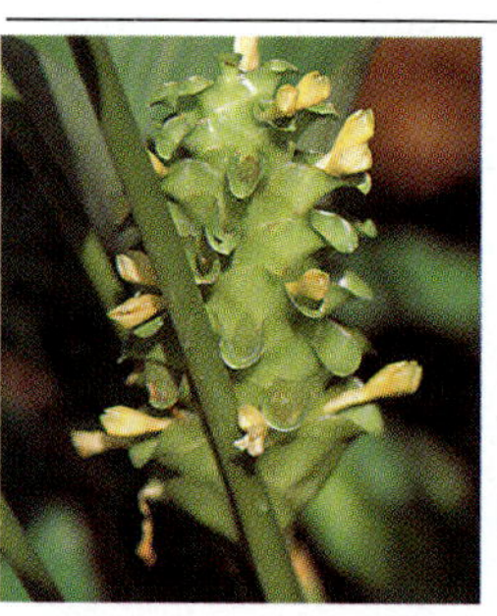

CALATHEA BURLE-MARXII 'Green Ice'

A fantastic plant growing 3'-4' high. Requires shade. Has big, pure-green leaves. Produces a shiny, green bracted inflorescence down in plant with delicate yellow flowers. Zone 10 and higher.
83100 Rhizome $10.95
83101 Growing Plant
(6" pot)..................$17.95

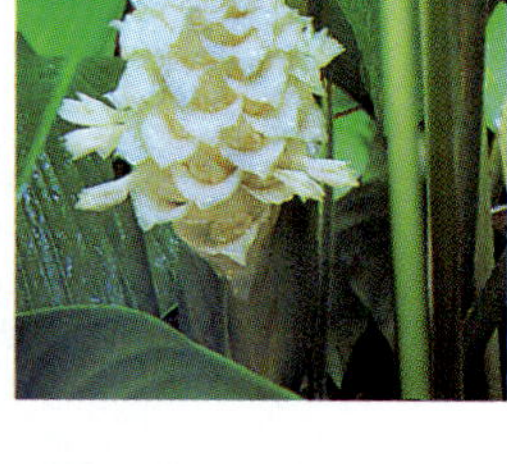

CALATHEA BURLE-MARXII 'White Ice'

A beautiful companion plant to 'Blue Ice' or 'Green Ice'. Grows 3'-4' high and requires shade. Produces a creamy-white bracted inflorescence with delicate flowers that nestles within the plant. Zone 10 and higher.
83300 Rhizome $17.95
83301 Growing Plant
(6" pot)....................$24.95

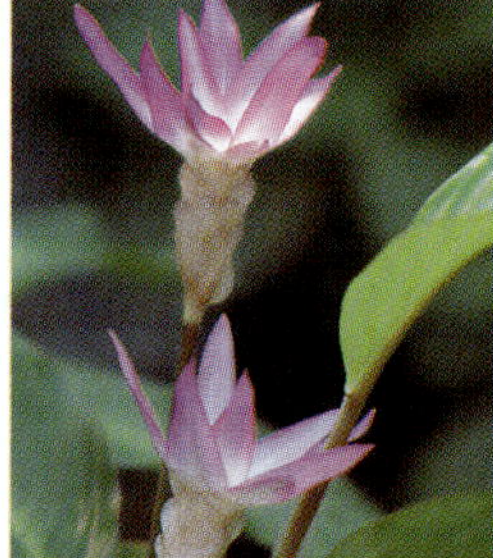

CALATHEA LOESNERI
'Lotus Pink'

A charming small (to 1') plant that does best in shady, humid conditions. Oval, slightly variegated, leaves. Pink flowers, resembling lotus blossoms, held 6" above leaves. Blooms July thru October. Good pot plant. Zone 9B and higher.
83000 Rhizome $10.95
83001 Growing Plant
(6" pot)....................$17.95

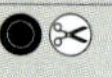 Full Sun   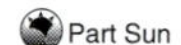 Part Sun   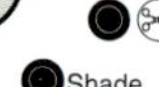 Shade   Extra Water   Fragrant   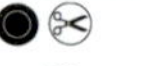 Cut Flower   N New

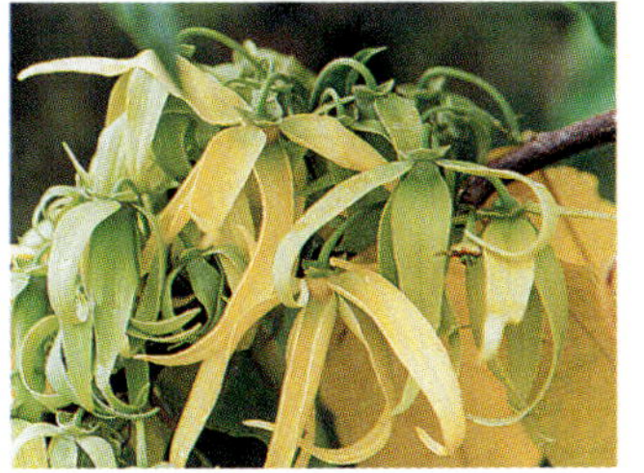

CANANGA ODORATA 'Ylang Ylang'

A magnificent tropical tree that produces seductively fragrant flowers. Prefers a moist, humus, rich soil. Large glossy green leaves. The flowers are long, twisted, drooping, greenish yellow petals appearing mostly in fall in thick clusters at the leaf axils and are followed by small greenish fruit. The Ylang Ylang (its Mayaysian name) is widely cultivated in the Comoros Island and Hawaii for the perfume industry. Zone 10 and higher. Full sun.

83251 Growing Plant (6" pot) $13.95

CLERODENDRUM BUNGEI 'Bridal Bouquet'

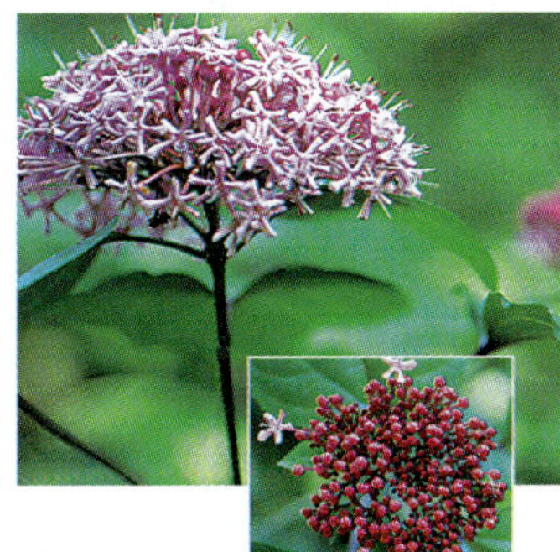

An easy-to-grow deciduous shrub. Native to China. Spreads readily by suckering. Large, serrate, widely oval, tropical leaves that are reddish and fuzzy underneath. Leaves can grow to 1' across. When leaves or stems are rubbed or bruised they produce a musky, scent. Large dense cymes (to 8") of reddish purple tubular flowers that are sweetly scented. Flowering occurs continuously all summer and into fall. Great plant for containers and defined areas with borders. Plants grow to 5'-7'. A once common southern plant that is making a comeback. Great to look at and possesses a good fragrance. Is cold hardy down to -20°F. Can be used in zones 5 and higher. A fantastic plant; butterflies can't resist it.

87001 Bareroot Plant in 6" pot $12.95

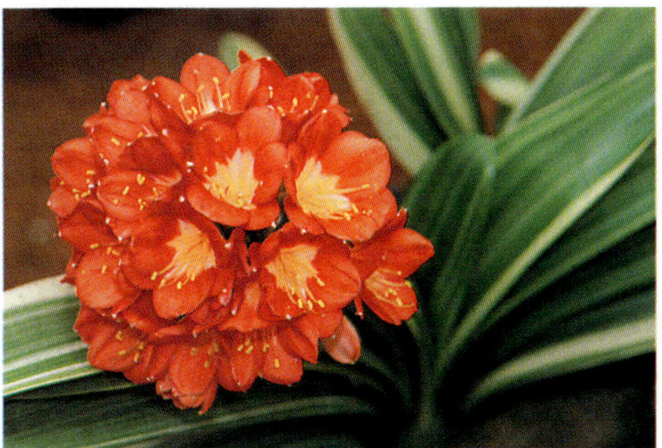

CLIVIA MINIATA 'Striped Beauty'

100% proofed variegated leaf plant. 99% of flowers will be wonderful hybrid orange. Rarely yellow or peach flowers may develop. First flowers will occur in 3-4 years, if well grown. Then flowers will appear regularly every year in February to April.

89402-3 (3 seed)............................$15.00	*89402-6 (6 seed)*............................$26.00
89402-9 (9 seed)............................$36.00	*89402-12 (12 seed)*......................$46.00
89400 Seedling Plant....................$19.95	
89401 Plant 18"-24" (Flower Proofed) $199.95	

We are currently growing more than 40 different Clivia miniata hybrids. Please inquire about names, descriptions and prices.

CLIVIA MINIATA 'American Yellow'

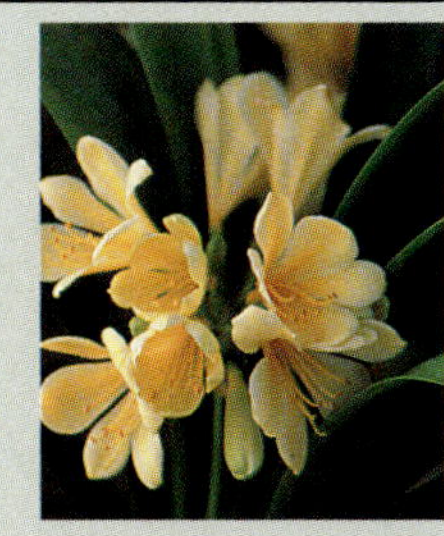

Yellow flowers once considered to be the 'holy grail' of Clivia. Now available after 30 years of careful selection at an unheard of price. Grow your own $1,000.00 Clivia for a few dollars. Seed are 85% true. Few will have orange flowers. Some may have peach-colored flowers. And a few might have variegated leaves. (Sold only in multiples of 3 seed.)

89412-3 (3 seed)............................$15.00
89412-6 (6 seed)............................$26.00
89412-9 (9 seed)............................$36.00
89412-12 (12 seed)......................$46.00
89410 Seedling Plant....................$19.95
*89411 Plant 18"-24"
(Flower Proofed)*........................$159.95

CLIVIA MINIATA 'Prince of Orange'

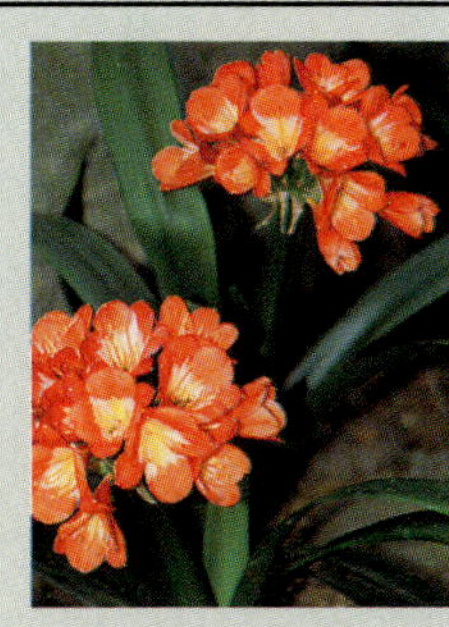

Deep orange flowers on wide dark green leaves make this an unforgettable plant obtained after 30 plus years of careful selection.

Seed are 90% true. A few will produce yellow flowers or peach flowers or have variegated leaves. (Sold only in multiples of 3 seed.)

89422-3 (3 seed)............................$9.00
89422-6 (6 seed)............................$16.00
89422-9 (9 seed)............................$23.00
89422-12 (12 seed)......................$28.00
89420 Seedling Plant..................$17.95
*89421 Plant 18"-24"
(Flower Proofed)*........................$59.95

 Full Sun   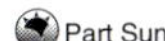 Part Sun   Shade   Extra Water   Fragrant   Cut Flower   New

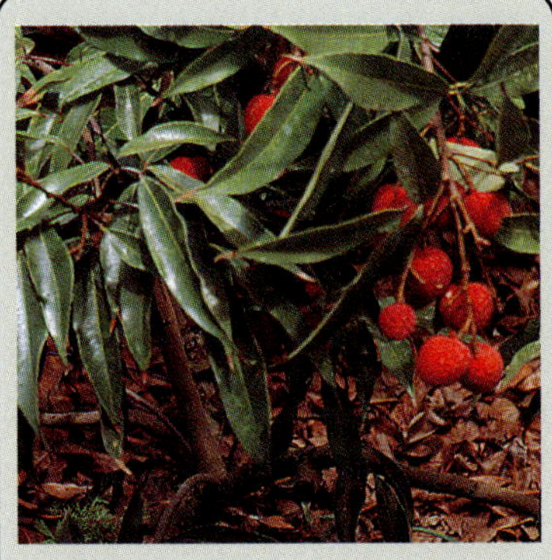

LYCHEE, LITCHI CHINENSIS 'Brewster'

A wonderful tasting fruit tree originally from Southern China. So long improved in cultivation that wild forms are unknown. Brewster is one of the cold hardiest forms (can take temperatures down to mid 20's for short periods) and is proven in container culture. Will flower and produce fruit in 1-2 years. Starts to flower in January and February with fruit in June and July. Slow growing in container (5-year old plant only 7'-8' tall). Even when not in bloom plant has great look with its dark green shiny foliage. Zone 9 and higher. 18"-24" tall plant in 6" pot.
89071 Growing Plant (6" pot)...$24.95

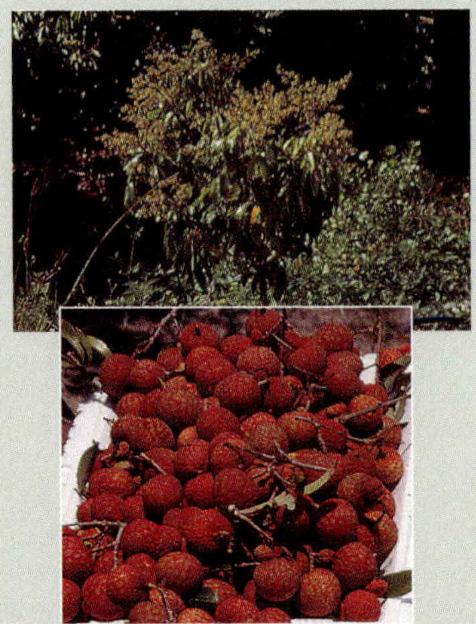

Top photo: young 'Brewster' in flower Lower photo: ripe fruit of 'Sweet Cliff' lychee

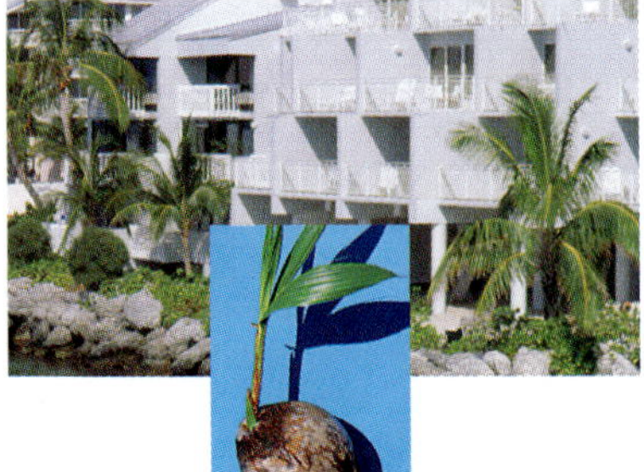

COCOS NUCIFERA 'Jamaican Tall' COCONUT

Real live coconut, sprouted from coconut husk. No plant is more tropical. This is the signature tropical plant. Can be grown outside and inside. Just don't let it freeze. Zone 10 and higher.
89030 (3-4 lb. coconut with 20"-30" leaves)..$14.95

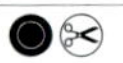

DRACAENA SANDERIANA 'Lucky Bamboo'

A wonderful "bamboo"-looking plant that can be grown in only water. Plant is considered to be lucky by many people of Southeast Asia. Comes as rooted stems of 3 different lengths that can be arranged in very attractive bundles and placed in small ceramic, glass or clay pots. Does not need soil. Thrives in low light indoors to medium light outdoors. Zone 10 and higher. Might be the easiest plant you can grow inside.
89500 (4"+ 6"—3 of each) $11.95
89510 (6"+ 8"—3 of each) $13.95
89520 (4"+ 6"+ 8"—2 of each) $12.95

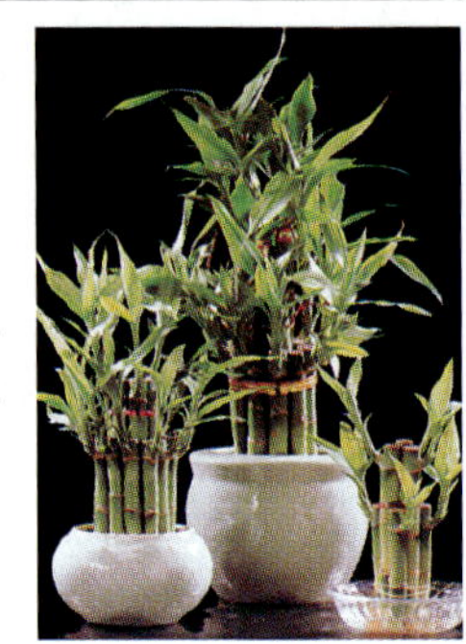

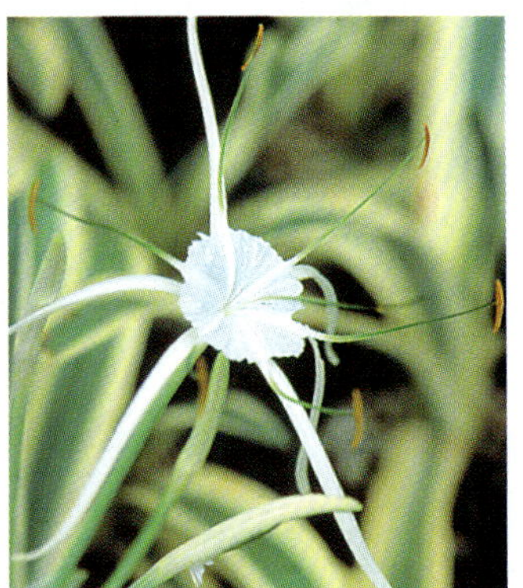

HYMENOCALLIS LITTORALIS 'Variegata' 'Variegated Spider Lily'

A unique plant that can tolerate the broadest possible range of growing conditions. It can grow in water, in wet boggy areas, or dry areas. Full sun to part shade. Magnificent white, fragrant flowers and dramatic striped foliage. Zone 8 and higher. Previously offered for $100 per plant.
84000 Rhizome $4.95
84001 Growing Plant (6" pot) $9.95

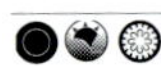

COCCOLOBA UVIFERA 'Sea Grape'

A tropical seaside plant that is always beautiful with or without leaves. The young leaves are small disks of burnished copper. Older leaves are the size of saucers and are a deep dark green with a wonderful veining pattern. The old leaves, following a hint of cold air, turn a brilliant red. Anyone who has been on a Caribbean, Bahamas, Central American or South Florida vacation has seen and admired the sea grape growing in the beachside sand.

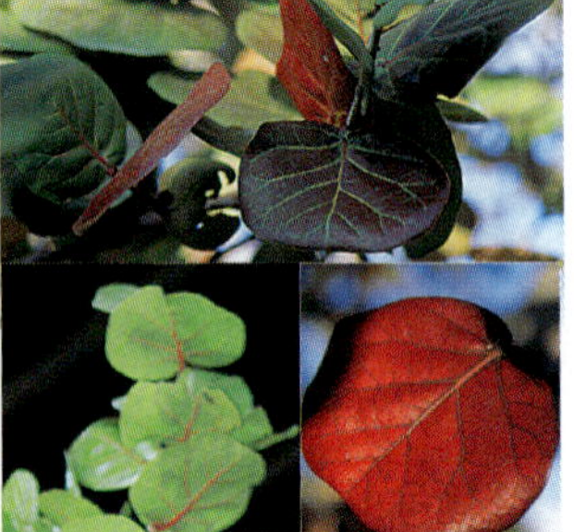

Zone 10 and higher. Fruit is delicious and can be used to make jellies, jams, or wines. Cut leaves are great as decorations or trays.
89031 Growing Plant (4" pot) $6.95

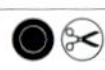

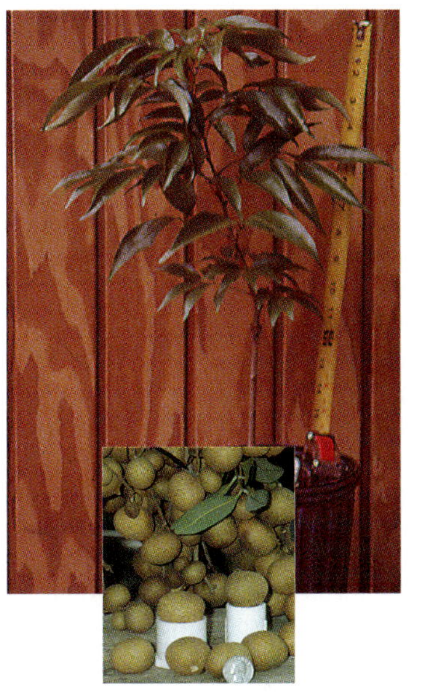

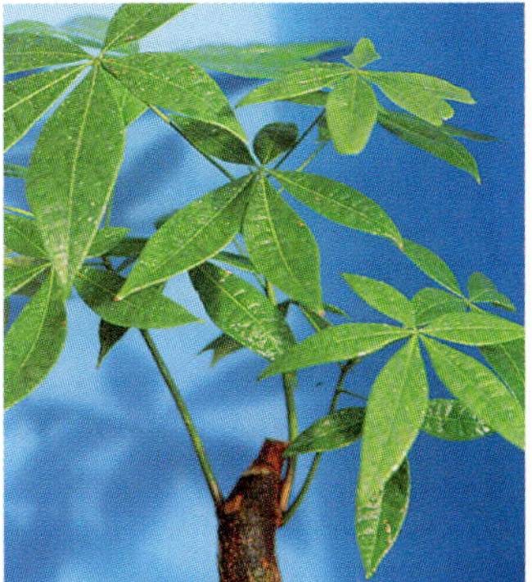

LONGAN, DIMOCARPUS LONGAN 'Kohala'

The 'Kohala' longan, a sweet tasting fruit tree, is one of the cold hardiest of the longans (tolerant of temperatures in mid-20s for short periods). Introduced to Continental U.S. from Kohala mountains on the Big Island of Hawaii where it grows up to 5,000' in elevation. It is the longan of commerce in Florida. Has proven itself in container culture. A fast grower but growth can be controlled by tip pruning (5-year old container plant could reach 9'-l0'). Blooms in February/March and fruits in August/September. Produces fruit 2 years after planting. Zone 9 and higher. Supplied as 18"-24" plants.
89081 Growing Plant (6" pot) $24.95

Orders Placed Through Our Web Site Receive a 15% Discount

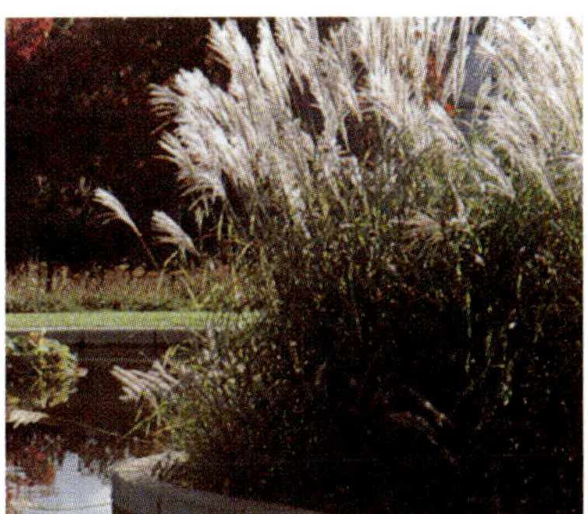

MAIDEN GRASS-MISCANTHUS SINENSIS 'Gracillimus'

A wonderful ornamental grass that is easy to grow. Makes fantastic flower plumes that dance in the slightest breeze. Excellent cut. Grows 5'-6' tall. Full sun. Hard freeze will kill tender grass stems, but plant will return from underground stems in spring. Clumping grass, doesn't run. Zone 8 and higher.
84561 Growing Plant (4" pot) $10.95

Photo with permission of John Greelee from *The Encyclopedia of Ornamental Grasses.*

PACHIRA AQUATICA 'Guiana Chestnut'

A fantastic houseplant that is taking Europe by storm. Has distinctive swollen, scaly trunk with green young stems topped with interesting finger-like leaves. In tropical areas will grow into a tree. Plant is native to Mexico and Northern South America. Restricted to a pot and pruned as a young plant, it becomes an attractive foliage houseplant. Grown in larger pot with appropriate water and fertilizer, plants produce numerous long stems that are covered with beautiful leaves. Zone 10 and higher.
84500 Growing Plant (6" pot) $12.95

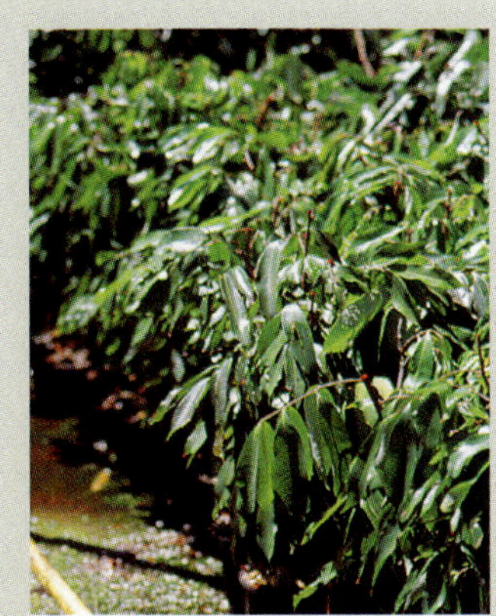

MIRACLE FRUIT SYNSEPALUM DULCIFICUM

A truly miraculous plant. Everything about it is unusual—its looks, its flowering, and the taste of its fruit (berries). A West African shrub that is slow growing with great looking dark green foliage the year round. Clusters of small white flowers occur in branch axils. Red berries are produced over an extended period that make sour things taste sweet. Chewing a small portion of the pulp of a single berry can change the taste of beer to apple juice, of lime to sweet lemonade, of grapefruit to orange, etc. Taste change lasts up to 2 hours. Has been used to treat cancer patients following chemotherapy to improve food taste and as a natural sweetening agent in place of sugar. Chemical proteins from the crushed berry coat the sour receptors on the tongue so everything tastes sweet. Unbelievable, has to be tried to be believed. Prefers 30-50% shade. Blooms from May-November and has fruit from June to December in Zone 9. In Zone 10 and higher plant is everbearing. Slow growing (5-year old plant, only 3' tall), makes it ideal for container culture; a 10-year old plant is only 4'-5'. Very heavy fruit producer; 6' plant produces as many as 300 berries at one time. Cold hardy down to 30°F for short periods of time. Zone 9 and higher. Supplied as a 10"-12" plant in a 4" pot.
89085 Growing Plant (4" pot)....$16.95

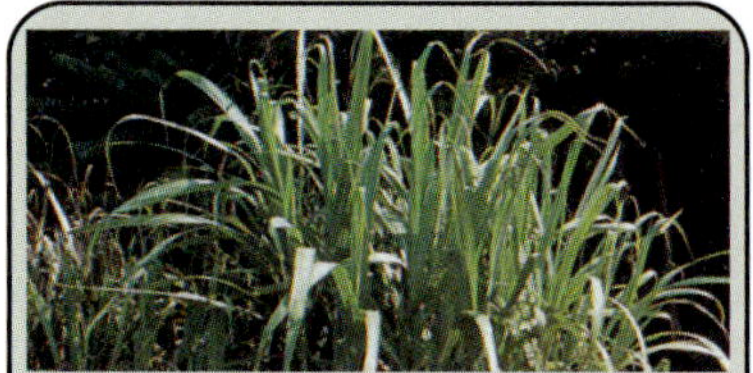

Photo with permission of John Greelee from *The Encyclopedia of Ornamental Grasses.*

SACCHARUM OFFICINARUM SUGARCANE 'LOUISIANA 384'

Real Louisiana sugarcane—never before offered in a mail-order catalog. A large grass (6'-9' tall) that yields sweet juice when eaten raw or crushed. When cooked can yield syrup. Louisiana is largest sugarcane producer in U.S. This is latest commercial variety ('384'), grown extensively throughout Southwest Louisiana. Prefers acid pH from 5.5–6.5. Needs full sun. Very fast grower. Zone 9 and higher. Can tolerate temperatures into low 20's for short periods of time when planted in ground. Makes nice accent or background planting.

89120 Sprouted Stalk (6" pot)....$11.95

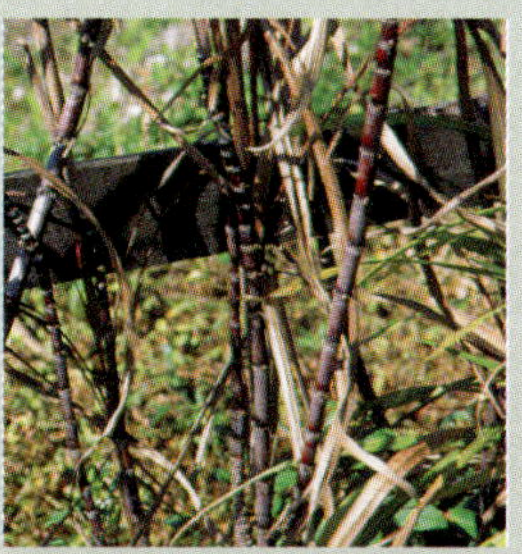

SACCHARUM OFFICINARUM SUGARCANE 'RED SUGARCANE'

Red sugarcane differs from Louisiana '384' by having a beautiful blackish maroon stem. Juice is slightly red and taste is different. The original Barbancourt rum from Haiti on the island of Hispaniola is said to have been made from red sugarcane. Dark shiny stem makes outstanding display. Does well in containers. Zone 9 and higher.

89125 Sprouted Stalk (6" pot)....$14.95

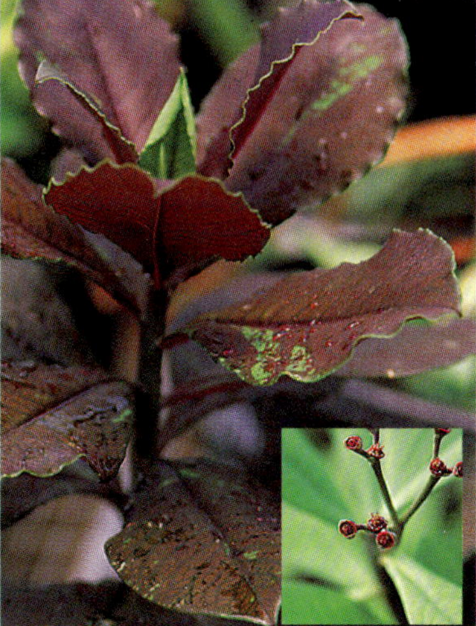

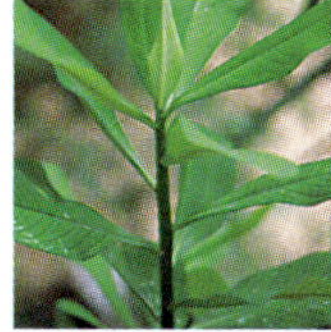

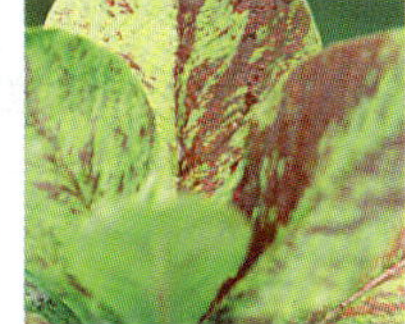

Top photo: Maroon stage;
Inset: Plant in bloom
Lower photos: green stage & mottled stage.

SYNADENIUM GRANTII 'CHAMELEON PLANT'

A very fast growing euphorb from East Africa. Has also been called 'Red Milk Bush' because of its red leaves and milky sap. A very easy-to-grow plant that has thick, leathery leaves. Grows very fast reaching 6'-7' in one growing season in Zone 9. Plant is uusual in that you can start off with a solid maroon or a solid green leaved form and it can change to a mottled form or go from green to maroon or maroon to green. Some older plants have all three colored leave stages on the same plant. Flowers are very small and inconspicuous. Makes a good pot plant. Zone 10 and higher. Medium shade to full sun. New.

89100 Growing Plant (6" pot)
(Maroon leaf stage).....................$10.95
89101 Growing Plant (6" pot)
(Green leaf stage) $10.95
89102 Growing Plant (6" pot)
(Mottled leaf stage) $10.95

TACCA CHANTRIERI 'Black Bat Plant'

A very unusual plant with attractive large (2'-3') mustard-like foliage that grows from an underground rhizome. Main feature of plant is strange unique flower that superficially resembles a flying bat with long whiskers. Other common names are: Cats Whiskers and Devil Flower. Prefers shade. Zone 10 and higher. A good container plant. And a great conversation piece.

89160 Growing Plant (6" pot) $14.95

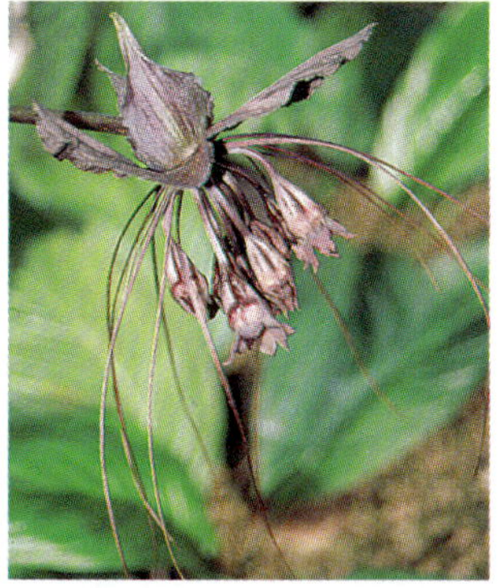

TACCA CHANTRIERI 'White Bat Plant'

Like the 'Black Bat Plant' except it has white flower resembling a flying bat. A great companion plant for the 'Black Bat'. Originally from Thailand. Not too many people have these exotic tropical plants. In limited supply. Zone 10 and higher.

89150 Growing Plant (6" pot) $19.95

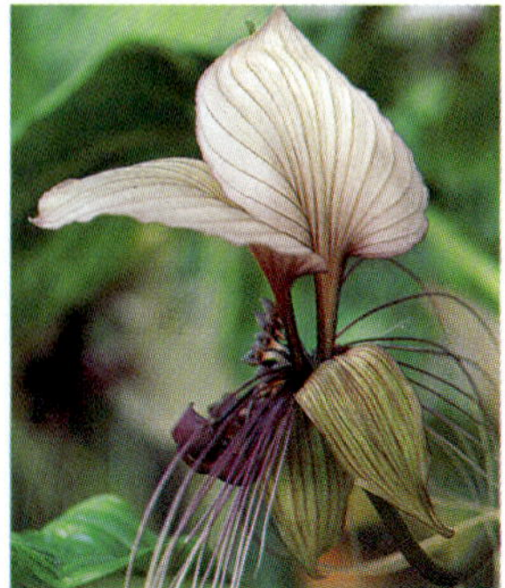

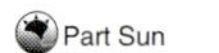 Full Sun   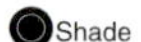 Part Sun   Shade   Extra Water   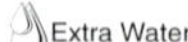 Fragrant   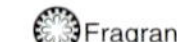 Cut Flower   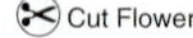 New

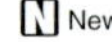

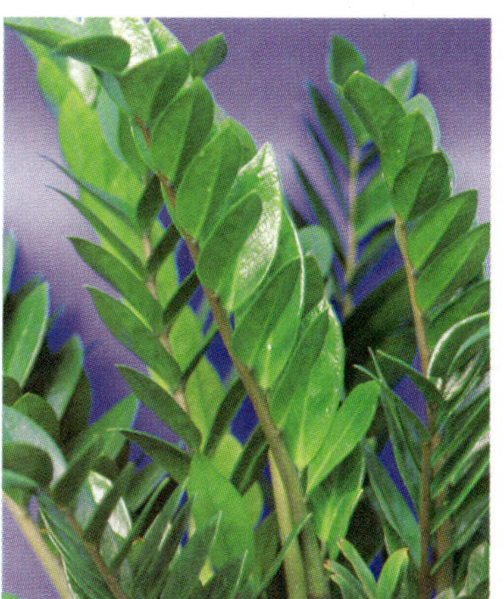

ZAMIOCULUS ZAMIOFOLIA 'Emerald Fronds'

An amazing aroid from Africa. Superficially resembles a cycad hence the genus and species names. Produces 2'-3' long pointed spears lined with alternating shiney dark leaves. Grows from an underground "tuber". Has tolerated sub-freezing temperatures down to 24°F planted outdoors and returned the following spring. Makes a great houseplant because it grows well in containers, can tolerate low humidity, low light and needs little water and little fertilizer. Full shade to medium sun. Zone 9 and higher. New.

89200 Growing Plant (6" pot) *$11.95*

Visit our Web Site : www.stokestropicals.com
E-mail us: info@stokestropicals.com

FULL SIZED FLORIST QUALITY TROPICAL PLANTS.

Because of the tremendous interest that we have received for certain proven indoor tropical plants, such as, ficus, palms, crotons, bird-of-paradise, and dracena, we are offering these plants for the first time. All of these plants will be shipped within 48 hours of receipt of order and payment. All will be shipped in separate boxes by USPS Priority Mail and can be shipped year-round because of special insulated packing. All will be in full size pots with correct soil mix. You just need to place inside your ornamental pot or other container and water and fertilize according to detailed cultural directions that are provided with each plant. **Because of soil we cannot ship to California, Arizona, and Washington.**

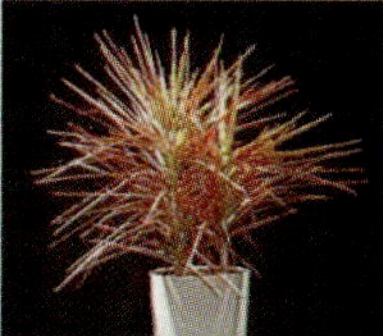

CORDYLINE TERMINALIS 'Colorama'

Best way to describe this one is HOT PINK. Colorama will light up any corner for you. Another top 10 air purifier according to NASA study. Let the potting soil dry to 1 inch before watering. Low to medium light. Comes 2 '- 3' tall. Hardy outside in Zone 10 and higher.

89935 (10" pot) *$40.00*

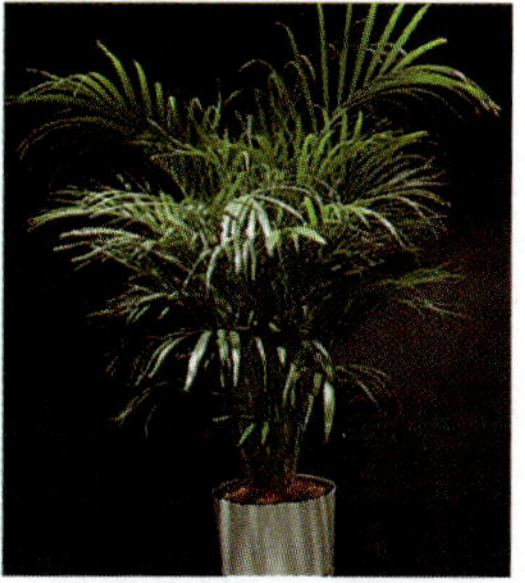

CHRYSALIDOCARPUS LUTESCENS 'Areca Palm'

Probably the most widely distributed indoor palm. Palms in general rank high in absorbing air pollutants, and this is one of the best. Very popular with those that like a dense full look. Keep soil moist. Medium to high light. Comes 3'- 4' tall. Hardy outside in Zone 10 and higher.

89955 (10" pot) *$42.00*

STRELITZIA NICOLAI 'White Bird of Paradise'

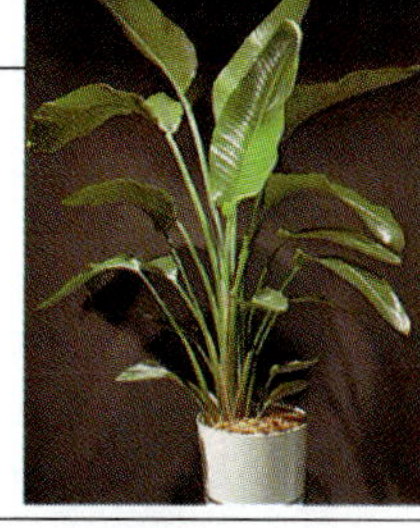

One of our favorites. When you see the graceful dark green leaves, it truly makes you think tropical. The "bird" dresses up any area. Keep moist but not wet and place in high light. Comes 3'- 4' tall. Hardy outside in Zone 10 and higher.

89920 (10" pot) *$45.00*

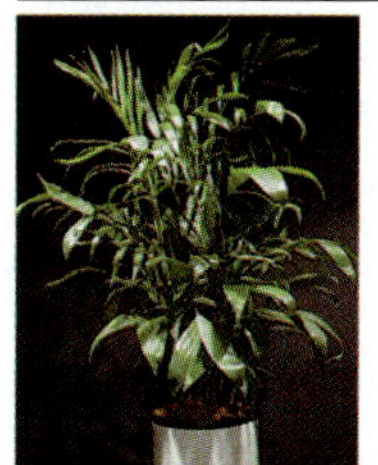

CHAMAEDOREA ELEGANS 'Parlor Palm'

This palm has a delicate look. Relatively small, but very full. Great in a decorative container as a centerpiece or on a pedestal. Let the top half of the potting soil dry between waterings. Low or medium light is fine. Comes 2'- 3' tall. Hardy outside in Zone 10 and higher.

89950 (10" pot) *$41.00*

FICUS BENJAMINA 'Ficus Tree'

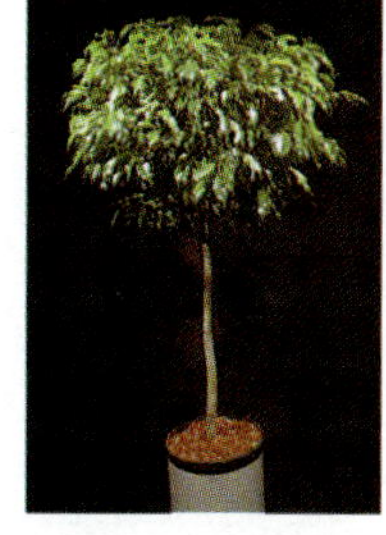

This is a favorite tropical tree to enjoy in your home or office. Deep green, shiny leaves radiate a healthy look. Keep moist in high light and you will enjoy this one for a long time. NOTE: Our Ficus are properly acclimated for indoors, and if kept near high light will experience little or no leaf loss. Comes 3'- 4' tall. Hardy outside in Zone 10 and higher.

89915 (10" pot) *$43.00*

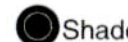 Full Sun 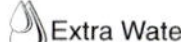 Part Sun ● Shade Extra Water Fragrant Cut Flower N New

TO ORDER CALL **1-800-624-9706**/24 HRS. OR VISIT OUR WEB SITE: www. stokestropicals.com

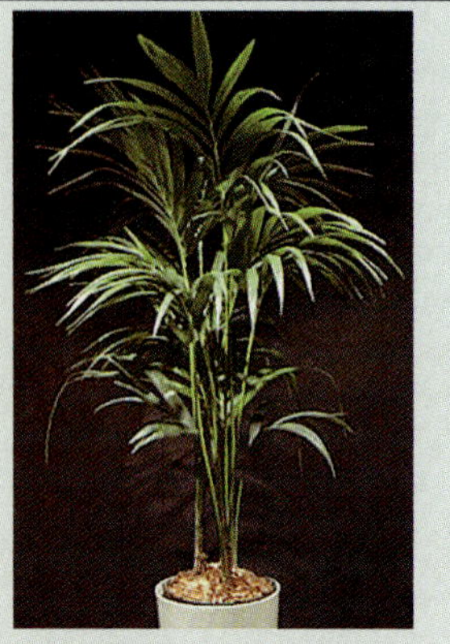

HOWEA FORSTERIANA 'Kentia Palm'

The cadillac of all indoors palms. Gracefully balanced, kelly-green, long-lasting. It is rare to find this palm in a home. Kentia is found mainly in malls, airports, hotels, and lobbies. As an added bonus, Kentia is one of the most efficient plants at absorbing contaminants from the air. For a tropical statement in your home, try one of our Kentia palms. Keep soil moist. Low, medium or high light will work. Comes 4' tall. Hardy outside in Zone 10 and higher.
89970 (10" pot) $65.00

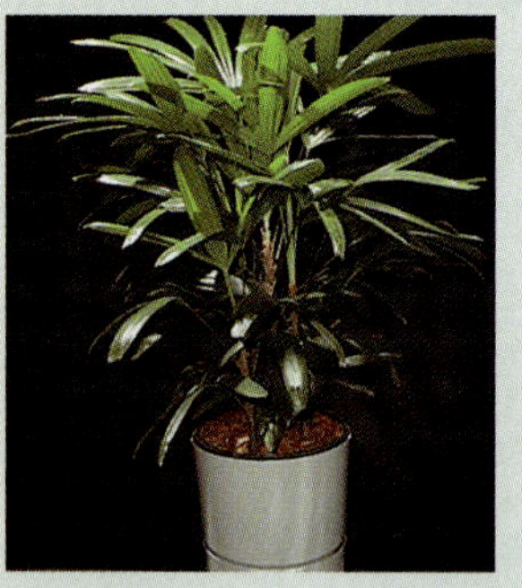

RHAPSIS EXCELSA 'Lady Palm'

This palm has been in cultivation for 300 years. Deep green color, balanced shape, slender leaves, and tough long-lasting nature make it a favorite. This palm is also rated very high as an air cleaner in NASA study. Keep moist. Medium to high light. Comes 3' tall. Hardy outside in Zones 9b and higher.
89965 (10" pot) $55.00

FICUS LYRATA 'Fiddle Leaf Fig'

What an eye catcher with its unusually large leaves. Very full bodied plant. Keep potting soil moist. Likes medium to high light. Comes 3'- 4' tall. Hardy outside in zone 10 and higher.
89910 (10" pot) $43.00

FULL SIZED FLORIST QUALITY TROPICAL PLANTS

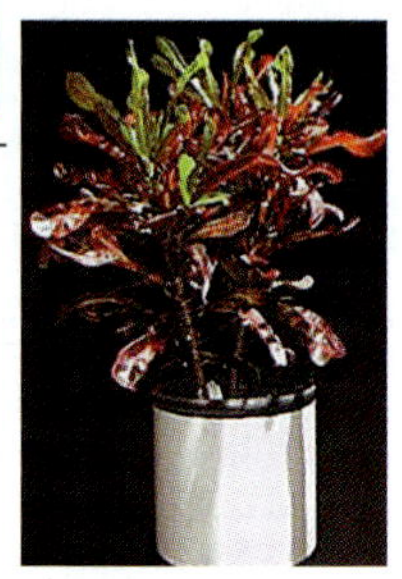

CODIACUM VARIEGATUM 'Mamey Croton'

Unusual, colorful, and tropical. This exotic will brighten up any room. It is hard to believe the bright, contrasting colors this tropical has. Keep moist but not too wet. Medium to high light is best. Comes 2'- 2½' tall. Hardy outside in Zone 10 and higher.
89930 (10" pot) $41.00

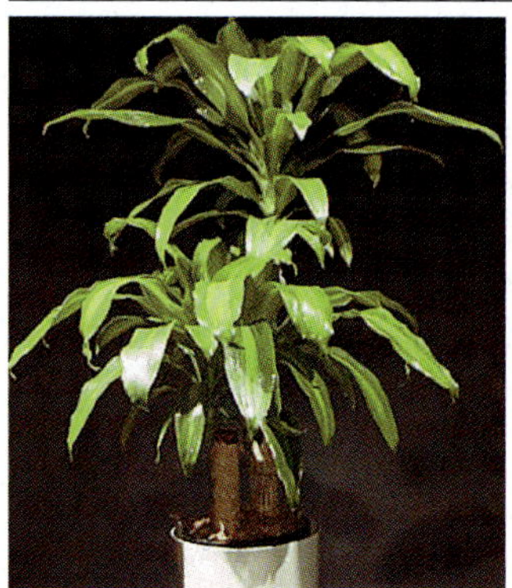

DRACAENA FRAGRANS MASSANGEANA 'Corn Plant'

Here is a living tropical ornament for your home or office. Two heavy canes with green-striped foliage. Another tropical that commands attention and questions from your visitors. Let the potting soil dry on top between waterings. Will do well in low light areas. Comes 3'- 4' tall. Hardy outside in Zone 10 and higher.
89945 (10" pot)..$43.00

CHAMAEDOREA HYBRID 'Florida Palm'

A NASA study lists this palm as the best for indoor purification. One of the most popular indoor palms. Let the top couple inches of the potting soil dry between waterings. Medium to high light will work. Comes 3'- 4' tall. Thrives in full shade; one of most commonly grown houseplant palms. Hardy outside in Zone 10 and higher.
89960 (10" pot) $53.00

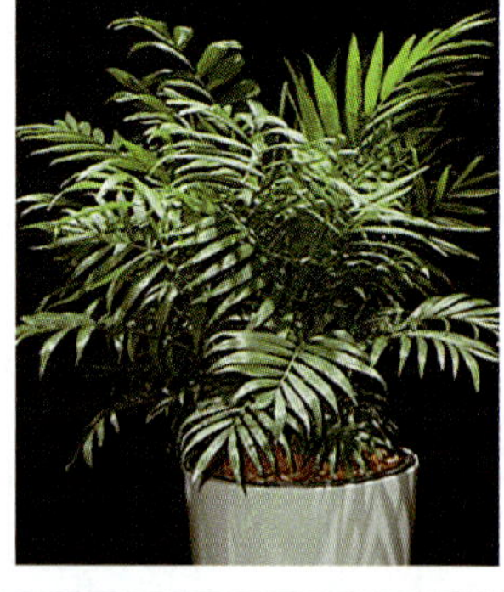

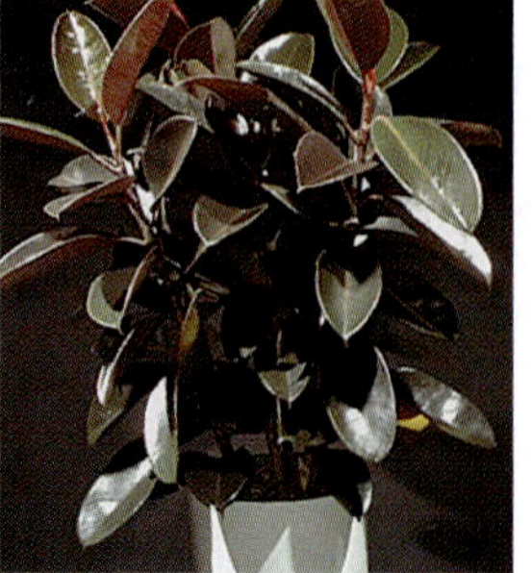

FICUS ELASTICA 'Burgundy Rubber Plant'

Deep rich burgundy colors with bright red top leaves. A living earth-tone ornament for your enjoyment. Extra durable plant and easy to care for. Keep soil moist. Medium to high light. Comes 2'- 3' tall. Hardy outside in Zone 9b and higher.
89940 (10" pot)..$42.00

SPECIAL PLANT COLLECTIONS

In all collections we reserve the right to make a substitution of an equal or more expensive plant that most closely resembles your original selection(s)

COLD HARDIEST COLLECTION — 5

Clerodendrum bungei	(Zone 5+)	87000
Musa basjoo	(Zone 4+)	11150
Plumeria sp. 'Sierra Madre'	(Zone 9+)	54291
Heliconia aff. Schiediana	(Zone 9+)	41170
Hedychium coronarium	(Zone 7+)	34900
Canna indica "India Prince"	(Zone 7+)	88000

Catalog price	$231.70
31019 Collection Price	$221.70
Save	**$10.00**

Only 1 collection per customer.

(rhizomes of ginger and canna and growing plants of all others)

BEST HUMMINGBIRD COLLECTION — 5

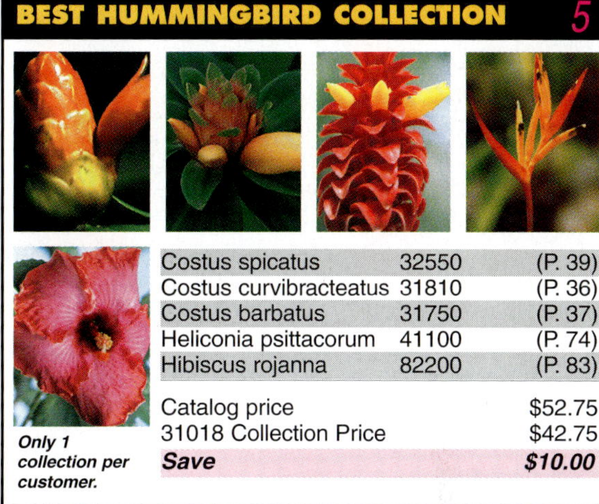

Costus spicatus	32550	(P. 39)
Costus curvibracteatus	31810	(P. 36)
Costus barbatus	31750	(P. 37)
Heliconia psittacorum	41100	(P. 74)
Hibiscus rojanna	82200	(P. 83)

Catalog price	$52.75
31018 Collection Price	$42.75
Save	**$10.00**

Only 1 collection per customer.

Only 1 collection per customer.   (rhizomes except Hibiscus in 4" pot)

WATER PLANT COLLECTION — 5

Alpinia aquatica	31000	(P. 30)
Canna sp. 'Bangkok Yellow'	88100	(P. 26)
Canna sp. 'Cleopatra'	88200	(P. 26)
Hedy. coronarium	34900	(P. 51)
Hymenocallis littoralis 'Variegata'	84000	(P. 118)

Catalog price	$29.95
82950 Collection Price	$37.75
Save	**$7.80**

Only 1 collection per customer.

BEST BUTTERFLY COLLECTION — 5

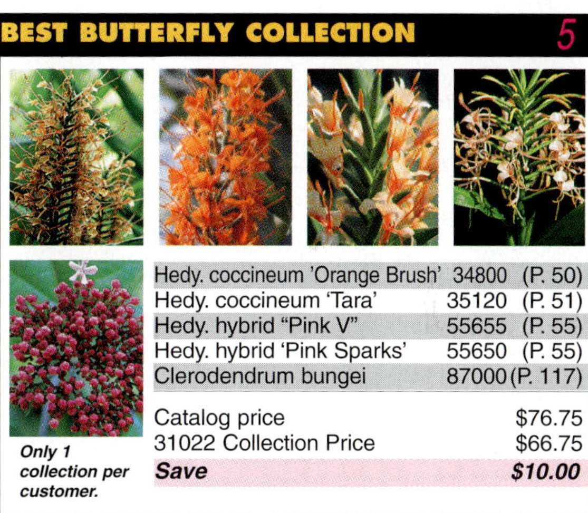

Hedy. coccineum 'Orange Brush'	34800	(P. 50)
Hedy. coccineum 'Tara'	35120	(P. 51)
Hedy. hybrid "Pink V"	55655	(P. 55)
Hedy. hybrid 'Pink Sparks'	55650	(P. 55)
Clerodendrum bungei	87000	(P. 117)

Catalog price	$76.75
31022 Collection Price	$66.75
Save	**$10.00**

Only 1 collection per customer.

RARE BROMELIAD COLLECTION — 4

Fudge Ripple	21050	(Page 112)
Gigantea Nova	21350	(Page 113)
Medium Rare	21100	(Page 112)
Mint Julip	21400	(Page 113)

Catalog price	$164.80
88900 Collection Price	**$154.80**
Save	**$10.00**

Only 1 collection per customer.

A SUPERIOR IDEA!

Consider making a donation of our rare exotic plants to your local botanical garden, zoo or aquarium. Your donation of rare plants will be a lasting memorial to you and your family. You will be benefiting your neighbors and your community by making available to them plants that would otherwise never be exhibited by your local botanical garden, zoo or aquarium. Plus you will be preserving rare plants that may ultimately become extinct by putting them in the care of professionals.

Here is what one person had to say about the pleasure of donating our rarest tropicals to his favorite botanical garden.

"When I first received the 1998 Stokes Tropicals Catalog I knew I wanted many of the unusual and interesting plants illustrated. As gingers grow especially well in the Santa Barbara climate, I ordered an extensive collection together with rare bananas. I was so pleased with the size of the plants and the quality that I ordered a similar collection and donated these to my favorite botanical garden, Lotusland, here in Montecito. I want my family, friends, and visitors to the garden to enjoy this rare collection as I do in the spectacular palm grove setting. I think that donating plants from your own garden or purchasing unusual plants to donate to your towns" gardens is a wonderful idea and I am pleased that Stokes Tropicals is encouraging us—the plant lovers."

Dr. Glynne Couvillion
Montecito, CA.

Bananas

Stokes Tropicals' Plants can be found in:

Special Plants

BOTANICAL GARDENS:

Bermuda Botanical Gardens	Hamilton, Bermuda
Boerner Botanical Gardens	Hales Corner, WI.
Botanica, the Wichita Gardens	Wichita, KA.
Brooklyn Botanical Gardens	Brooklyn, NY.
Buffalo & Erie County Botanical Gardens	Buffalo,NY.
Cape Fear Botanical Garden	Fayetteville, NC.
Cheyenne Botanic Gardens	Cheyenne, WY.
Chicago Botanical Gardens	Glencoe, IL.
Cleveland Botanical Gardens	Shaker Heights,OH.
Denver Botanic Gardens	Denver, CO.
Edelweiss Gardens	Robbinsville, NJ.
El Arish Botanic Gardens	N. Queensland, Australia
Fairchild Tropical Gardens	Miami, FL.
Franklin Park Conservatory	Columbus, OH.
Frederik Meijer Gardens	Grand Rapids, MI.
Harry P. Leu Gardens	Orlando, FL.
Krohn Conservatory	Cincinnati, OH.
L.H. Cohn Arboretum	Baton Rouge, LA.
Lewis Ginter Botanical Garden	Richmond, VA.
Longue Vue Gardens	New Orleans, LA.
Longwood Gardens	Kennett Square, PA.
Luthy Botanical Garden	Peoria, IL.
Lotusland	Montecito, CA.
Mercer Arboretum & Gardens	Houston, TX.
Minnesota Landscape Arboretum	Chanhassen, MN.
Missouri Botanical Garden	St. Louis, MO.
Moody Gardens	Galveston, TX.
New Orleans Botanical Gardens	New Orleans, LA.
New York Botanical Garden	Bronx, NY.
Norfolk Botanical Garden	Norfolk, VA.
Rip Van Winkle Gardens	New Iberia, LA.
Stonecrop Gardens	Cold Springs, NY.
Strybing Arboretum	San Francisco, CA.
Sugar Mill Botanical Gardens	Port Orange,FL.
Quail Botanical Gardens	Encinitas, CA.
Walt Disney World	Orlando, FL.

ZOOS:

Animal Kingdom (Walt Disney World)	Orlando, FL.
Bronx Zoo	Bronx, NY.
Brookfield Zoo	Brookfield, IL.
City of Idaho Falls Zoo	Idaho Falls, ID.
Denver Zoo	Denver, CO.
Houston Zoological Gardens	Houston, TX.
Lee Richardson Zoo	Garden City, KS.
Louisville Zoo	Louisville, KY.
Lowry Park Zoo	Tampa, FL.
Memphis Zoo	Memphis, TN.
Metro Richmond Zoo	Richmond, VA.
Riverbanks Zoo & Garden	Columbia, SC.
Sedgwick County Zoological Society	Witchita, KS.
St. Louis Zoological Park	St. Louis, MO.
Sea World	San Diego, CA.
Toledo Zoo	Toledo, OH.
Black Hills Reptile Gardens, Inc.	Rapid City, SD

AQUARIA:

New Jersey Aquarium	Camden, NJ.
Seaworld	San Diego, CA.

GARDEN NURSERIES:

Brookside Gardens	Wheaton, MD.
Country Gardens	Adel, IA.
Excelsa Gardens	Loxahatchee, FL.
Gateway Gardens	San Antonio, TX.
Hillwood Gardens	Washington, D.C.
Live Oak Gardens	New Iberia, LA.
Tropical Gardens	Livingston, TX.

NURSERY CENTERS:

American Aquatic Gardens	New Orleans, LA.
Charleston Aquatic Nursery	Johns Island, SC.
Charvet's Garden Centers	Metairie, LA.
Condon Gardens	Houston, TX.
Hebert's Nursery	New Iberia, LA.
Iberia Gardens & Nursery	New Iberia, LA.
Marshalls Nursery	Lafayette, LA.
Mulu Nurseries	Worcestershire, UK.
The Plant Gallery	New Orleans, LA.
Walker's Garden Center	Rome, GA.

UNIVERSITIES AND COLLEGES:

Andrews University	Berrien Springs, MI.
Albion College	Albion, MI.
Elizabeth City State University	Elizabeth City, NC.
Louisiana State University– Burden Research Center	Baton Rouge, LA.
Salisbury State University	Salisbury, MD.
Smith College Botanic Garden	Northampton,MA.
State University College at Geneseo	Geneseo, NY.
Tabor College	Hillsboro, KS.
Temple University	Philadelphia, PA.
University of Florida	Ft Lauderdale, FL.
University of Minnesota	Chanhassen, MN
University of Waterloo	Kitchener,Ontario,Canada

STOKES TROPICALS' CORPORATE GIFT DIVISION

STOKES TROPICALS' GIFT CERTIFICATES are ideal for gifts, awards and incentives. The certificates can be purchased for any dollar amount desired. Your recipients can then redeem them for items of their choice from our latest catalog. The order can be placed by telephone, fax, e-mail, internet or by mail. An easy gift idea with no guesswork for you and complete satisfaction for your recipient.

GIFTS FOR:	AWARDS FOR:	INCENTIVES FOR:
• Customers	• Service	• Sales
• Business Associates	• Safety	• Marketing Promotions
• Employees	• Attendance	• Production
• Retirements	• Performance	• Financial Marketing
• Holidays	• Company Outings	• Quality Control

Call 1-800-624-9706 or
E-mail: info@stokestropicals.com for details.

BOOKS ON TROPICAL PLANTS

BROMELIADS: A CULTURAL MANUAL

Edited by Mark Dimmitt
1992 44 pp.

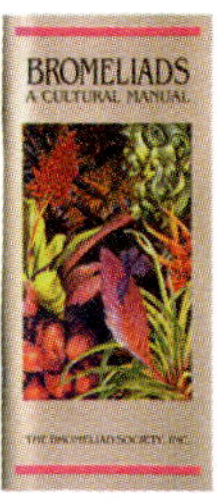

Outstanding color photos throughout. 4" (10cm) x 9", soft-cover. A handy inexpensive guide on the basic culture of the common genera of bromeliads. It includes a good bibliography and glossary. A booklet every bromeliad beginner should have.
71950..............................**$3.00**

EXOTIC TROPICALS OF HAWAII:HELICONIAS, GINGERS,ANTHURIUMS & DECORATIVE FOLIAGE

By Angela K. Kepler
1989 112 pp.

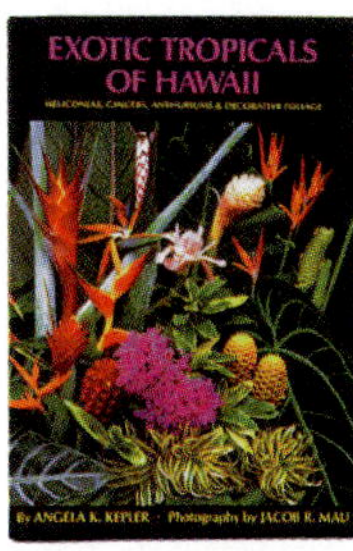

A great little book with lavish photography color photos throughout. 5³/₄" x 8¹/₂", soft-cover. Excellent coverage of Hawaii's exotic tropical plants. Emphasis is on heliconias and gingers but covers anthuriums, ornamental bananas, birds-of-paradise, bromeliads, calatheas, and other tropicals. Sections on "Care of Cut Flowers" and "Flower Arrangement". A must for the tropical plant enthusiast.
74500 .... **$13.00**

HELICONIA: AN IDENTIFICATION GUIDE

By Fred Berry and
W. John Kress
1991 334 pp.

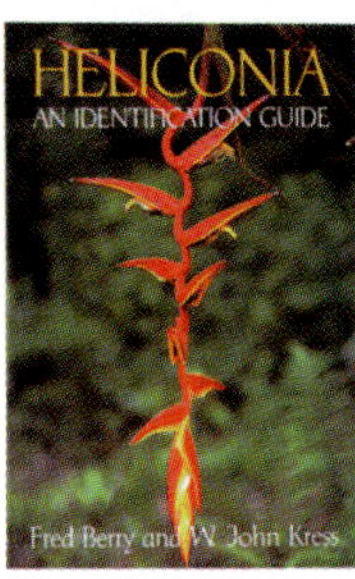

Excellent color photos throughout. 4⁷/₈" x 7⁵/₈", soft-cover. The bible on heliconia by two of the world's authorities on heliconia. Two hundred different varieties of heliconia are covered in this handy handbook-size publication. Chapters cover morphology, habitats and geographic distribution, breeding and hybridization, taxonomy, collecting heliconias in the wild, and an excellent pictorial guide for identifying the most common varieties, and more. Plus sources of information on heliconia, correct names, glossary and appendices on Cultivation and Commercial Production, and an Index of Taxa. An absolute must for the heliconia grower and enthusiast.
75000..........................**$21.00**

ORNAMENTAL GINGERS: A GUIDE TO SELECTION AND CULTIVATION.

By Timothy Sean Chapman
2nd Edition 1995 50 pp.
Six pages of good color photos of many ginger varieties— some seen for the first time. 8¹/₂" x 11", soft-cover. Contains much useful information on gingers heretofore unavailable in one source. Contains general information on growing, propagating, hybridizing, and gingers for cut flowers.

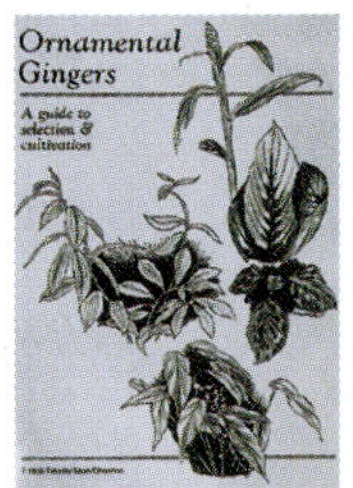

The most useful part of the book is the descriptions of genera and species of gingers.The author is a self-taught ginger expert and enthusiastic collector. For the ginger enthusiast this book is a valuable addition to the very limited literature on the subject of gingers.
76000..........................**$25.00**

THE EXOTIC PLUMERIA (FRANGIPANI)

By Elizabeth H. Thornton, andSharon H. Thornton
Revised 1985 55 pp.

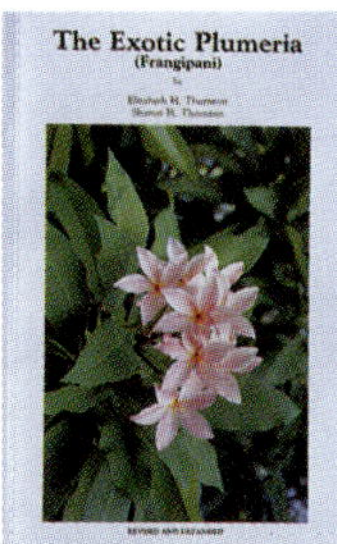

Excellent color photos throughout. 5³/₄" x 8³/₄", soft-cover. An excellent small book with chapters on propagation, pollination, cultivation, dormancy and winter storage, pests, diseases and more. Plus glossary, index to color photos, and bibliography. Doesn't cover the same territory as Eggenbergers' book and has photos of many unusual and rarely seen plumeria varieties. The serious plumeria collector will want the Thornton book.
77500..........................**$12.00**

HANDBOOK ON PLUMERIA CULTURE

By Richard M. and Mary Helen Eggenberger
3rd. Edition
1994 107 pp.

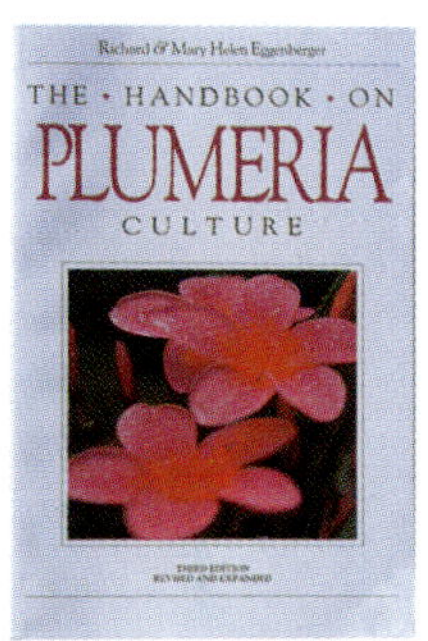

Excellent color photos throughout. 5³/₄" x 8³/₄", soft-cover. An excellent handbook that tells you everything you want to know about plumerias. Has chapters on nomenclature, historical data, major cultivars, Moragne hybrids, plumeria culture and more. Excellent descriptions and color photos of most popular commercial plumeria varieties. Plus a good glossary and bibliography. Written by two of the most knowledgeable experts on plumeria living today. A must for the plumeria enthusiast, serious plumeria collector, and grower.
77600..........................**$13.00**

THE HAWAII GARDENS TROPICAL EXOTICS

By Horace F. Clay and
James C. Hubbard
1977 266 pp.

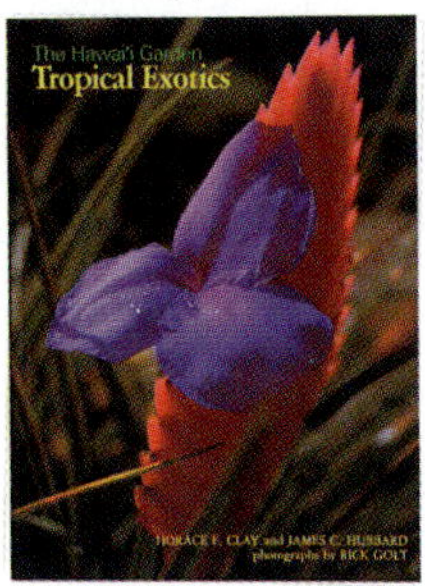

118 excellent full-page color photos of exotic tropical plants. The soft-cover book (8" x 11") covers 18 tropical plant families including: Bromeliaceae, Musaceae, Heliconiaceae, Zingiberaceae, and Costaceae. Includes useful information on habits, growing conditions, usage, propagation, pests and diseases, pruning, fertilizing and more on each of the 118 tropical plant species covered. One of the best tropical plant "coffee table books" out.

79000...........................**$28.00**

CURCUMAS OF THAILAND

By Dr. Surawit Wannakrairoj
1996 129 pp.

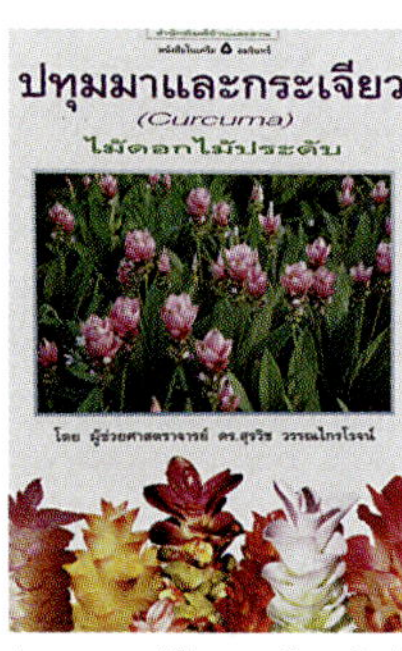

A magnificent book in hardcover 7" x 9¾" on the Curcumas of Thailand. Although it is written in Thai, it is still worth having for the 174 exquisite color photos of at least 38 different species and numerous more varieties and/or cultivars. Major emphasis is on *Curcuma alismatifolia* showing color pictures of several unique cultivars. Scientific and common names are in English. An absolute must if you like Curcuma gingers.

72000...........................**$25.00**

THE TROPICAL LOOK: AN ENCYCLOPEDIA OF DRAMATIC LANDSCAPE PLANTS

By Robert Lee Riffle
1998 428 pp.

A unique compendium of nearly 2,000 plants that evoke

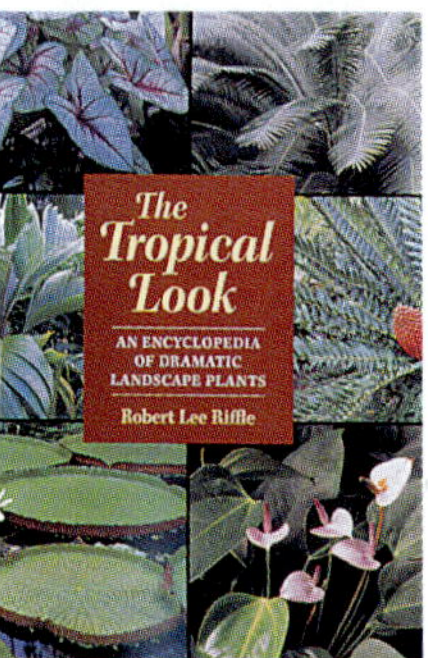

a tropical look of swaying palms, dripping banana leaves, vibrant frangipanis, and exotic fragrant gingers. Over 400 stunning photographs make the book a pleasure to use. Those who live in USDA hardiness Zones 8 and higher (minimum average temperature higher than 10°F—an area encompassing most of the southern and southwestern United States and the west coasts of the U.S. and Canada) will find a wealth of plants to chose from. Written by a passionate plantsman who seeks to spread the word about these important but underutilized plants. Book is hardcover 8¾" x 11¼".

73860...........................**$49.95**

HELICONIAS OF THAILAND

By Surawit Wannakrairoj
1995 218 pp.

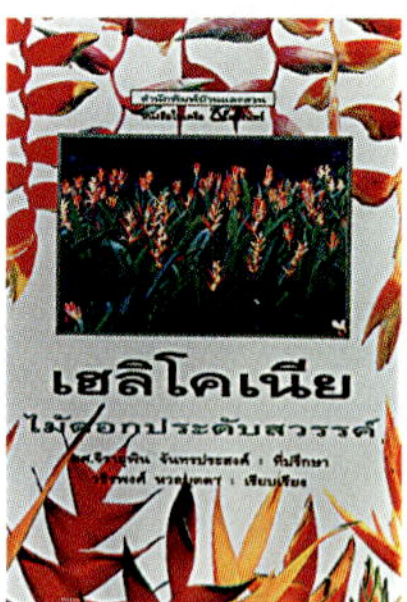

200 superb color photos of heliconias plus numerous line drawings and sepias of heliconias and heliconia parts. 7" x 93/4", hard cover. Text is in Thai, however scientific names are in Latin and common names are in English, which

makes it very useable to the Heliconia enthusiast and collector. Very good indices of scientific and common names make it reader friendly. A nice addition to Heliconia literature.

74000...........................**$35.00**

HIBISCUS HANDBOOK

By Sue J. Schloss, Editor
3rd Edition 1990 97 pp.

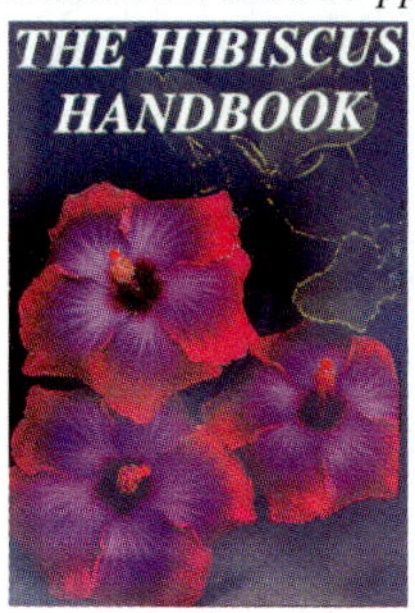

Plenty of color pictures and line drawings with good index. 7" x 9" Includes everything you could possibly want to know about growing hibiscus. You should have this book if you want to learn about hibiscus. A great beginner's book.

76040...........................**$13.00**

HIBISCUS CATALOGUE

By American Hibiscus Society Charitable Trust
2nd Edition, Feb. 1991 21pp.

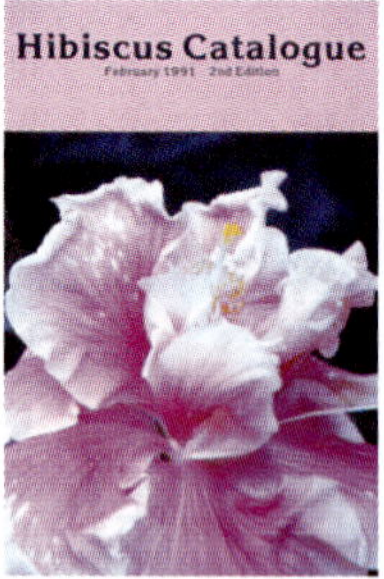

20 pages of full-color pictures of 180 Hibiscus cultivar flowers with descriptions. 8" x 11".

76020...........................**$8.00**

HIBISCUS ILLUSTRATED

By American Hibiscus Society Charitable Trust
3nd Edition, Nov. 1996 21 pp.

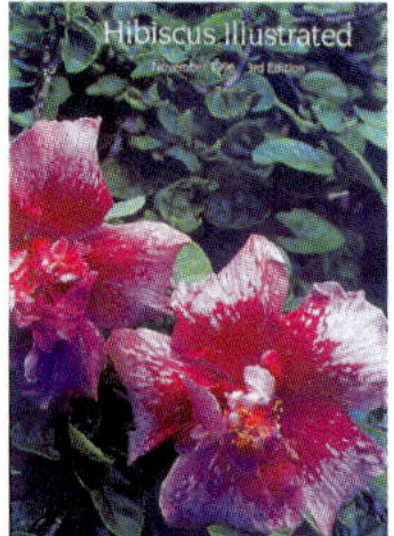

20 pages of full-color pictures of 180 Hibiscus cultivar flowers with full descriptions. 8"x 11".

76030...........................**$8.95**

HIBISCUS CATALOGUE

By American Hibiscus Society Charitable Trust
2nd Edition April 1989 13pp.

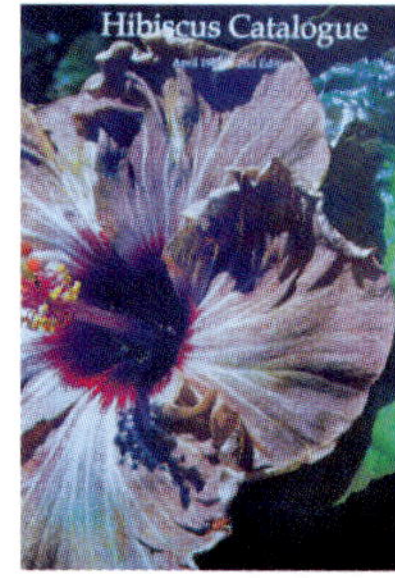

12 pages of full-color pictures of 144 Hibiscus cultivar flowers with descriptions. 8" x 11".

76010. ....**$6.00**

PALMER'S HIBISCUS IN COLOUR

By Stanley J. Palmer
1997 175pp.

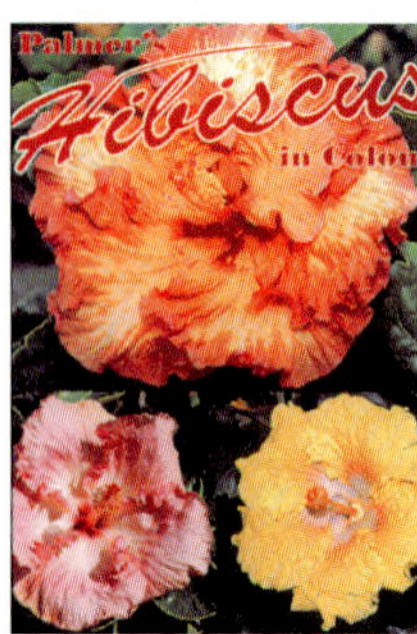

This 8" x 10⅝" hardcover book features a selection of the finest cultivars of the species Hibiscus rosañsinensis currently grown in Australia, U.S.A., South Africa, New Zealand and other places of the tropical and subtropical world. Includes information on bloom size, flower quality, bush size, growth habit, root stock, pod parent, and who hybridized the plant. Over 470 color photos. Easy to follow data on the successful culture of hibiscus. A must book for hibiscus lovers.

76050............................**$35.00**

TROPICALS

By Gordon Courtright
1988 155 pp.

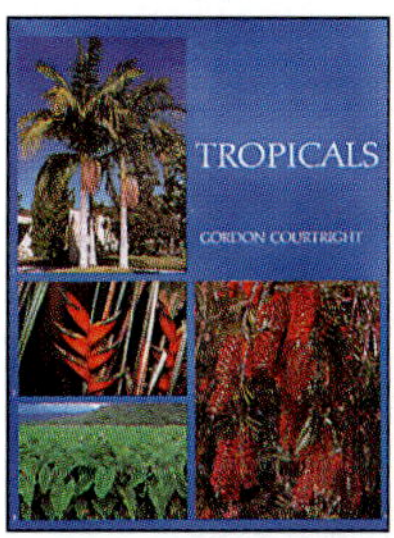

583 great color photos of a broad spectrum of tropical plants. 8 1/2" x 11", paperback. A counterpart to the author's Trees and Shrubs for Temperate Climates; it is designed for Zones 9,10, and 11. It is ideal for greenhouse gardeners who grow tender exotics under cover, and it is frequently used as an identification guide for plant lovers who travel to the tropics.

73750............................**$24.95**

GARDENING IN THE TROPICS

By R.E.Holttum and
Ivan Enoch
1991 384 pp.

An encyclopedia of tropical gardening with 650 color photos that will be of interest not only to gardeners in tropical and subtropical areas but also to greenhouse enthusiasts everywhere. 8 1/4" x 11 1/4", hard cover. Included are illustrated listings of herbaceous

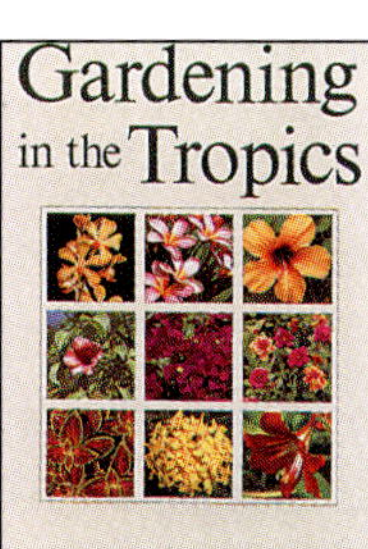

plants, shrubs and climbers, trees and palms, foliage plants and orchids. The fascinating fruits and vegetables of the tropics are covered extensively. Written for the mostly wet tropical climate of Malaysia, the book is also useful for the less steamy conditions of southern areas.

73900............................**$69.95**

THE BANANA LOVER'S COOKBOOK

By Carol Lindquist
1993 104 pp.

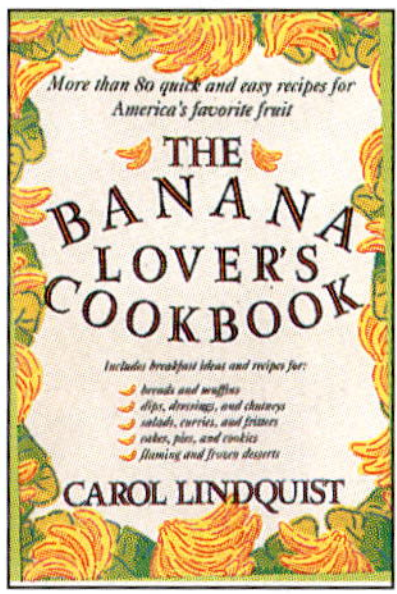

A delightful small book that tells you everything you want to know about eating and cooking bananas. Chapters on breakfast & brunch; muffins & quick breads; appetizers, condiments & dressings; soups, salads & sandwiches; hearty & savory dishes; cakes & cookies; puddings & pies; other desserts, frozen to flambeed; and kids' treats are included. Bananas are America's favorite fruit; 78 bananas are consumed per person annually. 7" x 9", paperback.

71100............................**$10.95**

THE SUBTROPICAL GARDEN

By Jacqueline Walker
(photos by Gil Hanly)
1996 176 pp.

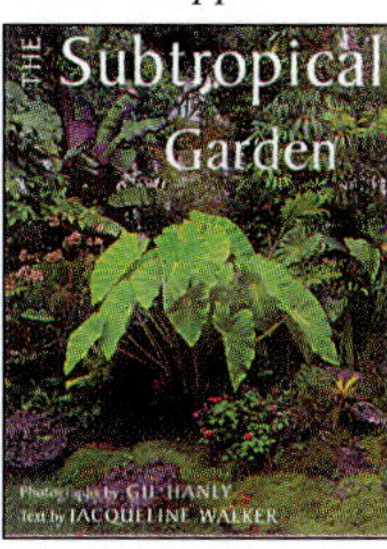

A tempting selection of palms, bamboos, shrubs, foliage plants, perennials, orchids and ferns suitable for gardeners in Zones 9 and 10–or adventurous souls in colder areas who want to garden on the edge, or use containers for overwintering indoors. Contains 197 superb color photos. 8 1/2" x 11", paperback.

73200............................**$24.95**

THE TROPICAL GARDEN

By William Warren
(photos by Luca Invernizzi
Tettonii)
1991 (reprinted 1994) 224 pp.

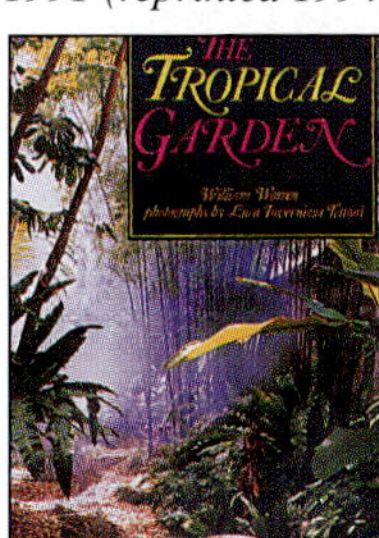

Lusciously photographed "coffee table" book that is a pleasure to browse. Begins with a brief history of tropical gardens, goes from the "Colonial Tropical Garden" to the "Contemporary Tropical Garden" and ends with an excellent Bibliography. In between, you are given a pictorial tour of some of the outstanding tropical gardens of the world. There are also sec-

tions on tropical plants, foliage plants, flowering shrubs, water plants, vines and creepers, ground covers and flowering trees, in addition to sections on various garden features. Book is hard cover, 9 5/8" x 12 1/2", with 365 color photos.

73500............................**$55.00**

FRESH FLOWERS: IDENTIFYING, SELECTING, AND ARRANGING

By Charles Marden Fitch
1992 256 pp.

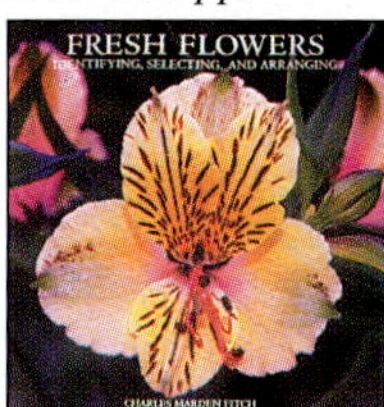

An indispensable color guide to identifying, selecting and arranging more than 200 of the most desirable flowers with 368 superb photos. This is a treasury for those who enjoy cut flowers. It features an illustrated identification section arranged by lookalikes for easy reference, an extensive chart keyed to the flower portraits with practical information like care and vase life, an inspiring primer on flower arranging for everyday living and special events, an illustrated portfolio of some fifty types of decorative foliage, and an overview of the methods used to bring us fresh flowers from all over the world. Book is hard cover, 9 1/4" x 9 1/2". A must for cut-flower lovers just for the pictures alone. The author is one of America's most accomplished photographers, and he displays a special affinity for tropical flowers.

79050............................**$39.95**

TROPICAL GARDEN PLANTS

(Formerly called Tropical Plants for Home and Garden)

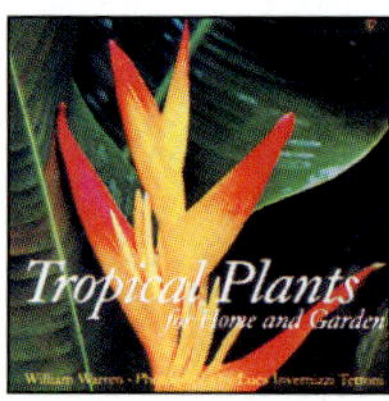

By William Warren (photos by Luca Invernizzi Tettoni) 1997 240 pp.

A veritable picture book of luscious tropical plants in all their glory. Packed with 449 color illustrations. More pictures than text. A supreme "coffee-table" book for the tropical-plant lover. Chapters on Ornamental Trees, Flowering Shrubs and Annuals, Foliage Plants, Vines and Creepers, Exotics, Ground Covers and other Plants for Similar Use, Water Plants, Palms and Palm-Like Plants, and Orchids. Plus it has a short Bibliography and good Index. Just a magnificent book that everyone who enjoys beauty should have. 9³/4"X 9³/4", hardcover.
73850...........................**$50.00**

HOT PLANTS FOR COOL CLIMATES: GARDENING WITH TROPICAL PLANTS IN TEMPERATE ZONES

By Susan A. Roth and Dennis Schrader 2000 228 pp.

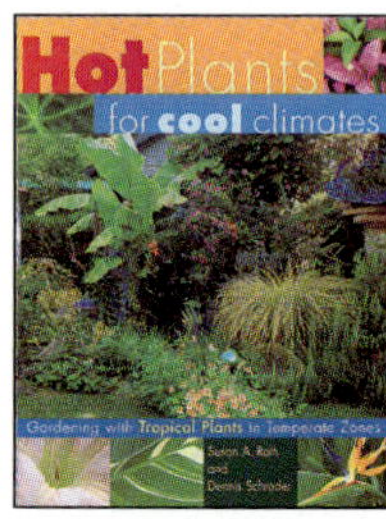

A brilliantly written book that tells you how to grow tropical and subtropical plants out of

climate. The book is 7" x 10", hardcover. It is full of well-chosen photographs showing how hot (weather) plants can thrive and actually define an environment in cool climates. But you don't have to live in a cool climate to make good use of the ideas and techniques amply illustrated in this great book. It has some fine chapters on: Sizzling Container Gardens, Hardy Plants for a Tropical Look, and Winter Survival Techniques plus some fine Appendices on Plant Lists and Sources of Tropical and Tropical-Looking Hardy Plants. A very good read.
71150...........................**$35.00**

GINGER (THE HERB LIBRARY)

By Kate Ferry-Swainson (Series Editor Deni Bown) 1999 80 pp.

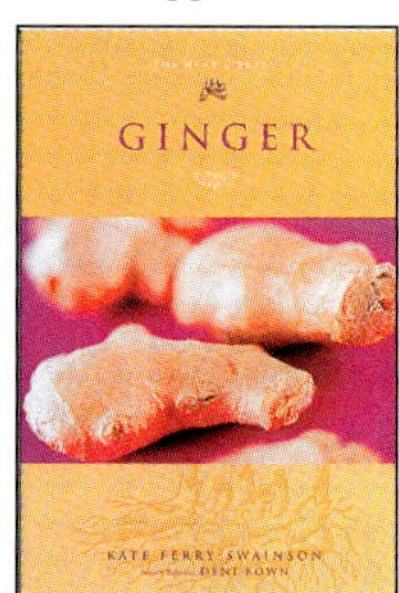

An amazingly interesting small book (5⁷/8" x 9", softcover) on the spice that derives from the edible ginger, Zingiber officinale. There are vastly interesting chapters on: History and Mythology, Remedies, Cosmetics and Scented Decorations, and Ginger Flavorings. Contains detailed recipes for preparing remedies, cosmetics, scented decorations, and ginger flavorings. This book can definitely make your life more healthy and pleasant. Plus a good number of Further Readings are listed for those that are interested in edible ginger. Very good color illustrations

throughout–many that are antique.
72500...........................**$12.95**

TROPICAL GARDEN DESIGN

By Made Wijaya 1999 208 pp.

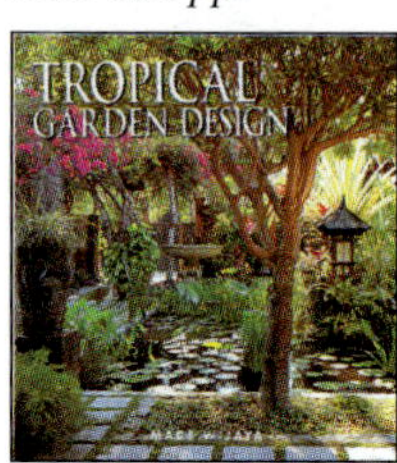

An absolutely fantastic book (10³/8" x 11" hardcover) by Southeast Asia's foremost landscape architect and designer, Made Wijaya. This is a retrospective of his wonderous work on more than 400 gardens in the tropical world, including the US ambassador's residence in Jakarta, the former Mustique estate of David Bowie, and his own tropical haven in Bali. The photography and illustrations are first class by a team of internationally acclaimed photographers. This book is an inspiration for gardeners everywhere; it is a glorious celebration of more than 20 years spent perfecting the art of tropical garden design. A coffee table book par excellence!
72650 ....**$50.00**

THE EXOTIC GARDEN: DESIGNING WITH TROPICAL PLANTS IN ALMOST ANY CLIMATE.

By Richard R. Iversen 1999 176 pp.

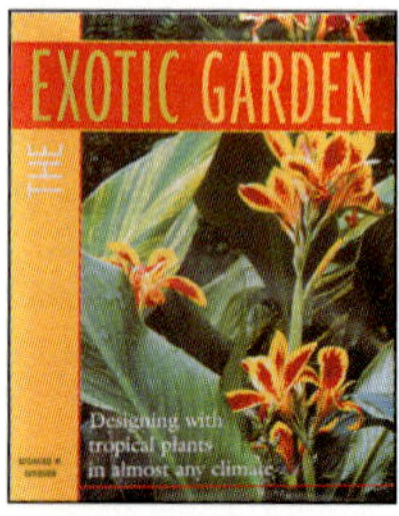

If you like tropical plants and you want to learn how they can be successfully incorporated into your landscape, Iversen's book is a must. There are chapters on Tropical Borders, Tropical Beds, Tropical Containers, Growing Tropical Plants, and more. With the current resurgence in interest in of using tropical plants in temperate landscapes, *The Exotic Garden* provides a primer on creating a tropical effect. A must for the professional landscaper as well as the adventurous home gardener. Book is hardcover, 8¹/2" x 11", with 236 color photos and 25 drawings.
73250...........................**$29.95**

HELICONIAS: LLAMARADAS DE LA SELVA COLOMBIANA

By John Kress, Julio Betancur, Beatriz Echeverry 1999 200 pp.

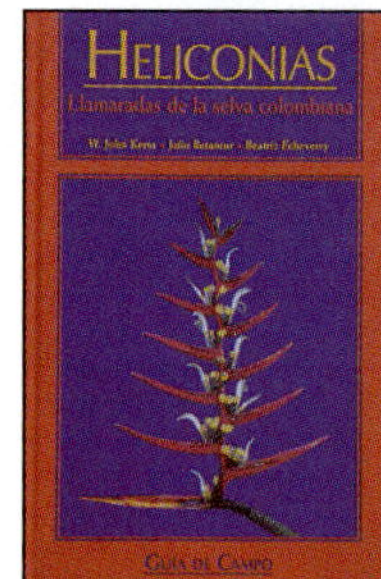

Filled with beautiful full color pictures of 91 species of heliconias with detailed descriptions and distribution in Columbia. Contains very useful glossary, comprehensive bibliography (253 references), and thorough index. For the serious heliconia enthusiast or collector, this wonderful little book is a must. John Kress is the world's foremost authority on heliconias. Hardcover, 5³/4" x 8¹³/16".
73950...........................**$40.00**

GINGERS OF PENINSULAR MALAYSIA AND SINGAPORE

By K. Larsen, H. Ibrahim, S.H. Khaw and L.G. Saw Edited by K. M. Wong 1999 137 pp.

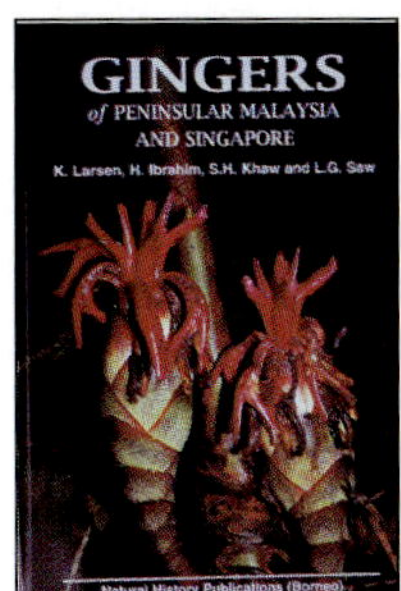

Currently the best book out on tropical gingers. Even though the gingers of Malaysia and Singapore are covered, don't be fooled these are the same plants that have been spread all over the world. Many of these same gingers are available to American and European gardeners at the present time. The book is literally filled with great color photos of both common and exotic gingers. And the text covers subjects on gingers heretofore seldom seen in print: plant structure in the ginger family, a checklist of peninsular Malaysian and Singapore gingers, glossary, references and general reading, index to scientific and common names, and much more. This book is an absolute must for anyone that likes gingers. Softcover, 6" x 8 $^{3}/_{8}$" filled with color photos and drawings.
73910............................$29.95

HAWAIIAN GARDENS ARE TO GO TO: A TREASURY OF TROPICAL PLANTS AND GARDENS.

By Clayton and Michele Oslund 1998 106 pp.

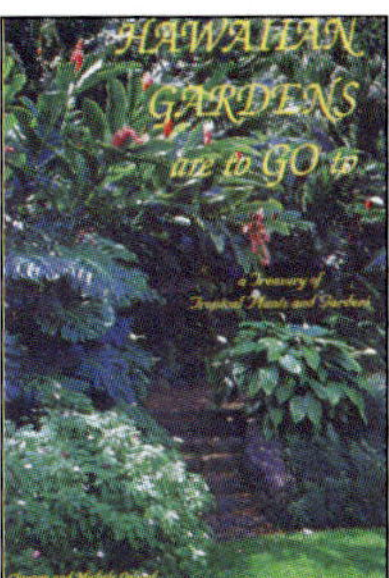

If you plan a real or a dream trip to Hawaii and you like tropical plants, this book is an absolute must. It is a pictorial journey through most of the Hawaiian gardens based on the experience of the authors guiding tours through 30 gardens and parks. Over 400 full-color photographs of rare and exotic plants and landscapes. Travel directions are included for all garden and park locations of the Big Island, Kauai, Maui, and Oahu. A spectacular book. Softcover, 8$^{1}/_{2}$" x 11".
74500............................$19.95

GROWING BOUGAINVILLEAS

By Jan Iredell 1994 96 pp.

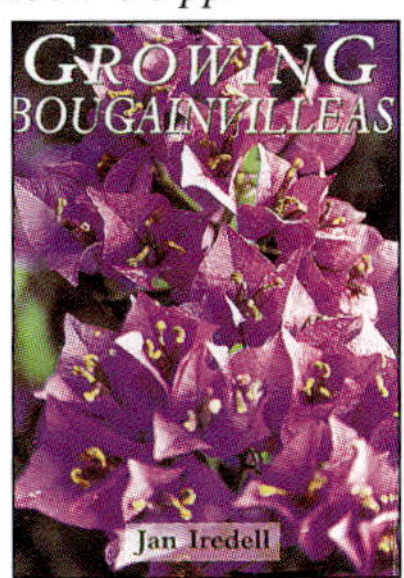

The best book available on bougainvilleas. It is a practical guide to growing and propagating these much-loved and diversely colored plants. It covers the history of the species and their early distribution, describes some of the many hybrids and cultivars, and gives valuable advice on how to grow and care for all bougainvilleas. Contains 85 wonderful color photos plus several colored illustrations. Whether you wish to grow one specimen plant or a large number of different cultivars as shrubs, climbers, standards, bonsai or even potted plants indoors, this book provides all the necessary information. Book is 7$^{1}/_{4}$" x 9$^{1}/_{4}$", softcover.
79010............................$25.95

BANANAS YOU CAN GROW

By James W. Waddick and Glenn M. Stokes 2000 128 pp. (Available April, 2000)

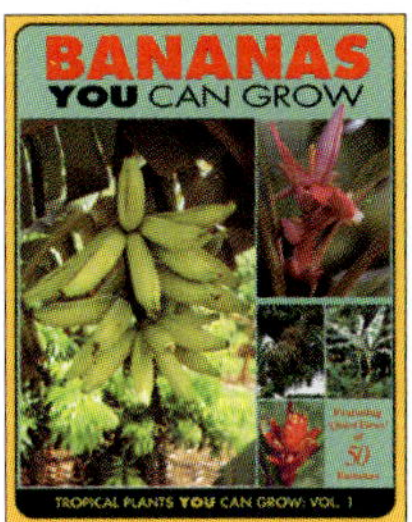

Brand new book for all gardeners wanting the latest information on gardening with bananas. Full color illustrations throughout with special sections on cultivation and propagation of bananas in the greenhouse, in containers, in the ground, and the landscape. The authors take in both northern gardener's concerns with "hardy" bananas and southern landscaping choices. Over fifty species and varieties are illustrated and compared. Multiple lists recommend the best bananas for different sites, edibility, cooking and more. Readings, plant sources and public gardens are also given. First book on bananas to cover all aspects for the home gardener. Book is softcover, 7$^{1}/_{4}$" x 9$^{1}/_{4}$".
71125............................$19.95

GIFT CERTIFICATES

Purchase a Stokes Tropicals' Gift Certificate as the ultimate gift for a birthday, special occasion, Christmas, Valentine's Day, Mother's Day, Father's Day, Graduation, Wedding, Anniversary, or other special reason. You choose the amount in increments of $25.00. Then the recipient selects the plant or product (book, logoed polo shirt, tropical painting, etc.) and we will ship directly to them.

We have gift certificates in the denomination of $25.00. Of course multiple gift certificates can be purchased. Certificate totals include shipping. For example, if the plant cost $19.00 and shipping is $5.95, then a $25.00 gift certificate would be adequate. If the cost of plant selected and shipping is less, then the difference will be refunded. Or if amount is more, then the difference will be billed to the gift certificate holder.

Gift Certificates make great gifts! The plants they buy last indefinitely, reminding one daily of the gift of thoughtfulness.

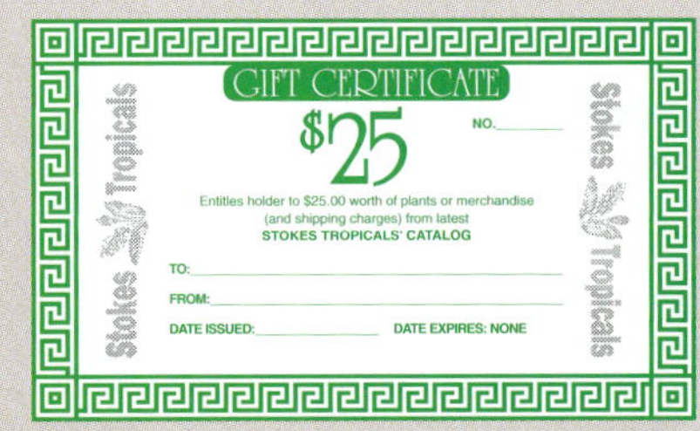

FERTILIZERS FOR TROPICAL PLANTS

These are the fertilizers we use to grow our tropicals. You can optimize your growing, flowering and fruiting of tropical plants by using our special blended fertilizers.Try them, if they don't work as good or better than any other fertilizer, just let us know and return unused balance for a refund. That's how sure we are!

STOKES TROPICALS' BANANA BLEND

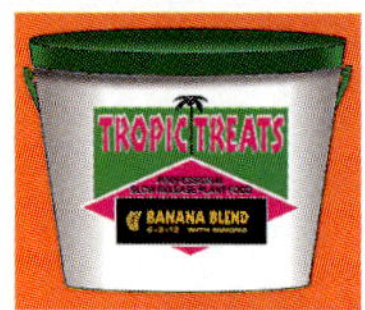

Controlled Release Fertilizer (3-Month Formula)

ANALYSIS 6-2-12 w/minors.

Uniquely formulated for best growth of Bananas. This total nutrient formula provides complete balance of all major and minor elements.

6000 (1 lb. Bucket)........$6.00
6001 (4 lb. Bucket)......$17.00

STOKES TROPICALS' BROMELIAD BLEND

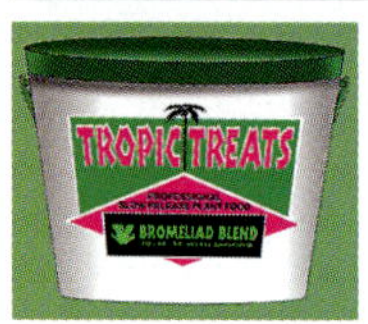

Controlled Release Fertilizer (3-Month Formula)

ANALYSIS 10-14-14 w/minors

Uniquely formulated for best growth of Bromeliads. This total nutrient formula provides complete balance of all major and minor elements.

6060 (1 lb. Bucket)........$6.00
6061 (4 lb. Bucket)......$17.00

STOKES TROPICALS' GINGER BLEND

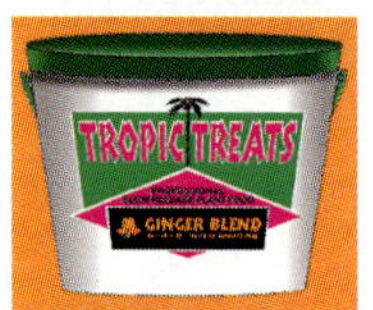

Controlled Release Fertilizer (3-Month Formula)

ANALYSIS 8-4-6 w/minors.

Uniquely formulated for best growth of Gingers. This total

nutrient formula provides a complete balance of all major and minor elements.

6020 (1 lb. Bucket)........$6.00
6021 (4 lb. Bucket)......$17.00

STOKES TROPICALS' HELICONIA BLEND

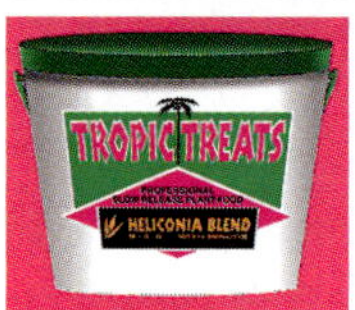

Controlled Release Fertilizer (3-Month Formula)

ANALYSIS 9-3-6 w/minors

Uniquely formulated for best growth of Heliconias. This total nutrient formula provides a complete balance of all major and minor elements.

6030 (1 lb. Bucket)........$6.00
6031 (4 lb. Bucket)......$17.00

STOKES TROPICALS' PLUMERIA BLEND

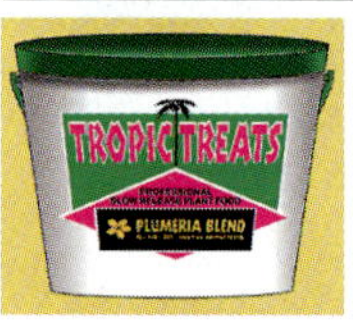

Controlled Release Fertilizer (3-Month Formula)

ANALYSIS 8-14-10 w/minors.

Uniquely formulated for best growth of Plumerias. This total nutrient formula provides a complete balance of all major and minor elements.

6040 (1 lb. Bucket)........$6.00
6041 (4 lb. Bucket)......$17.00

STOKES TROPICALS' HIBISCUS BLEND

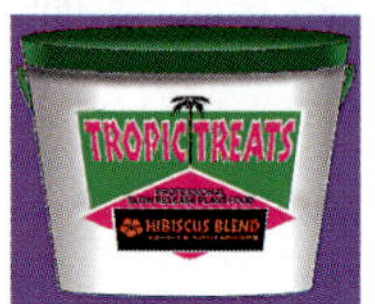

Controlled Release Fertilizer (3-Month Formula)

ANALYSIS 10-4-12 w/minors plus iron.

A special blend that has been determined by expert growers to be best for all Hibiscus to produce continuous blooms and lush foliage. Special blend consists of low phosphorus, high nitrogen and potassium with chelated iron.

6010 (1 lb. Bucket)........$6.00
6011 (4 lb. Bucket)......$17.00

DIRECTIONS FOR ALL FERTILIZERS ABOVE

Top dress container grown plant at the following rates:

CONTAINER SIZE — Each Gallon

APPLICATION—1 teaspoon per gallon every 3 months*

Apply over entire growing media surface. Avoid placing directly against plant trunk. Water thoroughly. For plants growing in the ground, apply at a rate of twice the above uniformly within the plant's drip line.

****FOR MONTHLY APPLICATION, USE AT 1/3 OF THIS RATE.***

STOKES TROPICALS' HUMIC ACID

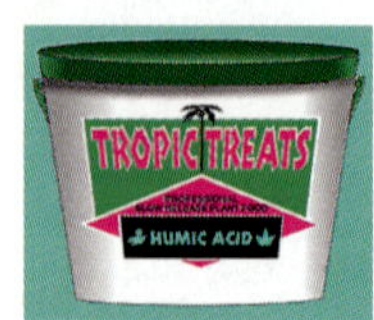

Stokes Tropicals' Humic Acid consists primarily of Humic

Acid but it also contains minor levels of minerals, gypsum and clays. Our special Humic Acid forms a unique complex with nutrients that are easily absorbed by the roots. The high carbon content stimulates beneficial soil organisms. Continued use improves the structure and organic content of the soil.

APPLICATION RATE:

For Container Plants: 2 teaspoons per gallon every 3 - 6 months. *For Plug Mix and Potting Soils:* 25 lbs. per 4 cubic feet or 6.75 lbs. per cubic yard. *For Lawn:* 300 - 500lbs. per acre. 500 lbs. for soil that only absorbs 2 - 3 inches deep. After using our Humic Acid, following year's application will absorb 14" - 15 " deep.

AVAILABLE IN:
6050 (1 lb. Bucket)........$3.00
6051 (3 lb. Bucket)........$7.50
Also 50 lb. bags and 2,000 lb. bulk bags (prices available upon request)

TROPIC TREATS' LIQUID FERTILIZERS

The only liquid formulas that supply calcium, magnesium, sulfur and all 10 trace elements, as well as N-P-K! Supply all the known essential plant mineral elements in one, easy-to-use liquid. These are the liquid fertilizers that we use to grow our tropicals both in greenhouses and outside in containers. We are offering these custom-blended fertilizers to our customers for the first time:

FLOWERING TROPICALS BLEND (7-9-5)

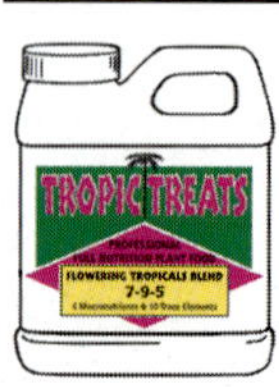

An excellent general purpose nutrient solution with 6 macronutrients and 10 essential trace elements that all our plants need. This growth formula will give your tropicals healthy leaf and stem growth; also works well for vegetables, fruits and lawns. Use as a rapid cure for nutrient deficiencies! Mixed at dilute concentrations Flowering Tropical Blend is quick acting as a foliar spray. It is ideal for poor soils and con-tainer- grown plants. The low soluble salts and slightly higher phosphorus makes this a great all-year tropical plant formula for those who don't want to switch formulas to promote flowering. Also works well on African violets, orchids and houseplants in general.

6070 (8 oz) bottle $5.00
6071 (Qt.) bottle $10.75

TROPICAL FOLIAGE BLEND (9-3-6)

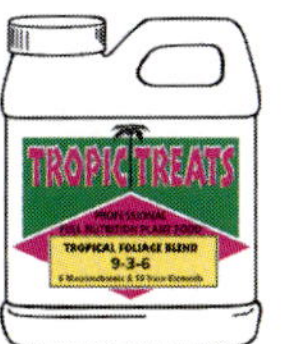

A tropical foliage for-mula with the 3-1-2 N/P/K ratio recom-mended by the Apopka R e s e a r c h Center in Florida for foliage production. Interiorscapers and exteriorscapers across the coun-try use this formula to maintain healthy, controlled foliage growth on plants (and trees). Works great on all our tropicals. It outperforms all others in low-light environments. The 3-1-2 ratio results in greater mineral uptake by foliage and flowering

plants, reducing harmful salt build up and eliminating defi-ciencies. Designed to be foliar applied for quick results. Will not burn foliage when properly applied.

6080 (8 oz) bottle $5.00
6081 (Qt.) bottle $10.75

TROPICAL PRO-TEKT (0-0-3)

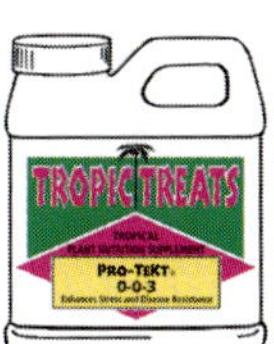

Supplies high-er levels of potassium and silicon to build strong cell walls in plants. Stron-ger cell walls are a protective barrier to pierc-

ing-sucking insects and invad-ing fungi. Use of Pro-Tekt reduces disease and insect prob-lems, increases stem strength, and leaf positioning, improves photosynthesis, and increases heat and drought tolerance. Use as a supplement with all Stokes Tropicals' fertilizers to reduce applications of insecticides and fungicides and dramatically increase heat and drought toler-ance (for interior and summer growing) for all plants. Even makes blooms last 20-30% longer. A fantastic addition to out fertilizer-nutrient-protec-tant armamentarium.

6090 (8 oz) bottle $5.00
6091 (Qt.) bottle $10.75

TROPIC TREATS' 1-YEAR INDOOR OR OUTDOOR PLANT FEEDER (16–8–10)

Feed your plants every time you water for one full year with Stokes Tropicals plant feeder. Fill the container and you don't have to fertilize again for a year.

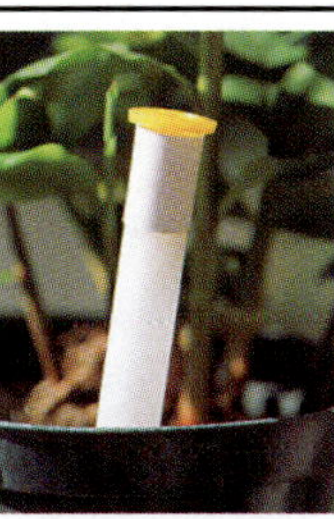

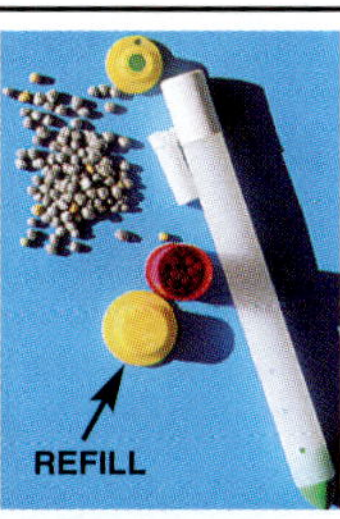

TROPIC TREATS 1-YEAR OUTDOOR PLANT FEEDER
6300-2 (2-pak) $7.00
6300-6 (6-pak) $16.00
6300 (Refills) (4-pak) $7.00
TROPIC TREATS 1-YEAR INDOOR PLANT FEEDER
6100-2 (2-pak) ....$ 6.00
6100-6 (6-pak) $15.00
6100 (Refills) (4-pak) ....$ 6.00

PLANT ZONE MAP

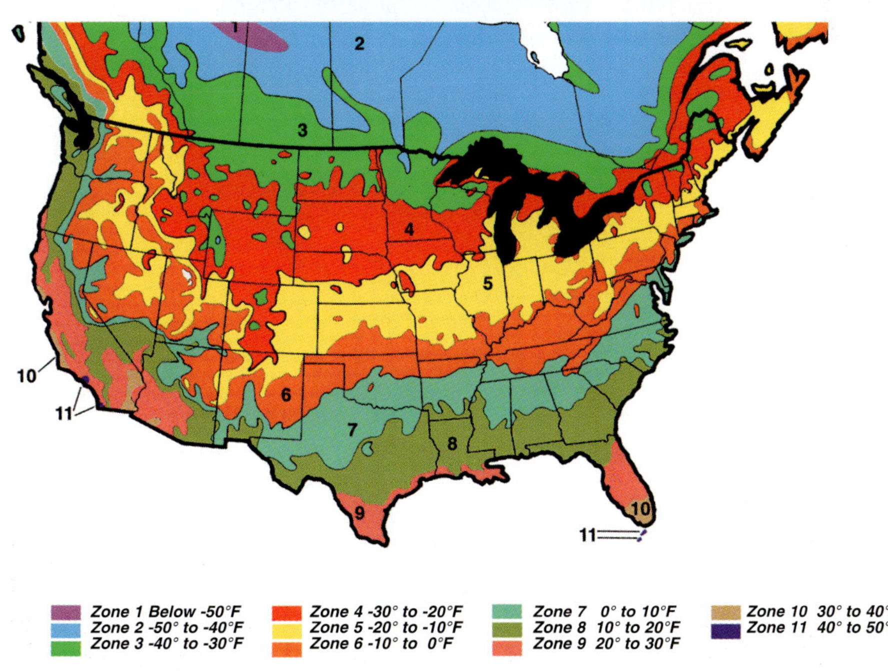

TROPIC TRENDS/*Garments & Gear*

The quality of Tropic Trends Garments & Gear begins with the selection of the finest materials, designs, and craftsmanship available. The product lines were developed to meet the wide range of lifestyles and preferences of today's discriminating consumer. The market for quality Embroidered Botanical Images is unlimited. Every niche is attracted to the style, comfort, and value of the Garments & Gear offered by Tropic Trends.

Tropic Trends product lines include traditional and contemporary leisure Garments & Gear, available in a range of fashion colors and designs.

COLLARED POLO SHIRTS

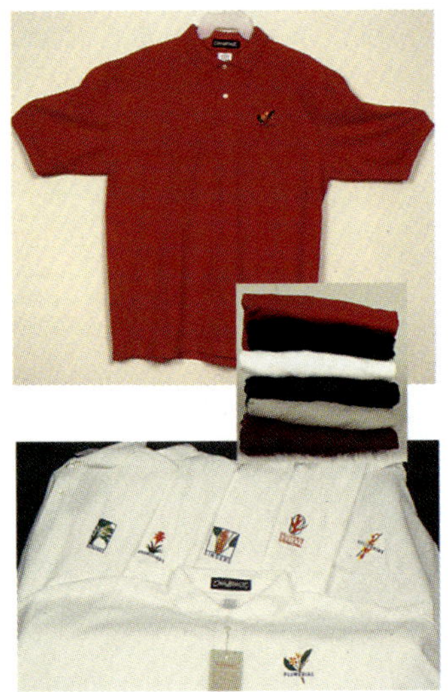

Look great and feel comfortable while taking care of your plants. Fashion knit collar, two button placket, felt cuffs and hemmed bottom. Made by famous shirt maker Outer Banks, 100% combed cotton.

Colors: Navy, White, Red, Beige, Black, and Burgundy

Sizes: Small, Medium, L & XL
600100 ....$35.00
Botanical Image embroidered on left chest.

Specify Image Number, Collared Polo Shirt Number, size, and Color when ordering.

GOLF/BASEBALL CAPS

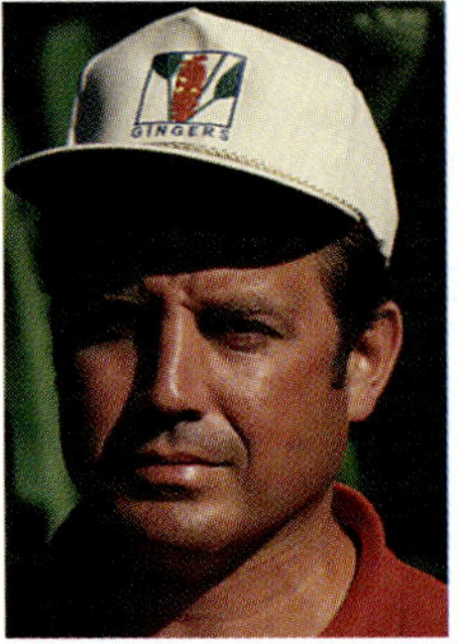

Golf/baseball cap with a b o t a n i c a l image embroidered on the front. Makes working or relaxing in the hot summer sun comfortable. One size will fit all. Available in all our embroidered Botanical Images.

Colors: Navy, White, Red, Grey, Beige
Sizes: One size fits all
600200 ....$14.00

Botanical Image embroidered to front panel.

Specify image number, item number, and color when ordering.

STRAW HATS

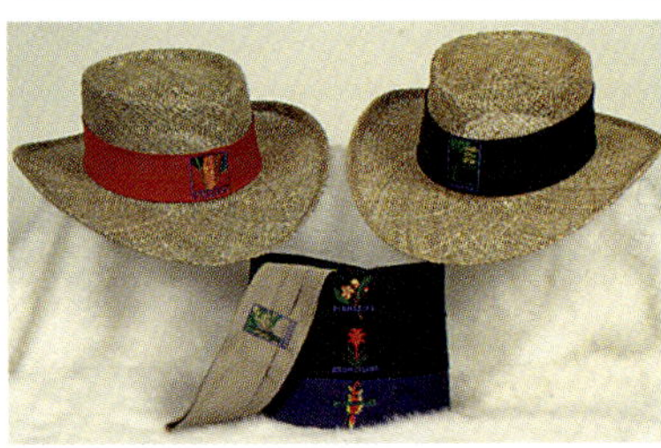

Unique Straw Hat with botanical image embroidered on front band. Very practical for gardening, travel, sports and dress. Brim protects ears, nose, and face from sun. One size fits all. Available in all our embroidered Botanical Images.

Color bands: Navy, Red, Black, and Green

Note: black band looks great with all Botanical Images.

Sizes: One size fits all
600300 ....$24.00

Botanical Image embroidered on hat band.

Specify Image Number, item number, and Color when ordering.

Embroidered apparel to suit your needs. We specialize in quality embroidery of botanical images on various garments. Check out some of our images of stock items. Additional images and/or custom images available with minimum orders. We have many botanical images available with minimum orders.

Images below are standard in stock items that can be ordered one at a time with any in stock Garments or Gear available.

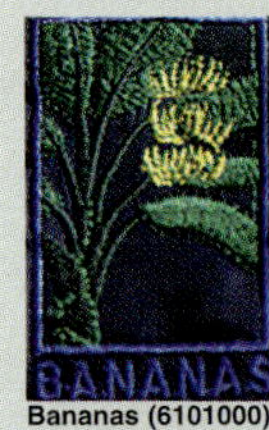
Bananas (6101000)

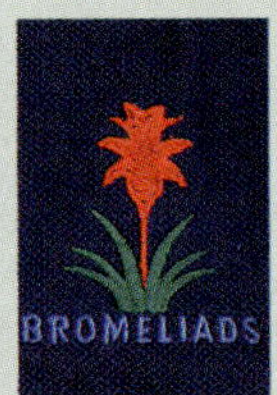
Bromeliads (6202000)

Gingers (633000)

Heliconia Rostrata (645000),

Heliconia Stricta with Heliconia Society International (644000)

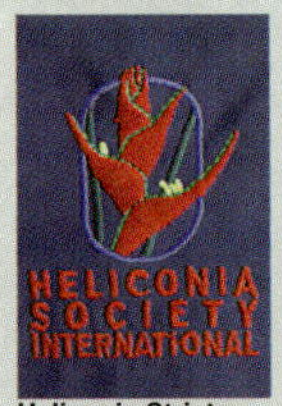
Plumeria (646000)

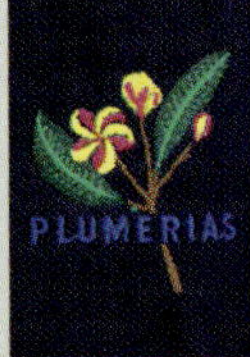

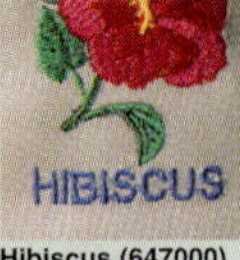
Hibiscus (647000)

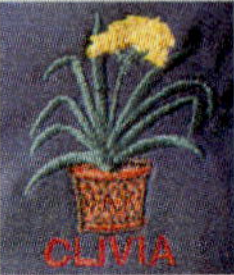
Clivia (648000)

OTHER LOGOS AVAILABLE
Azalea, Oak Tree, Orchids, Rose, Poinsettia, Tulip, or Custom.

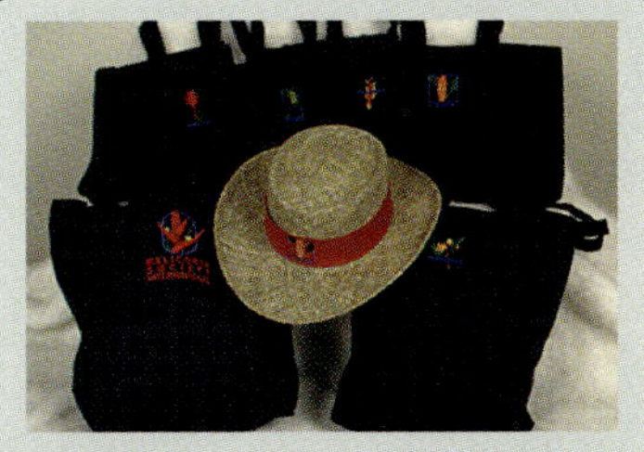

TOTES

Heavy cloth totes with large handles. Holds garden supplies, magazines, and many other items. Great for traveling. Colorful Embroidered Botanical Images. Great gift. Available in all our embroidered Botanical Images.

Colors: Navy and Washed Cotton

Size: 12"(30cm) x 12"(30cm)

600500 ....$15.00

Botanical Image embroidered to side of Tote.

Specify Image Number, item number, and Color when ordering.

BRIEF CASES

Great looking cloth briefcase made of

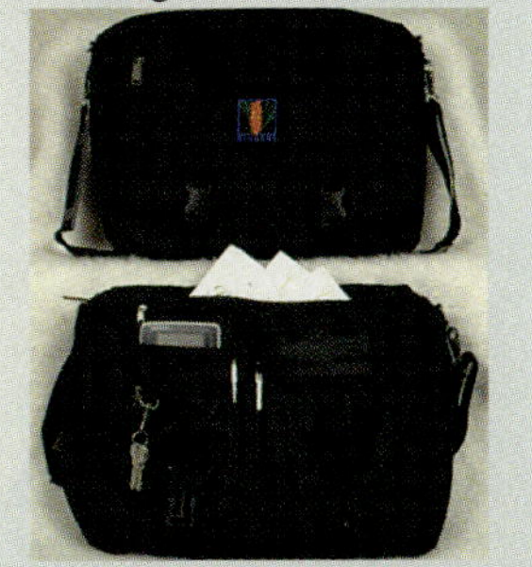

heavy nylon water repellent fabric that resists wear. Very utilitarian with six compartments, zipper sections, key ring, coin pocket, and pen pocket. Handles and shoulder straps. Great for traveling and for business. Colorful Embroidered Botanical Images. Makes excellent gift. Available in all our embroidered Botanical Images.

Colors: Black only

600600 ....$35.00

Botanical Image embroidered to side of Briefcase.

Specify Image Number, and item number when ordering.

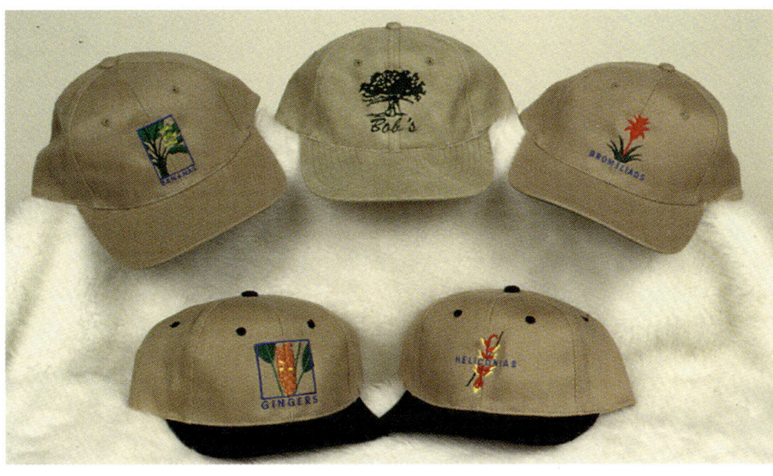

SIX PANEL CAPS

Fantastic cap with botanical image embroidered on front. Neat looking for the fashion conscious, very popular with both ladies and men. One size fits all. Available in all our embroidered Botanical Images.

Colors: All Tan, or Tan with Blue Brim

Sizes: One size fits all

600210 ....$16.00

Botanical Image embroidered on front of cap.

Specify Image Number, item number, and Color when ordering.

Just add your name to these items to utilize as a uniform or for promotional advertising for your business. Names added for $4.00 US. We can also Quote customized images and personalized garments.

GARDEN APRONS

Garden Apron with neck loop and waist tie. Two large front pockets for garden supplies, tools, pens, etc. Can also be used as a cooking apron for barbecues and in the kitchen. Colorful Embroidered Botanical Images. Great for a gift. Available in all our embroidered Botanical Images.

Colors: Navy, and Washed Cotton

Sizes: One size fits all

600700 ....$15.00

Botanical Image embroidered to front of Apron.

Specify Image Number, item number, and Color when ordering.

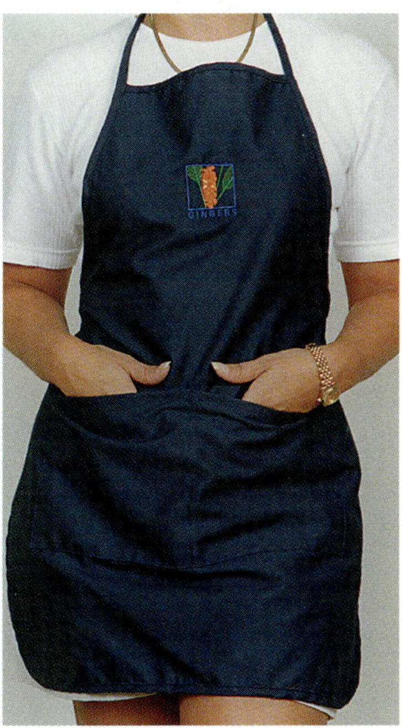

CALL 24 HRS. / 7 DAYS

TO PLACE AN ORDER:
1-800-624-9706

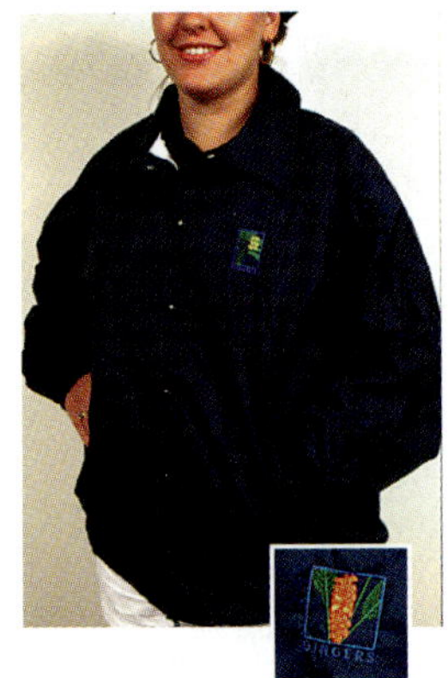

WINDBREAKERS

Nylon Windbreaker jacket. Great looking, lightweight nylon jacket with a cotton liner. Snap buttons on front. Great for traveling. Colorful Embroidered Botanical Images. Great gift. Available in all our embroidered Botanical Images.

Colors: Navy or Tan

Sizes: Medium – XL

600400 ....$45.00

Botanical Image embroidered on chest of jacket.

Specify Image Number, item number, size and Color when ordering.

GIFT CERTIFICATES

Purchase a Stokes Tropicals' Gift Certificate as the ultimate gift for a birthday, special occasion, Christmas, Valentine's Day, Mother's Day, Father's Day, Graduation, Wedding, Anniversary, or other special reason. You choose the amount in increments of $25.00 US. Then the recipient selects the plant or product (book, logoed polo shirt, tropical painting, etc.) and we will ship directly to them.

We have gift certificates in the denomination of $25.00 US .Of course multiple gift certificates can be purchased. Certificatescan be used for shipping. For example, if the plant cost $19.00 and shipping is $5.95, then a $25.00 gift certificate would be adequate. If the cost of plant selected and shipping is less, then the difference will be refunded. Or if amount is more, then the difference will be billed to the gift certificate holder.

Gift Certificates make great gifts! The plants they buy last indefinitely, reminding one daily of the gift of thoughtfulness.

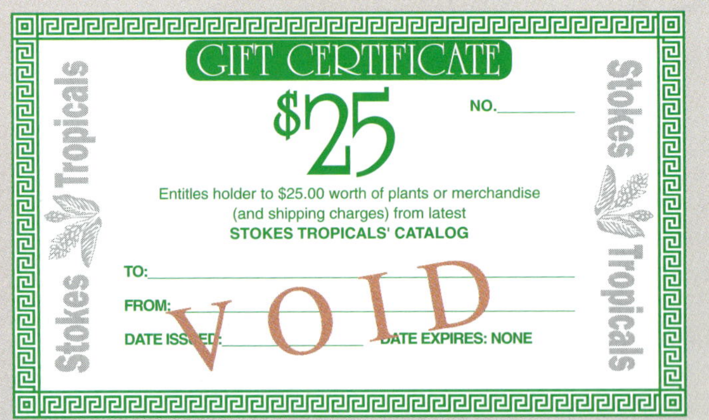

Put yourself or a friend on our mailing list. A phone call is all it takes to bring the beautiful STOKES TROPICALS' GUIDE/CATALOG into your home—or a friend's home. Free! For just $7.95 charged to your credit card or a personal check you get the guide/catalog with a guarantee of $7.95 free merchandise with your first purchase. So in effect the guide/catalog is free. Our guide/catalogs are becoming a collector's item because of their scientific value as a pictorial and descriptive reference of rare tropical plants. Guide/catalogs to foreign countries will be $7.95 & actual cost of postage.

STOKES TROPICALS' COTTON CANVAS GLOVES

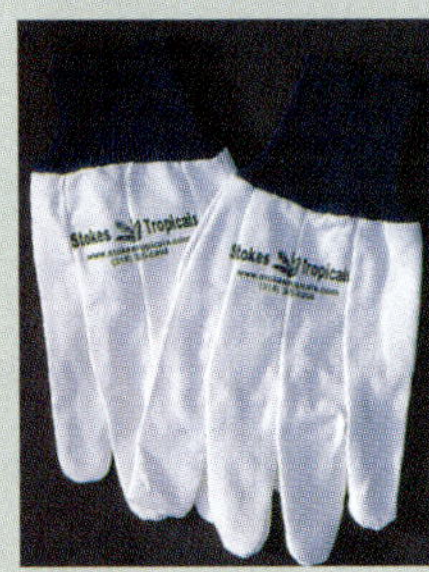

This multi-purpose glove is ideal for many of your work needs. One size fits most men and women except very large and very small hands. Gloves are 100% cotton with knit wrist bands and natural color. They are washable in cold water.

90560 ....$5.95
90560-6 (6 pair) $29.95

STOKES TROPICALS' PLASTIC SPRAY BOTTLE

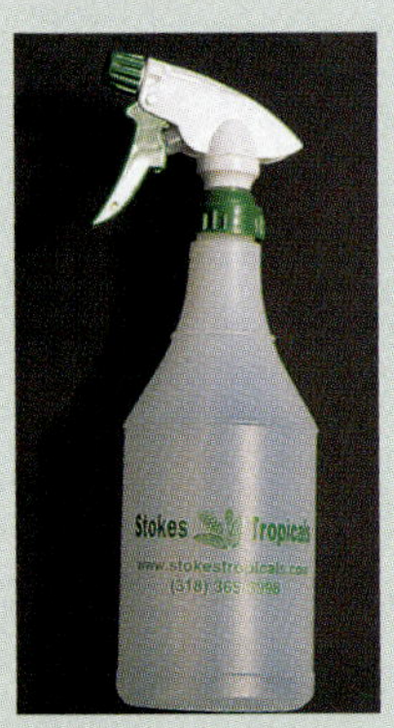

A multi-use spray bottle that can take care of many of your gardening and home needs. Easy to read measurements on side. Can be used to apply insecticides, fungicides, herbicides, soaps, or fertilizers. Can also be used to mist plant leaves with plain water.

90570 ....$4.95
90570-6 (six) $23.95

MULTI METER

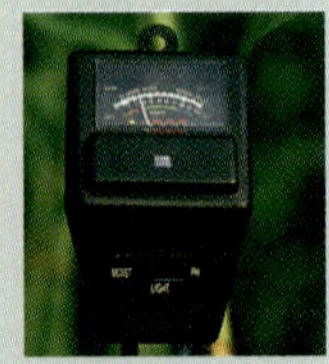

This meter has a 3-setting switch that lets you test light, moisture and pH for indoors and out. No battery required.

80100 ....$19.95

TO ORDER CALL **1-800-624-9706**/24 HRS. OR VISIT OUR WEB SITE: www. stokestropicals.com

TROPICAL PLANT SOCIETIES

BROMELIAD SOCIETY INTERNATIONAL (BSI)

The purpose of this society is to promote and maintain public and scientific interest in the research, development, preservation, and distribution of bromeliads, both natural and hybrid, throughout the world, and to promote fellowship.

BSI
c/o Carolyn Schoenau
P.O. Box 12981
Gainesville, FL 32604-0981
U.S.A.

Telephone: (352) 372-6589
Fax: (352) 372-8823
Email: BSI@nersp.nerdc.ufl.edu

Membership Classes:
Single $30.00
Dual (two memberships, one Journal, one address) $35.00
Fellowship $45.00
Life $800.00

Add:
$10.00 for U.S. FIRST CLASS mail
$8.00 for INTERNATIONAL
    SURFACE mail
$18.00 for INTERNATIONAL
    AIR mail

THE AMERICAN HIBISCUS SOCIETY (AHS)

The purpose of the American Hibiscus Society, is to encourage and promote the development and improvement of hibiscus and to collect, record and pass on information concerning hibiscus. It is non-profit and has its headquarters in Cocoa Beach, Florida.

The majority of its members are amateur gardeners. There are members in 40 states and 45 foreign countries. There are chapters located throughout Florida, Texas, Louisiana, the U.S., British Virgin Islands, and Washington D.C. (E-mail: seedpods@aol.com) or write for the nearest chapter. The Australian Hibiscus Society is affiliated. Members receive *The Seed Pod*, the quarterly publication of the AHS. There are a number of books published by the AHS covering all aspects of hibiscus culture–grafting, hybridizing, etc. —especially *The Hibiscus Handbook*, please see our books section beginnin on page 126.

To join the American Hibiscus Society (a non-profit organization) send US $17.50 for a year's membership and get the quarterly *The Seed Pod*. VISA and MasterCard are accepted. Mail to

AHS
P.O. Box 12073 W
St. Petersburg, Florida 33733-2073.

For non-U.S. air mail, add US $10. For further information contact Executive Secretary, AHS, P.O. Drawer 32150 W Cocoa Beach, Florida 32932-1540. Phone/fax: (407) 783-2576. E-mail ahsjeri@yourlink.net.

THE PLUMERIA SOCIETY OF AMERICA, INC. (PSA)

The purpose of The Plumeria Society of America is to promote interest in, and increase knowledge of, Plumeria history, hybridization, propagation and culture of Plumeria. The PSA promotes research into the history and development of Plumerias (also known by the name frangipani) and shares this knowledge with hobbyists and others interested in Plumerias. The PSA has an active research program and regularly underwrites Plumeria research activities worldwide. Additionally, as the International Registration Authority for Plumeria, the PSA maintains an international register of Plumeria names and associated information. The PSA is a nonprofit corporation with headquarters in Houston, Texas, USA. Officers and all participants are volunteers.

Membership dues are $15.00 (U.S.) per year. Membership includes a subscription to the Plumeria Potpourri, published 5 times a year, a membership directory and other announcements and bulletins. General membership meetings are the second Tuesday of January, March, May, July, and October in Houston, Texas

Additional information including membership applications may be requested from the address below or at their website www.theplumeriasociety.org

Mail Membership applications to:
Membership Committee
The Plumeria Society of America
P.O. Box 22791
Houston, Texas 77227-2791

HELICONIA SOCIETY INTERNATIONAL (HSI)

The purpose of HSI is to increase the enjoyment and understanding of Heliconia (Heliconiaceae) and related plants (members of the Musaceae, Strelitziaceae, Lowiaceae, Zingiberaceae, Costaceae, Cannaceae, and Marantaceae) of the order Zingiberales through education, research, and communication. Interest in Zingiberales and information on the cultivation and botany of these plants is rapidly increasing. HSI centralizes this information and distributes it to members.

The Heliconia Society International, a nonprofit corporation, was formed in 1985 because of rapidly developing interest around the world in these exotic plants and their close relatives. HSI is composed of dues-paying members. Officers and all participants are volunteers. Everyone is welcome to join and participate. HSI conducts a Biennial Meeting and International Conference (next meeting is in New Orleans, La., U.S.A. in July, 2000).

Membership dues are:
Individual - $35
Family - $40
Student - $10
Contributing - $50
Corporate (Company or Institution)- $100
Sustaining - $500
Libraries - $25

Membership fees constitute annual dues from July1 through June 30. All members receive the BULLETIN (usually published quarterly), the Membership directory, and special announcements.

Please send all inquiries regarding membership or Bulletin purchases to:
David Bar-Zvi
HSI Vice President for Membership
Fairchild Tropical Gardens
10901 Old Cutler Road,
Miami, FL 33156-4296

Phone (305)-667-1651
Fax (305)-661-8953

135

TO ORDER CALL **1-800-624-9706**/24 HRS. OR VISIT OUR WEB SITE: www. stokestropicals.com